An Aid to the MRCP PACES
VOLUME 2
STATIONS 2 AND 4

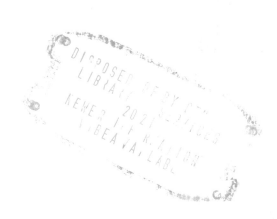

'MRCP; Member of the Royal College of Physicians . . .
They only give that to crowned heads of Europe'.
From *The Citadel* by A.J. Cronin

An Aid to the MRCP PACES

VOLUME 2
STATIONS 2 AND 4

D. Banerjee, R.E.J. Ryder, M.A. Mir & E.A. Freeman

Departments of Medicine, City Hospital, Birmingham
University Hospital of Wales and
University of Wales College of Medicine, Cardiff
and Department of Integrated Medicine,
Royal Gwent and St Woolos Hospitals, Newport

Blackwell
Publishing

© 1986, 1999 by Blackwell Science Ltd
© 2003 by Blackwell Publishing Ltd
Blackwell Publishing, Inc., 350 Main Street, Malden, Massachusetts 02148-5020, USA
Blackwell Publishing Ltd, 9600 Garsington Road, Oxford OX4 2DQ, UK
Blackwell Publishing Asia Pty Ltd, 550 Swanston Street, Carlton, Victoria 3053, Australia

First published as An Aid to the MRCP Cases 1986
Reprinted 1988, 1989, 1990, 1991, 1992, 1993, 1994, 1996, 1997
Second edition 1999 by Blackwell Science Ltd
Reprinted 2000, 2002, 2003
Third edition 2003 by Blackwell Publishing Ltd
Reprinted 2004

Library of Congress
Cataloging-in-Publication Data
An aid to the MRCP PACES/D. Banerjee . . . [et al.].—3rd ed.
        p. ; cm.
    Rev. ed. of: An aid to the MRCP short cases / R.E.J. Ryder, M.A. Mir, and E.A. Freeman. 2nd ed. c1999.
    Includes index.
    Contents: v. 2. Stations 2 and 4.
    ISBN 1-4051-0662-X (v. 2)
    1. Internal medicine—Examinations, questions, etc.   2. Diagnosis—Examinations, questions, etc.   3. Internal medicine—Case studies.   4. Diagnosis—Case studies.   5. Physicians—Licenses Great Britain—Examinations—Study guides.
    I. Banerjee, D. (Dev) II. Ryder, R. E. J. (Robert Elford John).
    Aid to the MRCP short cases.   III. Title: Aid to the Membership of the Royal College of Physicians Practical assessment of clinical examination skills.
    [DNLM: 1. Physical Examination—Examination Questions.
    2. Ethics, Clinical—Examination Questions.
    WB 18.2 A288 2003]
    RC58.A36 2003
    616'.0076—dc21

                                                                2002012013

ISBN 1-4051-0662-X

A catalogue record for this title is available from the British Library

Set in 9.5/12.5 pt Minion by SNP Best-set Typesetter Ltd.,
Hong Kong
Printed and bound in the UK by TJ International Ltd., Padstow

Commissioning Editor: Alison Brown
Editorial Assistant: Elizabeth Callaghan
Production Editor: Fiona Pattison
Production Controller: Kate Charman

For further information on Blackwell Publishing, visit our website:
http://www.blackwellpublishing.com

Contents

Preface

In clinical Stations 2 and 4 of the MRCP PACES exam (Practical Assessment of Clinical Examination), candidates are tested on their history taking and communication skills, and on their ability to abstract and provide the information not only to the examiners but also to patients, relatives and to other healthcare professionals. In an effort to test those skills that doctors are required to possess and execute daily in their clinical practice, and to endeavour to mimic the normal clinical environment, the Royal Colleges of Physicians have ordained that these Stations should resemble outpatient or inpatient hospital settings, and that candidates should be given the information in the form of a GP letter or a message as they would receive this in their normal clinical practice. Their ability to take a probing history and formulate diagnostic hypotheses, to respond to the anxieties and concerns of the patients and their relatives, to explain management plans, and to discuss sensitive prognostic and ethical issues is tested in both Stations by two examiners who have a preprinted mark-sheet for each scenario.

These are the tasks that all candidates approaching this exam will have performed many times, and seen being executed by their senior colleagues. However, until recently communication skills were neither taught as part of any formal syllabus nor tested in any examination. Consequently, many candidates will have had no formal teaching on communication skills, and hardly any would have had the experience of having a senior colleague sit in during history taking and afterwards discussing the conduct of the interview. The chief objective of this second volume is to fill this gap, and to provide a structured approach for candidates on the commonly occurring problems in clinical practice. We have included 50 scenarios in each Station that cover most of the problems that candidates are likely to encounter. They will find it profitable to play out these scenarios with other candidates to grasp the essentials and to polish their skills.

The Colleges set the standards that candidates have to achieve to become both proud collegiate members and good clinical practitioners. Our humble endeavour in the form of these two volumes is to translate those standards into a structured pathway for candidates to negotiate the hurdles of the PACES exam. Our experience in medical education, particularly after the publication of the first edition of *An Aid to the MRCP Short Cases*, has taught us that doctors who learn structured examination routines and good bedside behaviour for the exam tend to retain these habits. As many medical schools are changing the format of their exams to resemble the PACES, we hope that medical students will also find these volumes useful. Their success in the exams and their development into good clinicians providing first-rate service to medicine gives us much professional satisfaction.

Acknowledgements

We are extremely grateful to Mrs Jane Price, patient representative and advocate at Royal Gwent Hospital, Newport, who read the manuscript for Station 4 and contributed many invariable corrections and contributions.

Dev Banerjee
Bob Ryder
Afzal Mir
Anne Freeman

Introduction

I would have definitely benefited from more practice in history taking and in communication skills before the exam.
(see comments on Experience 15, p. 306)
Both the history section and the communication/ethics section are very rushed in the exam. It will feel very artificial because you will find there is too much to cover in 14 minutes (plus 1 minute thinking time and then 5 minutes questions) but persevere and be empathetic.
(see comments on Experience 22, p. 313)
I finished the history taking very quickly so had to sit in silence until time was up. That was awful!
(see comments on Experience 16, p. 307)

Stations 2 and 4 of the PACES examination are designed to be a comprehensive test of a candidate's ability to obtain an in-depth history, provide information to patients, and other relevant people, about sensitive issues such as malignant and sexually transmitted diseases, and their ability to discuss management and care plans with patients and allied medical staff.

Station 2 will assess your history taking skills. Two examiners will observe how you gather the appropriate and relevant facts from a patient, assimilate that information into either a diagnosis and/or a management plan, and then assess your discussion with them. During the 5-minute interval before you enter this Station, you will be given written instructions for the case you are going to see. This is often in the form of a letter from the patient's GP; thus, the Station simulates an outpatient clinic except that you will have two examiners, instead of two students, silently observing you. You will have 14 minutes with the patient and then 1 minute for reflection during which you must decide how you are going to present the crucial part of the history, which issues you will need to discuss with the examiners, and how you will suggest that you would respond to the referring letter.

Station 4 tests communication and ethics and your ability to guide and organize an interview with the subject (mostly an actor masquerading as a patient, relative or a healthcare worker). During the 5-minute interval preceding this Station you will receive written instructions summarizing the problem you will have to deal with. As for Station 2, you will have 14 minutes with the subject, in the presence of the examiners, during which you must explore and deal with the problem while providing emotional support whenever necessary, and

discuss further management. As the subject leaves the Station you will have just 1 minute to crystallize your thoughts for the 5-minute discussion with the examiners.

All three parties—the patient or an actor, the examiners and you—will each be given a preprinted sheet at both Stations. The patient will respond to your questions according to the brief, verbal as well as written on his or her sheet, the examiners will assess you according to their guidance notes, and you will have to complete your structured mark-sheet and hand it to the examiners at each Station. All this is done to ensure a level playing field for each candidate. Your sheet will form the basis for feedback to you should you fail to satisfy the examiners.

We have presented 50 scenarios for each of these two Stations which cover a diverse range of problems seen in clinical practice. For each scenario, we have given the information that might be written on the patient's sheet, and what the examiners' guidelines may look like which they will use to assess your interaction with the subject. We have also given some helpful hints before each Section but these will only prove useful if you have thoroughly prepared yourself for these tasks.

Doctors taking this exam need to have practised these skills and should have knowledge not only of the various clinical conditions likely to be encountered, but also of the myriad of ethical and legal issues which may arise. Doctors approaching the PACES exam, whether in the finals and/or in the higher exams, should make a purposeful preparation for it from the outset and, in the process, learn about structured clinical methods and good bedside behaviour.

Preparation
I would suggest that candidates need to have thought of the answers before they are asked, as the questions were really quite predictable.
(see comments on Experience 3, p. 287)

It is a well-known fact that the best preparation for passing the membership examination is to work on the firm of a good clinical teacher. In the real world of today, there are very few such teachers who would regard teaching as a worthwhile and rewarding pursuit, and those who are available are usually too busy to teach because of the increasing clinical and administrative demands. As one clinical tutor once ruefully remarked, 'In the past we used to teach students and now, in the current environment of political correctness and proper documentation, we spend our time talking about it!' More than ever the onus lies on the students to take due care of their learning programme and to make use of any learning opportunity (teaching sessions, clinical meetings, symposia, grand rounds, etc.) during their clinical duties.

History taking

The candidate mistimed the whole station; he raced through the history of presenting complaint in about 1 minute, proceeded to briefly take the rest of the history, and then realised he had 9 minutes left. The silence was broken by 'OK then, tell me about those palpitations again'.
(see Invigilators diaries — Stations 2 and 4, p. 324)

History taking is an art and cannot be acquired simply by reading books. Nonetheless, a book such as this can help you organize your approach to each symptom, select a battery of appropriate questions, interpret the information received, and narrow down the diagnostic hypotheses. It is important that students learn a structured approach from the very beginning during their clinical attachments, but it is never too late for postgraduate students to adapt and develop it.

There are 6–8 principal symptoms in each system and students should consult a book on clinical skills and master a battery of questions for each symptom, and then practise the art of asking these questions at every opportunity during their clinical training. Remembering the questions is easier than the art of asking them which can be improved by constant practice, self-criticism and by helpful criticism from a good teacher. A famous neurologist once said, during a teaching session, that diagnosing the cause of headache, the most common symptom in medicine, is like completing a jigsaw puzzle of asking 13 questions. Those who can only count 12 questions should consider asking the final question to the patient as to what he or she thinks is the cause of the headache. The same can be said about any other symptom such as chest pain or palpitations.

It is important to explore the presenting symptoms fully before going on to other aspects of the history taking. The examiners take a dim view of any candidate who skates back and forth from the presenting complaints to past or family history. It becomes easier to identify the chief areas of concern in other parts of the history, and the possible risk factors, only after adequately exploring the presenting complaints. Besides, it is imperative to let the patient ventilate fully his or her major concerns both in clinical practice and in the exam. A systems review will be necessary to find out if the patient has any other complaint which he or she has not mentioned.

During your clinical attachments and preregistration and senior house officer appointments, you should get into the habit of going over your notes each time you take a history, and judging whether you have covered all aspects of the history and assembled differential diagnoses. Once you have done that you should then prepare a summary of the problem(s) and the possible management plan and articulate it vocally to yourself. This habit will serve you well in any examination. As you prepare for the PACES exam, you should act out each history scenario from this book with a fellow candidate and discuss the conclusions and management plans. This will tighten up your history taking technique and your presentation skills. Remember, the examiners do not know you are clever; you have to demonstrate it. The exercise will also help make you a methodical and articulate clinician.

Communication skills and medical ethics

The patient said to the candidate, 'I'm worried this may be something serious.' The candidate replied 'That doesn't surprise me'.
(see Invigilators diaries — Stations 2 and 4, p. 324)

Unlike the history taking techniques, which are now taught from the very first year of medical training, the instruction on communication skills is still in its infancy. In the past, young doctors acquired these skills by osmosis from their senior colleagues whom they observed during their discussions with patients and relatives. Since 1995, communication skills have been incorporated in the new curricula that have been adopted by most medical schools in the UK. The Royal Colleges of the UK and the General Medical Council have all focused their attention on communication skills, and their assessment is now part of all major clinical examinations. As a result of this increasing emphasis on good communication, appropriate counselling skills and knowledge of ethics, one Station has been devoted to their assessment in the PACES examination. Most candidates approach this Station with some foreboding.

There are three main reasons why a candidate's heart may sink before entering the communication and ethics Station. First, unlike history taking, which has a long-established structure with subsets, communication skills are fluid and elastic and vary from problem to problem and from person to person. Although there are some recognized basic principles of a counselling interview as outlined at the beginning of Section E (p. 132), each problem, with its inherently unique circumstances, can impose its own constraints, which are different even when the same problem is discussed with another person.

Secondly, the multi-angled assimilative exercise of communication skills involves learning from tutors; talking to patients, relatives and other healthcare professionals; and studying the diverse range of ethical and legal issues that surround these problems. Unlike a clinical skill, which can be demonstrated by a tutor, communication skills cannot be imparted by a single demonstration or learned by one useful interview with a patient. It is a continuing learning process and most candidates are conscious that their technique and knowledge have some gaps.

Thirdly, even an apparently straightforward counselling scenario may present an unexpected hurdle, either because of its unique circumstances or because the interviewer forgot some simple principle. We know of a real-life incident when a consultant, during his round in a coronary care unit, was a witness to an unsuccessful cardiopulmonary resuscitation on one of his patients. As he and his entourage emerged from the door, the deceased patient's wife, who had just arrived, asked him about her husband. The consultant told her, as sympathetically as he could, that her husband had passed away. On hearing this the lady fainted, fell on the concrete floor before anyone could catch her, and sustained a nasty cut to her forehead. Sometime later, she charitably remarked, 'It was my own fault. I should have been sitting!' During a busy and eventful round, the consultant had forgotten to observe the basic principles of privacy and comfort which should be afforded to all recipients of bad news. He did not take the lady into a side room, get a nurse to sit with her to offer support and coffee, and then give her the bad news.

These considerations, apart from highlighting the concerns of the candidates, clearly reinforce a well-known fact that there is no shortcut to experience in acquiring communication skills. Medical students should grasp the fundamentals of communication, learn from personal and video demonstrations, and observe intently as many consultations as possible during their rotation through general practice and hospital placements when senior doctors speak to patients and relatives. They should seek permission to sit in on any interview between a senior clinician and a patient or a relative. As their training advances, and during their junior appointments, they should practise their own communication skills.

Candidates approaching this exam should have already gained some experience and they should use this book in developing it further and improving upon it. There are 50 scenarios on communication and ethics and we would suggest that two candidates should play out each scenario, one acting as the subject and the other the doctor, and then discuss the problem and the performance in the light of the examiner's information. After playing out each scenario they should discuss the various ethical and legal issues arising from it. We have provided relevant references to our sources of such information and candidates should look up these for themselves. Possession of adequate knowledge about the various aspects of each problem is essential in order to spare some thought and time to decide on the proper and appropriate kinetic behaviour (body language) in tune with that scenario. It is difficult to be thoughtful of a patient's sensitivities if you are struggling to recall information from distant and faded memory lacunae. Remember that even if all the points raised are addressed, the candidate will still fail if the overall impression of the examiners is of poor empathy and a hesitant interaction with the subject.

To sum up, those candidates who have acquired some personal experience of communication skills, who have studied and gained a thorough knowledge of these 50 scenarios, and who have been through them with fellow candidates would be leaving very little to chance. From our accumulated experience we have come to believe that no candidate passes the MRCP examination by pure luck, and a candidate who leaves gaps on the chance that the examiners may not explore them may be unsuccessful.

The examination

They are stone cold in expression and that often makes you think that you are doing badly but that's not always true.
(see comments on Experience 4, p. 289)

By the time you seriously consider taking the PACES examination, you should have gained enough experience in taking a history on almost any presenting complaint, obtained some instruction and experience in counselling and communication, studied several times a standard textbook on medicine and one on clinical skills, and have had many opportunities to summarize and present case histories in various forums. If, in addition, you were blessed with some critical appraisal of your presentations from senior colleagues and, in turn, you have constantly improved your performance by taking a comprehensive account of history and counselling scenarios, including preparing a succinct summary for presentation, then you have made the adequate preliminary preparation to study this book for your final preparation.

Study this book thoroughly; grasp the details of each scenario in the two main sections, play out each scenario with your fellow candidates and polish up your presentation. Get into the habit of summarizing the chief points in each scenario and practise presenting them to anyone who is prepared to listen and provide some helpful criticism. Practise speaking clearly and fluently in front of a mirror and into a tape recorder and play it back. When you have done all of this then you should feel confident and self-assured to enter the PACES exam.

Section D

A candidate, after seeing a patient with funny turns, gave no indication of any tests to be performed, any follow-up or any thoughts about the causes for the funny turns, ended the consultation by saying 'Thanks, we've finished now'.
(see Invigilators' diaries—Stations 2 and 4, p. 324)

Station 2
History Taking Skills

1 Abdominal swelling
2 Ankle swelling
3 Asymptomatic hypertensive
4 Back pain
5 Breathlessness
6 Burning of the feet
7 Chest pain
8 Cold and painful fingers
9 Cause of collapse?
10 Confusion
11 Cough
12 Diabetic feet
13 Difficulty in walking
14 Dizziness and feeling faint
15 Double vision
16 Dysphagia
17 Epigastric pain and nausea
18 Facial swelling
19 Funny turns
20 Haemoptysis
21 Headache
22 Hoarse voice
23 Hypercalcaemia
24 Hyperlipidaemia
25 Jaundice

26 Joint pains
27 Loin pain
28 Loss of weight
29 Lower gastrointestinal haemorrhage
30 Macrocytic anaemia
31 Neck lump
32 Painful shins
33 Painful shoulders
34 Palpitations
35 Personality change
36 Pins and needles
37 Polyuria
38 Pruritus
39 Purpuric rash
40 Pyrexia
41 Renal colic and haematuria
42 Tiredness
43 Tremor
44 Visual disturbances
45 Vomiting
46 Vomiting and forgetfulness
47 Weakness of an arm
48 Weight gain
49 Weight loss and chronic diarrhoea
50 Wheeze

Section D | **Station 2**

The history taking station in the PACES examination tests the candidates' ability to explore and probe the presenting complaint(s), gather and interpret information, formulate a plan of action, communicate it to the patient and then discuss the conclusions and management plan with the examiners. The cases presented in the exam, and in this book, are the ones that doctors encounter in their everyday clinical practice and the ones that candidates should be familiar with. Yet our information from various sources suggests that since the PACES examination was started many candidates have performed poorly both in this station as well as in station 4. It seems perverse that doctors, trained in the basic skill of medicine from the very first year of medical school, and experienced in taking histories from their patients every day, should perform poorly in it. A brief reflection over the reports received by us suggests three main reasons for this failure.

First, candidates are not used to having someone, particularly two senior doctors, sitting with them while they are taking a history. In the exam, many candidates become too conscious of the presence of the pair of examiners and they tend to use either a machine-gun approach by asking a lot of questions about a symptom without reflection, or skate from one aspect of the history to another in an effort to demonstrate their ability to focus on important issues. Candidates unwittingly stray into the areas that are not covered in the patient's information sheet. The patient/actor then falls on his or her own resources to manufacture some quick answers and both lose their way. This creates a bad impression both on the patient as well as the examiners and, in the process, candidates lose their grip on the main problem.

Secondly, most candidates who fail to satisfy the examiners have badly handled the presenting complaints. They do not approach the problem logically by creating a list of possible diagnoses from the given complaints, and they do not probe each complaint to narrow down that list to a probable diagnosis.

Finally, some candidates forget that in a history taking station there are three agencies to answer to; the patient who needs to know what is wrong with him or her and what the doctor proposes to do about it; the examiners who have to be satisfied about a plan of action; and the referring doctor who needs an answer to the problem posed in the letter. Many candidates who fail in this exam have made a bad job of their presentation.

For any hope of successfully negotiating this station, candidates have to be thoroughly prepared for this encounter by studying and acting out the scenarios in this book with their colleagues. The scenarios have been written in a form similar to the PACES exam. In each scenario, we have included a GP letter which you will be given outside the room, a patient information sheet which you will not see in the exam but which gives the patient all the necessary information to allow them to respond to your questions, and an examiners' information sheet which gives you a good idea about the main points that the examiners will be looking for and how they will assess you. We suggest that you study each scenario carefully and then act it out with a fellow candidate, keeping in mind the following important guidelines.

- Read the letter carefully and ascertain who is making the referral and the exact nature of their concern. At the end, you will have to answer that by offering a plan of action.
- Note the exact presenting complaints and write them down on a piece of paper to remind yourself as you progress through history taking.
- From the presenting complaints, consider the possible differential diagnoses that will need to be covered during the consultation. Based on this, formulate an approach as to how the consultation should be carried out, what relevant questions should be asked and in what order, and what issues should be tackled.
- Introduce yourself to the patient and explain the purpose of the interview, e.g. 'Your GP has written to me explaining that you are having some trouble with your breathing. I would like to ask you some questions, if I may, so that I can decide on a plan of action to investigate this problem.'
- The first question about the presenting complaint(s) is the most important one; it should allow the patient to talk freely, e.g. 'Tell me about it', or, 'Tell me all about your breathing difficulty and how it started.' This approach avoids leading the patient, allows him or her space and time to say what concerns him or her the most, and identifies the problem that the candidate will have to address at the end in explaining a plan of action to the patient. A fringe benefit of such an open-ended question is that the patient may say a bit more about what is on his or her information sheet. We know of one incident when a volunteer patient, who was probably inadequately briefed, regurgitated all that was on the information sheet in answer to this one question!
- Probe each complaint sequentially and get an idea of the impact of the symptoms on the patient and the family. Do not jump from one complaint to another without getting a good idea of the nature of each.
- Be attentive and do not lose eye contact with the patient. You may take notes but do not overdo it and do not appear to be taking a dictation.
- Verify and expand on any incidents that the patient may mention. For example, if the patient has uncontrolled asthma and says that he or she was admitted to the ITU last year, find out what his or her symptoms were at the time, what was the cause of the exacerbation, how long he or she was in ITU, and what treatment was given.
- Pace yourself. You have 14 minutes which should allow you to cover all aspects of the history. Do not rush through the consultation and find that you have 7 minutes of silence to endure which will seem like an eternity. The exam is not a test of whether you can see 10 new patients in one clinic session! Do not appear to be taking past history, drug history or social history only because you have some time left; make them an essential part of your consultation. In particular, take a comprehensive social history which may have some bearing on the patient's illness. Complete a brief systems review to ensure that you get the full picture and that you do not miss any symptom that the patient may not have considered important enough to mention.
- As you complete the consultation, ask the patient if there is anything you have not discussed or he or she has forgotten to mention.
- Make sure the queries in the referral letter have been addressed. Formulate a management plan and explain it to the patient in simple terms. Reassure him or her that a letter will go to the GP. Tell the patient about the follow-up arrangements that will be made. You will have to explain all this to the examiners during your discussion with them.
- Be polite and courteous throughout.

Case 1 | Abdominal swelling

Candidate information

You are the SHO in a general medical clinic. Mr David Brian has been referred to you by his GP.

Please read this letter (it should take no more than 2 min) and then continue with the consultation.

> Dear Doctor
>
> **Re: Mr David Brian, aged 53**
>
> Thank you for seeing Mr Brian urgently in your clinic. He gives a 4-week history of abdominal swelling. There is some discomfort from the swelling but no specific pain and he rarely drinks alcohol. On examination, he is thin, looks unwell, is not jaundiced and I suspect that he has ascites. Please see and advise.
>
> Your sincerely
>
> Dr G. Practitioner

You have 14 min until the patient leaves the room, followed by 1 min for reflection, before the discussion with the examiners. Be prepared to discuss the solutions to the problems posed by the case and how you might reply to the GP's letter.

Patient information

Mr David Brian is a 53-year-old musician who presents with a 4-week history of progressive abdominal swelling. He has noticed his abdominal wall to be tight and as a result he has some generalized discomfort but there is no specific pain. He has had loss of appetite, malaise and some wasting of the muscles of his limbs. He has no associated symptoms of jaundice, ankle swelling, haematemesis, melaena, change in bowel habit or vomiting. He has no other respiratory, cardiovascular or urinary symptoms. He has an unremarkable past medical history. He rarely drinks alcohol and has never had any liver disease in the past. He takes no medication except for occasional paracetamol for headaches. He has no risk factors for HIV or viral hepatitis. He has not been abroad recently and he lives with a partner. He has never smoked. He is concerned that he may have cancer.

Examiner information

1 Data gathering in the interview

A good candidate would be able to elicit:
- the details of the abdominal swelling particularly the time span, if the swelling was progressing, whether the swelling is generalized or focal and if there is any associated pain or discomfort
- other gastrointestinal symptoms which may indicate liver cirrhosis or abdominal malignancy, e.g. haematemesis, melaena, jaundice, change in bowel habit, inguinal lymphadenopathy

- systemic symptoms, e.g. loss of weight and appetite, fever, breathlessness as a result of the ascites and other clues to a malignancy elsewhere
- risk factors for liver cirrhosis, e.g. excessive alcohol consumption, viral hepatitis, drug-induced, auto-immune
- other causes of ascites, e.g. symptoms suggestive of acute or chronic pancreatitis, intra-abdominal sepsis/infection, congestive cardiac failure, hepatic vein thrombosis, nephrotic syndrome and tuberculosis
- any exposure to asbestos (peritoneal mesothelioma is a rare cause of malignant ascites)
- the impact of the illness on him and his work
- the concerns of the patient

2 Identification and use of information gathered

The candidate should be able to interpret the history and create a problem list. The objectives for the candidate are to:
- develop a list of possible differential diagnoses
- have a list of investigations
- explain the possible causes of the illness to the patient and explain the need to admit

3 Discussion related to the case

- Causes of abdominal swelling include obesity, gaseous distension, pregnancy in females, intra-abdominal masses, e.g. ovarian in females and fluid, i.e. ascites.
- In liver disease, ascites indicates a chronic or subacute disorder and does not occur in acute conditions (e.g. uncomplicated viral hepatitis, drug reactions, biliary obstruction). The most common cause is cirrhosis, especially from alcoholism. Other hepatic causes include chronic hepatitis, severe alcoholic hepatitis without cirrhosis and hepatic vein obstruction (Budd–Chiari syndrome). Portal vein thrombosis does not usually cause ascites unless hepatocellular damage is also present.
- Non-hepatic causes of ascites include generalized fluid retention associated with systemic disease (e.g. heart failure, nephrotic syndrome, severe hypoalbuminaemia, constrictive pericarditis) and intra-abdominal disorders (e.g. carcinomatosis, tuberculous peritonitis). Hypothyroidism occasionally causes marked ascites and pancreatitis rarely causes large amounts of fluid (pancreatic ascites). Patients with renal failure, especially those on haemodialysis, occasionally develop unexplained intra-abdominal fluid.
- A diagnostic tap of 50 mL should be obtained and sent for cytology, microscopy, acid alcohol fast bacilli (AAFB) and amylase. The presence of haemorrhagic ascites is in favour of malignancy, acute pancreatitis and abdominal trauma. Straw-coloured ascites is more commonly found in cirrhosis, infective causes, congestive cardiac failure, nephrotic syndrome, hepatic vein obstruction as well as malignancy.
- A neutrophil count of >250 cells/mm^3 is indicative of an underlying bacterial peritonitis justifying broad-spectrum intravenous antibiotic therapy in the presence of a fever.
- This case favours a diagnosis of a malignancy and the investigation of choice would be a computed tomography (CT) scan of the abdomen. Treatment of ascites in a patient with liver cirrhosis aims to reduce sodium intake and increase the renal excretion of sodium with a careful combination of diuretics and fluid restriction.

Comments on the case

This case tests the candidate's ability to generate a list of differential diagnoses for ascites. The patient is unwell and must be admitted for investigations.

Case 2 | Ankle swelling

Candidate information

You are the SHO on call in a cardiology clinic. Miss Vicky Daniels has been referred to you by her GP.

Please read this letter (it should take no more than 2 min) and then continue with the consultation.

> Dear Doctor
>
> **Re: Miss Vicky Daniels, aged 29**
>
> Thank you for seeing Vicky Daniels who works as a cleaner at the local law courts. She has had asthma for 2 years treated with budesonide and Bricanyl inhalers and chest pain off and on. However, her breathlessness and chest pain have worsened over the last 2 months and she now has ankle swelling. I would appreciate your help.
>
> Yours sincerely
>
> Dr G. Practitioner

You have 14 min until the patient leaves the room, followed by 1 min for reflection, before the discussion with the examiners. Be prepared to discuss the solutions to the problems posed by the case and how you might reply to the GP's letter.

Patient information

Vicky Daniels is a 29-year-old domestic cleaner at the local law courts who has had a 2-year history of breathlessness and chest pain. Up to 2 years ago she was reasonably fit and well but she remembers that, after a lower respiratory chest infection, she began to get more breathless with a feeling of tightness in the chest. At that time it was felt she may have asthma and, as there is a strong family history, she was started on budesonide 200 μg b.d. and Bricanyl (prn (as required)) turbohalers. Unfortunately, her dyspnoea has progressed so much that walking upstairs or up a slight incline is a real effort. The chest pain is usually central, non-pleuritic, without radiation and is occasionally exertional. It usually eases with resting. She also complains of extreme tiredness and ankle swelling over the last 2 months and she has now stopped working. There are no obvious relieving or precipitating factors or any known allergy to the common household allergens. She has no orthopnoea, syncope, palpitations, cough, sputum, haemoptysis, rash or arthropathy and there are no gastroenterological or neurological symptoms. There is no previous history of pulmonary emboli, congenital heart disease, chronic lung disease, scleroderma, systemic lupus erythematosus (SLE) or HIV infection. She takes no medication apart from the inhalers. She has never smoked, she drinks on occasions and lives with her mother who also has asthma. There are no pets in the house. She is obviously very worried about her progressive breathlessness and is desperate for help.

Examiner information

1 Data gathering in the interview

A good candidate would be able to elicit:
- the chronology of the symptoms
- the exact features of the dyspnoea and the chest pain with particular reference to her exercise ability. Does the chest pain sound anginal or pleuritic (pulmonary emboli)?
- the recent onset of ankle swelling; which leg, how far up the leg and whether putting on shoes is difficult
- other respiratory symptoms, e.g. haemoptysis (chronic pulmonary emboli), chronic cough and sputum (chronic lung disease, e.g. bronchiectasis), cardiovascular symptoms, e.g. syncope and palpitations (congenital heart disease, mitral valve disease)
- the full asthma history—is this really asthma? Whether there is any evidence of diurnal symptoms of cough and wheeze, allergy to common household allergens (e.g. cats, house dust mite, pollen), if the inhalers have helped the symptoms, and on what basis did the GP diagnose asthma (serial peak flows vs. clinical)
- past medical history of congenital heart disease, mitral valve disease, chronic lung disease, thrombo-embolic disease, collagen-vascular disease such as scleroderma and SLE
- drug history, e.g. appetite suppressors such as fenfluramine
- family history of primary pulmonary hypertension
- the impact of the illness on her life, family and work
- any recent air travel which may have exacerbated symptoms (pregnancy does too in primary pulmonary hypertension and mitral stenosis)
- her concerns

2 Identification and use of information gathered

The candidate should be able to interpret the history and create a problem list. The objectives for the candidate are to:
- assemble a list of differential diagnoses
- have a list of investigations to be arranged urgently and explain these to the patient
- address any concerns
- arrange follow-up as soon as possible to discuss the results

3 Discussion related to the case

- This case tests the ability of the candidate to have a list of differential diagnoses for ankle oedema, breathlessness and chest pain in a young, non-smoking, previously fit woman. The possibilities are primary pulmonary hypertension (a rare condition that favours young females) or secondary pulmonary hypertension (e.g. recurrent pulmonary embolism), chronic lung disease (e.g. bronchiectasis), congenital heart disease, collagen-vascular disease (e.g. scleroderma or SLE), HIV infection, drug-induced especially from weight-reducing appetite suppressors or other rarer causes (e.g. veno-occlusive disease).
- In the absence of any secondary causes, this case is most likely to be primary pulmonary hypertension. Investigations would include: chest X-ray showing enlarged central pulmonary arteries and clear lung fields, ECG revealing right axis deviation and right ventricular hypertrophy, an echocardiogram demonstrating right ventricular enlargement, a reduction in left ventricular cavity size, and abnormal septal configuration consistent with right ventricular pressure overload, full lung function testing for impaired diffusion and hypoxaemia, ventilation–perfusion scan to rule out pulmonary emboli and cardiac catheterization (with care) to characterize the disease and to exclude an underlying cardiac shunt as the cause.
- Management is challenging and the patient should be looked after by a cardiologist with a specialist interest. Reduction in pulmonary vascular resistance with short-acting vasodilators, e.g. nitric oxide, intravenous adenosine or intravenous prostacyclin may determine who will respond better to high-dose oral calcium-channel blockers, e.g. nifedipine and diltiazem. Recent trials have shown the benefit of long-term intravenous administration of prostacyclin. In those who do not respond, heart and lung transplantation may need to be considered.

Comments on the case

This lady presents with three symptoms, i.e. dyspnoea, chest pain and ankle swelling. Hence the candidate must be prepared to take *three* clear histories with a view to looking for a link between them.

Case 3 | Asymptomatic hypertensive

Candidate information

You are the SHO in a general medical clinic. Mr Tom Walker has been referred to you by his GP.

Please read this letter (it should take no more than 2 min) and then continue with the consultation.

> Dear Doctor
>
> **Re: Mr Tom Walker, aged 49**
>
> Thank you for seeing Mr Walker whom I found to have a blood pressure (BP) of 180/95 mmHg. I started him on bendrofluazide 2.5 mg o.d. but his BP continues to be elevated. He smokes 15 cigarettes a day and drinks 16 pints at the weekends. Past medical history includes anxiety attacks and mild asthma, for which he takes a salbutamol inhaler on a PRN basis. He is a self-employed painter and decorator. Please see and advise.
>
> Yours sincerely
>
> Dr G. Practitioner

You have 14 min until the patient leaves the room, followed by 1 min for reflection, before the discussion with the examiners. Be prepared to discuss the solutions to the problems posed by the case and how you might reply to the GP's letter.

Patient information

Mr Tom Walker is a 49-year-old, slightly overweight painter and decorator who is currently asymptomatic with no relevant symptoms such as chest pains, palpitations, headache, dyspnoea, blurred vision, sweating, tremors, weight change or urinary problems. On a recent visit to the GP for a Well-Man clinic appointment, a BP of 180/95 mmHg was recorded and he was started on bendrofluazide 2.5 mg o.d. Subsequent BP measurements by the GP have shown no improvement. However, Mr Walker does admit to poor compliance with the bendrofluazide as a result of impotence being a side-effect. He does occasionally have episodes of anxiety that may manifest as irritability, difficulty in sleeping and worry. These have been amplified by a recent reduction in contractual painting and decorating work. He does also admit to high levels of anxiety when visiting his GP. Other past medical history includes mild asthma usually triggered by coryzal illnesses but at present this is stable without any nocturnal symptoms and he rarely needs to take his inhaler. He tends to lead a sedentary lifestyle, smokes 15 cigarettes a day and drinks heavily, particularly at the weekends—about 8 pints of beer a day. He lives with his wife and has two children who have left home. His father had hypertension. He does admit that the impotence persists even when the bendrofluazide is not taken and that this has caused some marital strife.

Examiner information

1 Data gathering in the interview

A good candidate would be able to elicit:

- whether a raised blood pressure has been found before. (If a female patient presents with a history like this, do not forget to ask about pregnancy-induced hypertension.)
- any relevant symptoms, e.g. headache, chest pains, palpitations, dyspnoea, ankle oedema, blurred vision, sweating, tremors, weight change, urinary symptoms
- symptoms of the anxiety disorder and obvious triggers, e.g. anxiety when meeting doctors
- previous medical history including ischaemic heart disease, hypercholesterolaemia, renal disease, peripheral vascular disease, diabetes mellitus, endocrine and thyroid disorders
- family history of hypertension, heart disease, hyperlipidaemia and endocrine disorders
- drug history, especially the bendrofluazide with particular reference to side-effects (ask about the impotence and its impact), corticosteroids, sympathomimetics, liquorice
- the use of the salbutamol inhaler—overusage can cause shakes and tremors
- detailed smoking and alcohol history
- lifestyle, i.e. physical exercise, diet
- work history
- social history, particularly any marital problems

2 Identification and use of information gathered

The candidate should be able to interpret the history and create a problem list. The objectives for the candidate are to:

- be aware of the possible causes of the hypertension
- decide if anxiety or the non-compliance to antihypertensives or the 'white-coat' effect may be contributing to the hypertension
- appreciate the reasons for non-compliance, particularly the side-effects of the bendrofluazide
- have an understanding of any marital strife and work problems that may be exacerbating the anxiety

3 Discussion related to the case

- This case tests the ability of the candidate to judge the possible causes of raised blood pressure, i.e. 'white-coat'-induced, anxiety-provoked, essential or secondary causes, e.g. renal (diabetic nephropathy, chronic glomerulonephritis, adult polycystic disease, renovascular disease and chronic tubulointerstitial nephritis), endocrine (Conn's syndrome, adrenal hyperplasia, phaeochromocytoma, Cushing's syndrome and acromegaly), cardiovascular (coarctation of the aorta) and drug-induced (oral contraceptive pill, steroids).
- The candidate must be able to: (a) address the issues of compliance; (b) assess other cardiovascular risk factors; (c) discuss moderating alcohol consumption with smoking cessation and improving health, e.g. diet and exercise; (d) probe sensitively into the circumstances generating the anxiety; and (e) discuss the importance of blood pressure control. This should encourage improved compliance.
- The candidate must have a plan of investigations such as routine tests especially urea and electrolytes (U/E), lipids, urine dipsticking, fundoscopy, chest X-ray, ECG and 24-h ambulatory blood pressure monitoring.
- There may be no relevant symptoms unless hypertension has resulted in end-organ damage.
- The candidate must be able to discuss with the examiners: (a) the interpretation of 24-h ambulatory BP monitoring; (b) the WHO criteria for defining hypertension with or without the presence of diabetes; (c) discuss the impact of the Framingham USA study on outcomes; (d) the causes of secondary hypertension, e.g. renal, endocrine, drug-induced and pregnancy-induced; (e) the complications of hypertension; (f) relevant retinal changes seen on fundoscopy; (g) drug treatment including side-effects; and (h) the management of malignant hypertension.
- Follow-up will have to be arranged to discuss the results of the 24-h ambulatory measurements. The consideration of anxiety control, e.g. relaxation training through a psychologist may be made.

Guidelines from the British Hypertension Society (1999) are as follows.

- In all hypertensives and borderline hypertensive people first of all use non-pharmacological measures such as weight reduction, reducing alcohol and dietary salt intake, anxiety control or 'stress management'.
- Initiate antihypertensive drug therapy in people with sustained systolic blood pressure (BP) ≥ 160 mmHg or sustained diastolic BP ≥ 100 mmHg.
- Decide on treatment in people with sustained systolic BP between 140 and 159 mmHg or sustained diastolic BP between 90 and 99 mmHg according to the presence or absence of target organ damage, cardiovascular disease or a 10-year coronary heart disease (CHD) risk of $\geq 15\%$ according to the Joint British Societies CHD risk assessment programme/risk chart.

- In those with diabetes mellitus, initiate antihypertensive therapy if systolic BP is sustained ≥140 mmHg or diastolic BP is sustained ≥90 mmHg.
- In non-diabetic hypertensive people, optimal BP treatment targets are: systolic BP <140 mmHg and diastolic BP < 85 mmHg. The minimum acceptable level of control (Audit Standard) recommended is <150/<90 mmHg. Despite best practices, these levels will be difficult to achieve in some hypertensive patients.
- In diabetic hypertensive people, the optimal BP targets are: systolic BP < 140 mmHg and diastolic BP < 80 mmHg. The minimum acceptable level of control (Audit Standard) recommended is <140/<90 mmHg. Despite best practice, these levels will be difficult to achieve in some people with diabetes and hypertension.
- In the absence of contraindications, or compelling indications for other antihypertensive agents, low-dose thiazide diuretics or beta-blockers are preferred as first-line therapy for most hypertensive people. In the absence of compelling indications for beta-blockade, diuretics or long-acting dihydropyridine, calcium antagonists are preferred to beta-blockers in older subjects.
- Other drugs that reduce cardiovascular risk must also be considered. These include aspirin for secondary prevention of cardiovascular disease and primary prevention in treated hypertensive subjects over the age of 50 years who have a 10-year CHD risk ≥15% and in whom blood pressure is controlled to the Audit Standard. Statin therapy is recommended for hypertensive people with a total cholesterol ≥5 mmol/L and established vascular disease, or a 10-year CHD risk ≥30% estimated from the Joint British Societies CHD risk chart.

Comments on the case

This is a common case where a patient may not have a specific symptom complaint. 'Hypertension' is not a presenting complaint, and the candidate must state that the patient is asymptomatic when presenting the case to the examiners. Many patients attend specialized clinics after an objective measurement finding, e.g. raised blood pressure, abnormal urine analysis or an abnormal chest X-ray. However, the case tests the candidate's ability to scrutinize and explore more deeply into the history and particularly about hidden symptoms, i.e. the impotence, the psychology of non-compliance (commonly neglected by candidates), the complex social background and other health issues that would facilitate a primary prevention programme.

Case 4 | Backpain

Candidate information

You are the SHO in a general medical clinic. Mrs Janet Reardon has been referred to you by her GP.

Please read this letter (it should take no more than 2 min) and then continue with the consultation.

> Dear Doctor
>
> **Re: Mrs Janet Reardon, aged 63**
>
> Thank you for seeing this lady. She has complained of a continuous back-ache for the last 6 weeks. She is otherwise well. I have tried her with co-codamol without much success. Please see and advise. I wonder if she has osteoporosis.
>
> Yours sincerely
>
> Dr G. Practitioner

You have 14 min until the patient leaves the room, followed by 1 min for reflection, before the discussion with the examiners. Be prepared to discuss the solutions to the problems posed by the case and how you might reply to the GP's letter.

Patient information

Mrs Janet Reardon is a 63-year-old divorcee who was previously a bank clerk. She gives a 6-week history of backache. There was no obvious precipitant to this ache, e.g. falls, trauma, lifting, etc. The pain is localized to the mid-vertebral thoracic area and radiates circumferentially along one of the ribs on the right side and around to the front. The pain is sharp and constant and is worse on coughing, sneezing and twisting. The pain interrupts her sleep if she twists in bed and there has been only little relief with co-codamol. There are no pains in her joints, especially the neck, hands and hips. There is no history of any sciatic pain. There are no other symptoms such as fever, malaise, weight loss; or any respiratory or abdominal symptoms although she does feel more tired than usual. She has no past history of note apart from one admission for a lower respiratory tract infection 5 years ago. She has not had an oophorectomy. She smokes 20 cigarettes a day and does not drink alcohol. She does not take any medication and in particular has never taken oral corticosteroids. She has been postmenopausal for 14 years and never took hormone replacement therapy (HRT). She lives alone in a bungalow. She is concerned that she may have osteoporosis as there is a strong family history of this (mother and elder sister).

Examiner information

1 Data gathering in the interview

A good candidate would be able to elicit:

- the full details of the backache especially the site of the pain, nature and character, radiation, precipitating and relieving factors and any history of trauma or falls
- if the pain is worse after coughing, sneezing or movement
- any pains in other joints or evidence of sciatica, claudication or neck pain
- other symptoms, e.g. fever, malaise, weight loss, respiratory or abdominal symptoms
- any symptoms suggestive of neoplasia
- any history of trauma
- any details in the history suggesting the possibility of risk factors for osteoporosis, e.g. early menopause, history of oophorectomy, family history of osteoporosis, smoking, nutrition, corticosteroid therapy and other possible endocrine or rheumatological diseases
- drug history, including HRT
- smoking history
- a detailed account of the impact of the pain on her life
- particular concerns, especially the possibility of a diagnosis of osteoporosis

2 Identification and use of information gathered

The candidate should be able to interpret the history and create a problem list. The objectives for the candidate are to:

- determine a list of differential diagnoses of osteoporosis with or without vertebral body collapse/compression, intervertebral disc disease (e.g. herniation), metastatic bone disease, myeloma, Paget's disease, infection (e.g. septic arthritis or chronic brucellosis)
- confirm the diagnosis by arranging the appropriate investigations as mentioned below
- address the pain control
- discuss the possibilities of osteoporosis and the therapeutic options (pharmacological and non-pharmacological)
- discuss smoking cessation, diet and general exercise

3 Discussion related to the case

- This case tests the ability of the candidate to take a detailed history, to consider the possibility of osteoporosis and to guide the history around the risk factors for osteoporosis. Another possibility, which may commonly present this way, is intervertebral disc disease. It is important to explore the possibility of metastatic disease especially from a pulmonary or breast malignancy; this patient is a heavy smoker. Myeloma is probably unlikely but still must be acknowledged as a possibility.
- A plan of investigations should include biochemical markers, e.g. bone profile, serum immunoglobulins, full blood count (FBC), liver function tests (LFT) and X-rays of the thoracic and lumbar spine which may show fractures (although unreliable to evaluate bone density). Bone densitometry, such as dual energy X-ray absorption scanning (DEXA), is being increasingly used to investigate osteoporosis. Isotope bone scans may be considered to look for fractures and metastatic deposits. If bone densitometry is normal, a magnetic resonance imaging (MRI) scan of the thoracic and lumbar spine should be considered to look for intervertebral disc disease.
- For discussion, the candidate must be able to define osteoporosis as a bone density of more than 2.5 standard deviations below the young adult mean value for individuals matched for sex and race. The candidate must be able to discuss the risk factors, investigations and management, especially pain control, the role of oestrogen therapy and biphosphonates, diet and smoking cessation.
- The management of osteoporosis includes risk factor reduction, particularly reviewing corticosteroid therapy and prevention of falls. A large body of clinical trial data indicates that various types of oestrogens reduce bone turnover, prevent bone loss and induce small increases in bone mass of the spine, hip and total body. The effects of oestrogen are seen in women with natural or surgical menopause and in late postmenopausal women with or without established osteoporosis.
- The effect of oestrogens on fracture frequency is less well determined. Only epidemiological databases indicate that women who take oestrogen replacement may have a 50% reduction, on average, of osteoporotic fractures including hip fractures. The beneficial effect of oestrogen is greatest among those who start replacement early and continue the treatment; the benefit wanes after discontinuation such that there is no residual protective effect against fracture by 10 years after discontinuation. Long-term oestrogen use may be associated with an increase in the risk of venous thromboembolism and gallbladder, uterine and breast cancer although, in observational studies, oestrogens have been associated with a significant reduction in myocardial infarction. However, the evidence is not totally convincing and ongoing trials may provide further information in the future.

Comments on the case

In this case the examiners will expect the candidate to take a detailed history of the backache, including the impact of the symptoms on the patient's life, while acknowledging the possibilities of other diagnoses. Do not assume the patient has osteoporosis just because this is what the GP is considering as most likely; keep an open mind and do not forget about pathological fractures. The candidate also needs to explore the patient's fears about osteoporosis and so the consultation will involve discussing a plan of management with some counselling on the subject.

Case 5 | Breathlessness

Candidate information

You are the SHO in a general medical clinic. Mr Alan Smith has been referred to you by his GP.

Please read this letter (it should take no more than 2 min) and then continue with the consultation.

Dear Doctor

Re: Mr Alan Smith, aged 76

Thank you for seeing this ex-smoker who has had asthma for 5 years. Recently he has been complaining of increasing breathlessness and wheeze. His peak flow was 150 L/min in the surgery. He is on beclomethasone and salbutamol inhalers. Please see and advise.

Yours sincerely

Dr G. Practitioner

You have 14 min until the patient leaves the room, followed by 1 min for reflection, before the discussion with the examiners. Be prepared to discuss the solutions to the problems posed by the case and how you might reply to the GP's letter.

Patient information

Mr Smith is a 76-year-old man who first presented to his GP 5 years ago after a lower respiratory tract infection manifesting as wheeze, purulent sputum and breathlessness. Then his peak flow rate was 170 L/min. He continued to complain of breathlessness and wheeze and he was started on regular salbutamol and beclomethasone inhalers by the GP after he suspected asthma. He had not been seen at the practice until 4 weeks ago but now he is complaining of breathlessness after 50 m, difficulty with stairs and inability to walk to the post office to collect his pension. Other symptoms include wheezing on exertion, mucoid sputum every day and fatigue. The symptoms of wheeze and breathlessness do not vary during the day. He gets woken twice at night as a result of the cough. He has no chest pain or ankle swelling. There are no obvious triggers such as pollen, house dust mite, cat dander, pollution, smoke or cold air. He had one infective exacerbation last year but he did not visit his GP for help. His past medical history includes a duodenal ulcer 15 years ago. He has no known drug allergies and he has no pets at home. He lives with his wife in a terraced house and she does most of the shopping. He has previously worked as a welder and smoked 20 cigarettes a day from the age of 15 years up to 5 years ago. He does not drink alcohol. His main concerns are that he is getting more and more breathless without much relief from the inhalers and that he is unable to go out to meet his family or his friends for social events.

Examiner information

1 Data gathering in the interview

A good candidate would be able to elicit:
- how his chest complaints first presented 5 years ago
- his premorbid state before this, i.e. exercise tolerance, symptoms of cough/wheeze/sputum, activities of daily living
- how rapidly his symptoms have deteriorated
- a detailed account of the present symptoms, i.e. breathlessness (over what distance on the flat before he stops, up an incline), ability to do stairs, cough/wheeze/sputum and their variability during the day
- an idea of the number of exacerbations per year, winter exacerbations, worse after coryzal illnesses?
- any allergic factors, e.g. triggers such as pollen, exercise, smoke, pets, house dust mite, history of allergic rhinitis and/or eczema
- inhaler history; type (i.e. multidose inhaler vs. turbohaler vs. accuhaler) and technique. Previous use of prednisolone and, if so, any improvements in symptoms and any side-effects
- occupational history, any exposure to agents at work, e.g. isocyanates, platinum salts, hardening agents, soldering fluxes
- smoking history (calculate the pack years, i.e. one pack of 20 cigarettes per day for 1 year is 1 pack year), age when started
- drug history, e.g. use of non-steroidal anti-inflammatory drugs (NSAIDs), diuretics, etc.
- impact of disease both physical and psychosocial, i.e. on dressing, washing, housework, sleep, how often he gets out of the house, ability to attend social events, the impact on the family, embarrassment of using inhalers especially in public
- his concerns, e.g. does he panic when he cannot get his breath, does he expect his chest to get worse, does he feel embarrassed by having to use inhalers in public?

2 Identification and use of information gathered

The candidate should be able to interpret the history and create a problem list. The objectives for the candidate are to:
- explain what chronic obstructive airways disease (COPD) and asthma are
- address the worsening symptoms
- confirm the correct diagnosis by arranging the appropriate investigations

- consider different inhaler devices if the inhaler technique is poor
- give general health advice such as exercise, nutrition and vaccination (influenza and pneumococcal)

3 Discussion related to the case

- This case tests the ability of the candidate to differentiate the diagnosis of asthma from COPD. COPD typically presents with progressive symptoms (usually in the presence of a smoking history) without variable daily symptoms and no obvious allergen allergy, i.e. triggers that are typical in asthma. A proportion of patients may have both COPD and asthma. The suboptimal peak flow on its own should not lead to the diagnosis of asthma.
- The candidate should have a plan of investigations, e.g. chest X-ray, FBC, ECG, full lung function tests including spirometry, lung volumes, diffusion, flow volume loops, reversibility of forced expiratory volume in 1 s (FEV_1) to salbutamol, oxygen saturation on air, serial peak flows and follow-up to discuss these results.
- British Thoracic Society guidelines define COPD as a chronic, slowly progressive disorder characterized by airway obstruction ($FEV_1 < 80\%$ predicted and $FEV_1 : VC$ ratio $< 70\%$), which does not change markedly over several months, together with symptoms such as breathlessness on moderate exertion and cough $\pm$ sputum. Presenting features of acute exacerbations include worsening symptoms of a previously stable condition, increased wheeze/dyspnoea/sputum volume and purulence. In deciding whether to treat a patient at home or at hospital, one should ask if the patient is unable to cope at home, whether there is cyanosis, reduced consciousness, moderate breathlessness, poor general condition, poor level of activity and poor social circumstances (all of which should favour hospital admission). Initial treatment is to achieve an arterial Pa_{O_2} of at least 6.6 kPa without a fall in pH to below 7.26 (secondary to a rise in Pa_{CO_2}). A pH of below 7.26 is predictive of a poor outcome. For patients aged over 50 years the maximum initial inspiratory oxygen concentration should be 28% via a Venturi mask which delivers the most predictable levels of inspired oxygen. Nebulized bronchodilators, i.e. beta-agonists (salbutamol 2.5–5 mg or terbutaline 5–10 mg) and an anticholinergic (e.g. ipratropium bromide 0.25–0.5 mg) should be given. Antibiotics should be considered in the presence of two or more of the symptoms of increased breathlessness, increased sputum volume or purulent sputum.

- Patients with stable COPD who have a Pao_2 of <7.3 kPA, with or without hypercapnia, and an FEV_1 of <1.5 L should receive long-term oxygen therapy (LTOT) which must be given for at least 15 h daily at an oxygen flow rate set between 2 and 4 L/min. If the Pao_2 is between 7.3 and 8.0 kPa, and there is evidence of pulmonary hypertension (e.g. peripheral oedema), LTOT should be considered. LTOT is of proven benefit in those with hypoxaemia, hypercapnia and pulmonary hypertension. Blood gas tensions should be measured with supplemental oxygen to ensure that the set flow is achieving a Pao_2 of >8 kPa without an unacceptable rise in $Paco_2$.

- Checking inhaler technique is essential in the management of patients with COPD and asthma. Typically, the most common inhaler, the metered dose inhaler (MDI), has the following instructions: (a) remove cap and shake inhaler; (b) breathe out gently; (c) put mouthpiece in mouth (with the inhaler upright) and at the start of inspiration (slow and deep) press the canister down and continue to inhale deeply; (d) hold breath for 10 s, then breathe out; and (e) wait about 30 s before taking another inhalation. Other inhalers include the turbohaler, autohaler and accuhaler. The candidate will be expected to acknowledge the importance of chlorofluorcarbon (CFC) vs. non-CFC inhalers.

- Patients with stable asthma are treated according to the 5-step guidelines (British Thoracic Society). Essentially, step 1 is the occasional use of relief bronchodilators; step 2 is the addition of a low-dose corticosteroid inhaler; step 3 is the addition of a long-acting beta-agonist *or* increasing the dose of the corticosteroid inhaler; step 4 is high-dose corticosteroid inhalers and a long-acting beta-agonist, with the possible addition of sustained-release theophylline; and step 5 is starting oral steroids. The best possible results to be aimed for are reduction in the following: symptoms, need for bronchodilators, and an improvement in activity of the peak flow rate with minimal side-effects from medication.

Comments on the case

The candidate will be expected to take a full history to decide if the patient is describing asthma or COPD. It is not uncommon for a patient to be labelled as asthmatic when in fact he has COPD. Do not be swayed by the GP's previous diagnosis of asthma—keep an open mind. Patients with COPD often have a wheeze and this patient really presented 5 years ago with an exacerbation of COPD rather than asthma. The candidate will be expected to address the patient's concerns and to have a clear idea about management.

Case 6 | **Burning of the feet**

Candidate information

You are the medical SHO in clinic. Mr Jeremy Duncunson has been referred to you by his GP.

Please read this letter (it should take no more than 2 min) and then continue with the consultation.

Dear Doctor

Re: Mr Jeremy Duncunson, aged 52

This man complains of burning pains in his legs which stop him from sleeping. He has type 2 diabetes mellitus and his last HbA1c was high at 8.5%. Recently, he has been found to have hypertension with a BP of 176/78 mmHg, proteinuria and a raised cholesterol (6.5 mmol/L with HDL-cholesterol 2.2 mmol/L and triglycerides 2.33 mmol/L). His current medication is metformin 500 mg t.d.s. and aspirin 75 mg o.d. I have started him on lisinopril and simvastatin. Unfortunately, he drinks excessively. Please advise on diagnosis and management.

Yours sincerely

Dr G. Practitioner

You have 14 min until the patient leaves the room, followed by 1 min for reflection, before the discussion with the examiners. Be prepared to discuss the solutions to the problems posed by the case and how you might reply to the GP's letter.

Patient information

Mr Jeremy Duncunson is a 52-year-old unemployed previous car attendant who has had diabetes mellitus for the last 8 years. His most recent problem is a 4-month history of pains in both feet and shins. These pains are burning and stabbing in nature and are at their worst at night while in bed. He finds sleeping quite irksome with his legs covered with the pressure of the bed clothes and the heat of the bed. Recently, they have been keeping him awake for half the night. During the day he is aware of the burning but, if he is occupied, he manages to ignore it. Tight socks and shoes also aggravate the pain. The pain is not exacerbated by walking and he has found no comfort from simple analgesics. He has no weakness in his legs and no obvious feeling of 'walking on cotton wool' or losing his balance if walking in the dark. He has no ulcers on his feet. He does not have any other systemic symptoms of note. He attempts to follow a diabetic diet and he tests his own glucose levels at home which have been around 9 mmol/L. He is treated with metformin 500 mg t.d.s. and additionally he takes aspirin 75 mg o.d. He does not have any past history of coronary artery disease but recently the GP has found a raised blood pressure, a high blood cholesterol level and protein in the urine. For these he has been started on lisinopril and simvastatin. He attends the eye clinic but has not needed laser therapy. He lives alone and stopped smoking 5 years ago (15 cigarettes a day) but he does drink on average about 4 pints a night at the local public house. His excessive alcohol intake does not compromise his diet and he is not malnourished. He is concerned, with the feet particularly, about the possibility of vascular disease. He is also concerned about the protein in the urine as the GP has told him that this may be a sign of diabetic kidney disease.

Examiner information

1 Data gathering in the interview

A good candidate would be able to elicit:
- the exact details of the burning pains in the feet; which foot, which part, shins and/or calves
- when the pains are worse, i.e. night time, walking, tight shoes/socks; whether he has to pull away the bed sheets to relieve the pain and whether there is a pressure effect from the bed sheets. ?Help from simple analgesics
- other symptoms such as muscle weakness, wasting, sensory problems, e.g. a feeling of walking on cotton wool, losing balance when walking in the dark or when he has his eyes closed
- impact on his life, e.g. sleep quality
- other neurological symptoms, any backache
- a history of peripheral vascular disease, ?any suggestion of claudication
- diabetic history; has control worsened or improved
- smoking, alcohol and nutritional history (vitamin deficiencies)
- other systemic symptoms suggestive of a neoplasm
- drug history including those that can cause peripheral neuropathy, e.g. isoniazid, chemotherapy drugs
- social history
- concerns of the patient, especially with regard to the proteinuria

2 Identification and use of information gathered

The candidate should be able to interpret the history and create a problem list. The objectives for the candidate are to:
- give a differential diagnosis including neuropathic pain (probably in this case caused by poorly controlled diabetes)
- stress the importance of treating blood pressure and cholesterol levels as a primary prevention measure and to discuss possible targets
- discuss with the patient possible medical treatments

for the neuropathy including improved glycaemic control and foot care
- discuss strategies to cut down his alcohol consumption

3 Discussion related to the case

- A clinical diagnosis of neuropathy is usually sufficient but if in doubt nerve conduction studies could be considered. Investigations for other non-diabetic causes of neuropathy should be considered, e.g. alcohol, vitamin deficiency, pernicious anaemia, myeloma, drugs, uraemia, carcinoma, infections (syphilis). Other causes of leg pain include peripheral vascular disease and spinal or nerve root problems.
- It is important to understand the risks of future sensory loss and diabetic foot ulceration.
- Discussion of alcohol abstinence is necessary as alcohol may also be contributing to his neuropathy and bad diabetic control.
- Discuss treatment for the neuropathy including improved glycaemic control, analgesia, possible use of other pain control options such as antidepressants (imipramine or amitriptyline), anticonvulsants (carbamazepine or gabapentin) or opiates. If pain persists then referral to the pain management team may be necessary to consider transcutaneous electrical nerve stimulator (TENS), lidocaine or mexiletine injections or spinal stimulation.
- The discussion should focus on the management of peripheral neuropathy as requested in the GP's letter; however, the GP also mentions cholesterol and blood pressure levels. Targets for BP control in a patient with uncomplicated type 2 diabetes would be to treat above 150/85 mmHg with a control target of <140/80 mmHg; in the presence of proteinuria targets would be lower, <130/75 mmHg. Cholesterol should not be treated in isolation but as part of cardiovascular event prevention. Previously, a risk of myocardial infarction above 30% over 10 years would have been set as a target; however, as the cost of statins falls this target is expected to reduce to 20 or even 15%.

- Other modes of diabetic neuropathy include symmetrical sensory polyneuropathy which is characterized by loss of vibration and temperature sensations. Unrecognized trauma brought about by ill-fitting footwear is a common problem leading to ulceration. Neuropathic arthropathy (Charcot's joints) sometimes occurs in the ankles.
- Other neuropathies include a painful neuropathy such as in this case. These are typically burning in sensation, worse at night and the pressure from bedclothes may be extremely distressing. Good long-term glycaemic control is essential for its management but, in some patients, the neuropathy is resistant to therapy. Mononeuritis multiplex, diabetic amyotrophy (asymmetrical wasting of quadriceps) and autonomic neuropathy are other neuropathies seen in diabetes mellitus.

> **Comments on the case**
>
> This case tests the ability of the candidate to differentiate diabetic neuropathies (of which there is more than one) with other non-diabetic causes. The candidate must have a list of differential diagnoses thought out before starting the consultation so that the history taking can be guided appropriately. In this case, the diabetes is most likely the principal cause but alcohol may be making an important contribution.

Case 7 | Chest pain

Candidate information

You are the SHO in a cardiology clinic and you are seeing Mr Brian Daniels who has been referred to you by his GP.

Please read this letter (it should take no more than 2 min) and then continue with the consultation.

> Dear Doctor
>
> **Re: Mr Brian Daniels, aged 61**
>
> Thank you for seeing Mr Daniels who had a coronary angioplasty with stenting of his right coronary artery 3 years ago. Since then he has been fine and was discharged from your care 9 months ago. For the last 4 months, however, he has been suffering again from chest pain. This does not necessarily occur on exertion but can occur at rest. I have increased his nitrates but his pains persist. I wonder if his stent is not functioning adequately. Please see and advise. His medication includes: aspirin 75 mg, ISMN 60 mg b.d., atenolol 50 mg o.d. and simvastatin 20 mg.
>
> Yours sincerely
>
> Dr G. Practitioner

You have 14 min until the patient leaves the room, followed by 1 min for reflection, before the discussion with the examiners. Be prepared to discuss the solutions to the problems posed by the case and how you might reply to the GP's letter.

Patient information

Mr Brian Daniels is a 90-kg, 61-year-old, previous HGV driver who presented acutely 3 years ago with an inferior myocardial infarction. He suffered from postinfarct angina which occurred on exertion, especially when going up stairs. Then the chest pain was typically dull in nature and central with radiation to the shoulder. An angiogram soon after revealed a right coronary artery occlusion which was subsequently stented. He has been pain-free since then and has been leading an active independent life until 4 months ago when the pain recurred. This pain radiates to the throat but is different from the previous angina in that it is burning and worse after meals and occurs at night time and not during exertion. The pain may last for up to 2 h at a time. There is occasional nausea during the pain and he has been woken up in the night with a feeling of choking. There are no other symptoms of note, e.g. orthopnoea, dyspnoea, cough, sputum, haemoptysis, ankle oedema, loss of weight or other abdominal symptoms. He used to smoke 10 cigarettes a day until his myocardial infarction and he drinks approximately 5 pints per week. There are no other cardiovascular risk factors apart from a raised cholesterol of

6.8 which was found 3 years ago. He lives with his wife who has rheumatoid arthritis and he is the main carer for her. He stopped driving HGV vehicles at the time of his infarct and has not worked since. His concerns are that his angina may have returned.

Examiner information

1 Data gathering in the interview

A good candidate would be able to elicit:
- a history of the events 3 years ago and compare these with the present history
- how long the current chest pain has been present
- where the chest pain occurs
- if the pain is constant or intermittent
- the nature of the pain, e.g. sharp, stabbing, burning, band-like heaviness or dull
- if it radiates anywhere, e.g. to the arm, neck, jaw or back
- if it is worse on exertion and, if so, how many metres can he walk on the flat? Ask about stairs and walking up an incline. Does the pain occur at rest? Does the pain stop after stopping exertion and does it return when restarting exertion?
- any other features which may bring on the pain, e.g. hunger, eating, breathing, positional (e.g. lying flat in bed)
- other symptoms during chest pain, e.g. dyspnoea, cough, palpitations, nausea, syncope, epigastric pain, choking, etc.
- relevant risk factors, e.g. hypertension, diabetes mellitus, hyperlipidaemia, cerebrovascular disease
- full drug history and side-effects, e.g. headaches, impotence
- smoking and alcohol history
- family history
- the impact of the symptoms on his life and his ability to care for his wife

2 Identification and use of information gathered

The candidate should be able to interpret the history and create a problem list. The objectives of the candidate are to:
- distinguish the symptoms suggestive of oesophageal reflux from those of angina
- have a plan of relevant investigations to look for oesophageal reflux
- discuss the possibility of recurrence of the angina and arrange appropriate investigations and follow-up

- address the pain symptoms
- explore if any help can be provided to help with the care of the wife

3 Discussion related to the case

- This case tests the ability of the candidate to take a thorough history with assessment and analysis of the possible differential diagnoses, i.e. angina vs. oesophagitis.
- A plan of management has to be outlined in the consultation and this may include routine FBC, U/E, lipid profile, resting ECG, chest X-ray. In order to distinguish ischaemic pain from oesophageal reflux pain, an exercise ECG test is recommended and, if this is normal, a trial of proton-pump inhibition should be considered.
- The candidate must be prepared to discuss the management of oesophageal reflux. He or she must be able to discuss further investigations such as upper gastrointestinal endoscopy, 24-h intraluminal oesophageal pH monitoring and the treatment: pharmacological vs. non-pharmacological.
- Similarly, the candidate must be able to discuss the patient's management if the exercise ECG test is positive, i.e. further angiography and secondary prevention.

> **Comments on the case**
>
> This case highlights how important it is to obtain a thorough history of the previous events which would enable the candidate to compare the past symptoms with the present ones. The candidate should not fall into the trap of assuming the patient has angina. It can be very disheartening for the examiners to see the candidate set off at the start of the consultation following a 'biased' history without scrutiny and without giving a thought to other possibilities. Always have an idea of differential diagnoses and ask the relevant questions that would enable you to probe into each possibility.

Case 8 | Cold and painful fingers

Candidate information

You are the SHO in a general medical clinic. Mrs Brenda Normanton has been referred to you by her GP.

Please read this letter (it should take no more than 2 min) and then continue with the consultation.

> Dear Doctor
>
> **Re: Mrs Brenda Normanton, aged 52**
>
> Thank you for seeing Mrs Normanton who has been complaining of cold, painful fingers for the last year. Her past medical history is unremarkable except for an episode of winter bronchitis last year. She smokes 30 cigarettes a day. She takes no regular medication. Please see and advise.
>
> Yours sincerely
>
> Dr G. Practitioner

You have 14 min until the patient leaves the room, followed by 1 min for reflection, before the discussion with the examiners. Be prepared to discuss the solutions to the problems posed by the case and how you might reply to the GP's letter.

Patient information

Mrs Brenda Normanton is a 52-year-old woman who owns a fish shop in the local market. She gives a 1-year history of painful, cold fingers occurring most days. When exposed to cold temperatures, e.g. when handling fish stored in ice, her fingers start off pink, then turn white and then eventually to a dark blue, cyanotic colour which is associated with pain (especially on rewarming). Initially her index and middle fingers of both hands were the only ones affected but now all the others except the thumbs are involved. She has noticed her toes to be constantly cold but they do not discolour like her fingers. There is some associated numbness but when the episode is over after rewarming, the fingers look normal with normal sensation. She has tried wearing gloves but prefers not to at work. Her only other symptom is a chronic cough with whitish sputum in the mornings. She had acute bronchitis last winter which needed a course of antibiotics. She has no dyspnoea, chest pain, gastrointestinal symptoms, arthralgia, claudication or skin rashes. She takes no medication such as beta-blockers and although she was given a salbutamol inhaler during her exacerbation, she does not take this as she feels the inhaler does not help her cough and sputum. There is no past history of connective tissue disorders such as scleroderma or SLE, no blood dyscrasia or any other history of peripheral vascular disease. She smokes 30 cigarettes a day and has done so since the age of 15 and she has never considered giving up. She drinks 2 pints of beer in the evenings and she lives with her husband. She has three children who have all grown up and there is no relevant family history of note. Her work revolved around her fish shop which is her life-long passion. Her main concerns are her painful fingers and that the work precipitates this. She is also worried that she may lose her fingers.

Examiner information

1 Data gathering in the interview

A good candidate would be able to elicit:

- which fingers are affected, the colour changes and the presence of pain, numbness and burning. Whether the toes, earlobes or tip of the nose are also affected and if the thumbs are spared?
- frequency of the attacks
- precipitating factors, especially the cold; are the attacks more frequent during winter?
- does wearing gloves help?
- whether the fingers are normal between attacks
- any other associated symptoms, especially peripheral vascular disease, e.g. claudication or symptoms suggestive of connective tissue disorders (e.g. scleroderma, SLE, dermatomyositis), rheumatoid arthritis such as dyspnoea, dry cough, reflux, arthralgia, rashes
- history suggestive of cervical spine problems, neurological disease such as syringomyelia, carpal tunnel syndrome, or blood dyscrasias, e.g. cryoglobulinaemia, myeloproliferative disorders, Waldenström's macroglobulinaemia
- past history of trauma, e.g. vibrational injury, electric shocks, cold injury
- past history of chronic bronchitis and exacerbation, ischaemic heart disease
- full medication history, e.g. whether she has had beta-blockers and chemotherapy drugs such as bleomycin, vinblastine and cisplatin
- full smoking history
- working history and precipitating factors at work
- family history of Raynaud's disease
- concerns of the patient, particularly the worry of losing any of the fingers

2 Identification and use of information gathered

The candidate should be able to interpret the history and create a problem list. The objectives for the candidate are to:

- identify the possibilities of a secondary cause for her symptoms; if not, the patient most likely has Raynaud's disease (idiopathic)
- identify the precipitating features, particularly at work
- discuss smoking cessation and its benefits with the patient
- explain general measures for avoiding attacks, such as wearing gloves at work (keeping fingers warm)
- reassure that in idiopathic cases there is no long-term damage and it is rare for finger tips to be amputated because of gangrene

3 Discussion related to the case

- This case tests the ability of the candidate to differentiate secondary causes of Raynaud's phenomenon from idiopathic Raynaud's disease.
- Common secondary causes include connective tissue disorders, peripheral vascular disease, drug-induced, neurological, trauma-induced and blood dyscrasias.
- If there is no suggestion of a secondary cause then there is no specific investigation required; angiography of the digits is not indicated.
- Management is smoking cessation, keeping hands warm, and occasionally nifedipine 10 mg t.d.s. may be helpful.

Comments on the case

This case stresses the importance of taking a history, particularly of precipitating factors at work, possible secondary causes and a smoking history. The candidate will be expected to provide smoking cessation advice to this patient.

Case 9 | Cause of collapse?

Candidate information

You are the SHO in a general medical clinic and Mr John Weston has been referred to you by his GP. Mr Weston is accompanied by his wife.

Please read this letter (it should take no more than 2 min) and then continue with the consultation.

> Dear Doctor
>
> **Re: Mr John Weston, aged 53**
>
> Thank you for seeing Mr Weston so soon. He was found by his wife unconscious in a chair after a meal last week. The wife was the only witness and tells me that he was unconscious for at least 3 min. He is a known insulin-dependent diabetic and takes Mixtard insulin 34 units a.m. and 36 units p.m. He is not on any other medication. Please see and advise.
>
> Yours sincerely
>
> Dr G. Practitioner

You have 14 min until the patient leaves the room, followed by 1 min for reflection, before the discussion with the examiners. Be prepared to discuss the solutions to the problems posed by the case and how you might reply to the GP's letter.

Patient information

Mr John Weston is a 53-year-old unemployed man who had an episode of collapse last week which was witnessed by his wife. He is normally fit and well and leads an independent life. During this acute episode, he had sat down in the armchair after an evening meal and, according to his wife, he went grey, became unconscious and was unrousable for about 3 min. The meal itself had been uneventful, i.e. no choking, etc. There were no obvious limb movements, aura, tongue-biting or incontinence. After about 2 min he became flushed and it was another 5 min before he regained full consciousness. His wife did a blood sugar during the recovery and this was 11. He was alert and orientated by this time but had a slight headache. There was no limb weakness or dysphasia. Mr Weston did not want to visit casualty but did agree to see the GP the next day. At present, Mr Weston feels fine with no more similar episodes and no current history of chest pain, palpitations, dyspnoea, limb weakness or numbness. He has been a diabetic for 12 years, initially presenting with polyuria and polydipsia. Despite initial oral medication (full tolerable doses of gliclazide and metformin), he was switched over to insulin after 1 year. He regularly visits the hospital diabetic clinic and has had one episode of laser therapy to both eyes. His last hypoglycaemic attack was 2 months ago. These normally present with a feeling of faintness and dizziness but rarely with any loss of consciousness. He had taken the correct dose of insulin before the meal and his blood sugars are normally between 6 and 10. There is no other previous history of cardiovascular or neurological disease or head trauma. Apart from the insulin, he takes no other medications or illicit drugs. He drinks 3 pints a day and occasionally has spirits at the weekend. There is no family history of seizures. He lives with his wife who is obviously concerned that Mr Weston may have had a fit. He does not drive.

Examiner information

1 Data gathering in the interview

A good candidate would be able to elicit:
- at what time of day was the collapse and were there any preceding symptoms
- if he felt light-headed, nauseated or sweaty just before collapsing
- if he remembers collapsing on to the floor
- was the patient sat down at the moment of the collapse? If so, this may point away from a vasovagal cause
- if he lost conciousness and for how long
- if he went a particular colour, e.g. white, blue, grey
- his colour on recovery
- if there were any jerking movements of his limbs or face? If so, which limbs and which part of the face? Where did the jerking movements start and where did they spread to?
- did he bite his tongue? Was he incontinent of urine? Did he injure himself?
- did he regain consciousness gradually? Was he confused or alert? Did he have a headache, difficulty in speaking, weakness or aches in his limbs?
- if he has had any previous similar episodes
- a detailed history of the diabetes, especially the insulin treatment, previous hypoglycaemic episodes and their characteristics
- a detailed cardiovascular and neurological history, ascertain the possibility of a neurological or a cardiovascular cause of the collapse, e.g. dysrhythmia, dysphasia or weakness
- full alcohol and drug (including illicit) history
- past history of trauma
- a family history of seizures
- the concerns expressed by Mr and Mrs Weston

2 Identification and use of information gathered

The candidate should be able to interpret the history and create a problem list. The objectives for the candidate are to:
- differentiate the possible causes of the collapse, e.g. cardiac dysrhythmia, seizure, alcohol-related collapse,

transient ischaemic attack, hypoglycaemia, vasovagal and possibility of intracranial lesion
- explain the possible reasons for the collapse
- explain that the cause is not totally clear
- give a list of investigations needed to determine the cause
- address any concerns the couple may express

3 Discussion related to the case

- This case tests the candidate's ability to differentiate the above stated causes. A plan of investigations would include routine FBC, U/E, LFT, gamma glutamyl transferase (GGT), calcium, HbA1c, and blood glucose. This should be followed by a resting ECG, chest X-ray, 24-h ECG recording, echocardiogram, EEG and CT scan of the head.
- The candidate should be able to discuss the strengths and weaknesses of each diagnosis. This case, on balance, suggests a cardiac cause for the collapse.
- The candidate should be able to discuss with the patient a management plan if the results of tests are normal, i.e. consideration of exercise ECG test.
- The candidate should be able to discuss further management if a cardiovascular or neurological cause is found.

Comments on the case

This case illustrates how important it is to have a witness when the patient has passed out. There may well be a partner giving a history in the exam. Be sure to be able to obtain a thorough description of the events and to make sure you consider in detail each possible diagnosis. Do not assume this was a seizure. It is important to have an idea of the nature of any previous hypoglycaemic attacks. Be sure to have a plan of management as the couple are understandably concerned.

Case 10 | Confusion

Candidate information

You are the SHO in the care of the elderly clinic. Mr George Watkins has been referred to you by his GP and is accompanied by his daughter.

Please read this letter (it should take no more than 2 min) and then continue with the consultation.

> Dear Doctor
>
> **Re: Mr George Watkins, aged 82**
>
> Thank you for seeing this elderly man who has been getting progressively confused and forgetful over the last year. He lives alone and his past medical history includes a cerebrovascular accident (CVA) 7 years ago. His present medication is only a daily dose of 75 mg aspirin . His daughter is concerned that this may be Alzheimer's disease. Please see and advise.
>
> Yours sincerely
>
> Dr G. Practitioner

You have 14 min until the patient leaves the room, followed by 1 min for reflection, before the discussion with the examiners. Be prepared to discuss the solutions to the problems posed by the case and how you might reply to the GP's letter.

Patient information

Mr George Watkins is an 82-year-old retired tool mechanic who presents with increasing confusion and forgetfulness over the last year. The daughter, who lives four houses away, accompanies him. She tells you that her father has been slightly frail since his CVA 7 years ago. This affected his right arm and leg but he made a good recovery, so much so that he has managed to live alone. He manages most of his own affairs (with shopping help from the daughter) and he walks with a stick. He has had a tendency to forget certain things since the CVA but for the last year Mr Watkins has had difficulty in knowing what day or month it is and, more worryingly, has left the gas cooker on by mistake on two separate occasions. Occasionally, he gets the names of his daughters the wrong way round. There have been two occasions when the neighbour found him wandering outside the house at midnight. The confusion and forgetfulness have deteriorated rapidly during the last 6 months but he remains continent with appropriate emotions. There has been no recent history of falls, strokes, decreased consciousness or tremor. He does not take any other medication apart from aspirin (although he does forget to take this now and again) and he does not drink alcohol. He lives alone (widowed for 5 years) in a two-storey house and normally does his own cooking on a gas cooker. Until recently the daughter only did the shopping but, during the last 3 weeks, she has had to do all the cooking and most of the household chores.

Examiner information

1 Data gathering in the interview

A good candidate would be able to elicit:

- how long ago the symptoms were first noticed and how these symptoms have progressed, gradually or with sudden, worsening episodes?
- if the patient has any insight into the symptoms?
- a few examples of the confusion and forgetfulness
- whether he forgets what day or time it is
- whether he forgets where he is or does he lose his way around or outside his house
- whether he forgets who his daughter is
- long- and short-term memory, i.e. remote vs. recent events
- problems in concentrating, personal hygiene, emotions, continence
- any history of head trauma, seizures, vascular symptoms, e.g. diplopia, vertigo and neurological symptoms, e.g. abnormal gait, decreased consciousness, ataxia, peripheral neuropathy, tremor
- history of the stroke, recovery and any physical, psychological and social problems as a result of that
- drugs, e.g. benzodiazepines and barbiturates; and an alcohol history
- psychiatric illnesses, particularly depression
- social history with risk assessment, e.g. boiling water, cooking (gas), heating
- the input from the daughters and how the situation has affected their lives, e.g. family, work, etc.

2 Identification and use of information gathered

The candidate should be able to interpret the history and create a problem list. The objectives for the candidate are to:

- decide if the symptoms fit clinically with Alzheimer's dementia
- have a plan of investigations, i.e. dementia screen (see below)
- explain in depth the possible diagnoses and their impact
- address any concerns of the family
- offer possible referral to a specialist with a specific interest in dementia (e.g. at a memory clinic) who may be able to offer a multidisciplinary care package

3 Discussion related to the case

- This case tests the candidate's ability to take a detailed history from a relative. The presence of dementia is diagnosed clinically but can be aided by using psychometric testing. The historian has to be someone who knows the patient well. Clinical features such as disturbance in higher cortical function including memory, comprehension, learning capacity, language, orientation, apraxia, agnosia and an inability to plan and organize must be looked for. Behavioural changes such as wandering, agitation and aggression are common, as is depression.
- Investigations would include: FBC, U/E, LFT, glucose, calcium, vitamin B_{12}, thyroid-stimulating hormone (TSH), thyroxine (T_4), syphilis serology, chest X-ray and CT scan of the head to confirm cerebral atrophy or to exclude other intracranial pathology, e.g. tumour, multi-infarct dementia, chronic subdural haematoma.
- The candidate should be able to discuss the pathophysiology of Alzheimer's disease, the other types of dementia such as multi-infarct dementia, Parkinson's disease, Creutzfeldt–Jakob disease, Pick's disease and others, e.g. toxic (alcohol), post-trauma, endocrine (e.g. hypothyroidism) and vitamin deficiency (vitamin B_{12}).
- The candidate should be able to discuss the pharmacological management of Alzheimer's disease, particularly acetylcholinesterase inhibitors such as donepezil.

Comments on the case

This case highlights the importance of taking a detailed history from the relative, particularly with regard to the impact of the disease on the family. As dementia is a clinical diagnosis, the importance of looking for features of Alzheimer's disease in the history cannot be overemphasized. There has to be a plan of management addressing the disease, treating any associated behavioural disturbances and caring for the family; without which the candidate will be failing both the patient and the family. The relative may ask for a prognosis and future management; if you feel this will put you out of your depth then it is wise to refer to a specialist who has a multidisciplinary approach to managing such patients.

Case 11 | **Cough**

Candidate information

You are the SHO in a chest clinic. Mrs Indira Shah has been referred to you by her GP. *Please read this letter (it should take no more than 2 min) and then continue with the consultation.*

Dear Doctor

Re: Mrs Indira Shah, aged 42

Thank you for seeing this lady who has recently returned from visiting relatives in India. She has been complaining of a cough for nearly 9 months. She is otherwise fit and well. She has hypertension for which I started ramipril a year ago. This was stopped soon after the cough started and she was then given amlodipine 10 mg o.d. instead. I have tried her on a salbutamol inhaler for the last 2 months but her cough persists. A recent chest X-ray has been reported as showing normal lung fields. Please see and advise.

Yours sincerely

Dr G. Practitioner

You have 14 min until the patient leaves the room, followed by 1 min for reflection, before the discussion with the examiners. Be prepared to discuss the solutions to the problems posed by the case and how you might reply to the GP's letter.

Patient information

Mrs Shah is a 42-year-old lady of Indian origin who has lived in the UK for 25 years. She returned from a 2-week holiday in India 4 weeks ago. Until 9 months ago she was fit and well leading an active, independent life as a shop assistant. However, she developed a cough which is worse at night time and is increasing in severity, so much so that now she has occasional episodes of urinary incontinence and poor sleep quality. The cough persisted during her trip to India. The cough is associated with occasional mucoid phlegm (never purulent) and there is no evidence of blood. There is no wheeze or breathlessness but she does feel tired if she walks up an incline. Her only other symptom is occasional heartburn, particularly after a large meal, which is relieved by Gaviscon. There is no loss of weight or appetite, ankle swelling, chest pain or fever. She is a known hypertensive and was started on ramipril 1 year ago. The cough started 3 months after this but, despite discontinuing the ramipril, the cough has persisted. There is no contact or family history of tuberculosis. There is no other past medical history of note, such as allergic rhinitis, or any history suggestive of an inhaled foreign body. There are no pets at home and she has never smoked. Her husband does not smoke either. There are no obvious allergic triggers at home or work. Her medication now includes amlodipine 10 mg o.d. and a salbutamol inhaler which has not been of any help although her inhaler technique is good. She lives with her two sons and husband who owns a shop. She is particularly concerned with the poor sleep quality and the incontinence and together these are causing family strife.

Examiner information

1 Data gathering in the interview

A good candidate would be able to:

- obtain a detailed history of the cough with particular reference to the start of treatment with an angiotensin-converting enzyme (ACE) inhibitor
- confirm when the cough is worse, e.g. night time, morning
- confirm any associated sputum, haemoptysis, dyspnoea, orthopnoea, wheeze and fever and pay particular attention to the history of heartburn
- look for any other possible aetiology of cough, such as allergic rhinitis/sinusitis (postnasal drip), asthma, tuberculosis (?contact history in the UK and India)
- elicit a smoking and occupational history
- elicit any allergic history, especially common household allergens, e.g. cats, dogs, pollen, house dust mite, mould
- elicit a detailed drug history, including ACE inhibitors and any other drugs which may cause a pneumonitis, e.g. amiodarone
- determine the impact of the cough on the patient and the family, with particular importance paid to the poor sleep pattern and urinary incontinence

2 Identification and use of information gathered

The candidate should be able to interpret the history and create a problem list. The objectives for the candidate are to:

- decide a possible cause for this cough
- explain the possible differential diagnoses of a cough with a normal chest X-ray and to reassure that there is no evidence of lung cancer, pneumonia or tuberculosis on the X-ray
- sympathize with the patient with regard to the impact of the symptoms on her and the family
- have a plan of investigations
- stress that there will be no immediate curative treatment for the cough until the results of all the investigations are available

3 Discussion related to the case

- This case is a common dilemma presenting to respiratory physicians and it tests the ability of the candidate to structure the history towards finding an aetiological cause for the cough. This patient probably has gastro-oesophageal reflux to explain the night time cough, particularly with a history of heartburn. Other possibilities include: (a) asthma which may not necessarily manifest with wheeze; (b) postnasal drip as a result of allergic rhinitis or sinusitis; (c) ACE inhibitor induced—it is still possible for symptoms to persist beyond 9 months after discontinuation of treatment; and (d) chronic bronchitis which again is doubtful as she has never smoked and there is no obvious strong occupational history such as working with coal fires. Tuberculosis must always be considered as a cause of a chronic cough but there are no typical symptoms suggestive of this and reassuringly the chest X-ray was normal. An inhaled foreign body (e.g. a pea) should also be considered but the chest X-ray in such a case would be expected to show some radiological changes such as collapse, consolidation or effusion.
- Investigations should always start with a chest X-ray to rule out other obvious causes of a cough (associated with radiological abnormalities) such as pneumonia, lung neoplasm, sarcoidosis and heart failure. Simple investigations such as serial peak flow monitoring should be the next line of investigation, looking for any diurnal variation which would be suggestive of asthma. If sinusitis is strongly suspected then a CT scan of the sinuses may be useful. Other invasive investigations, such as 24-h intraluminal oesophageal pH monitoring or bronchoscopy, may be reserved until trials of corticosteroid inhalers for asthma, proton-pump inhibition for oesophageal reflux or nasal corticosteroid sprays for allergic rhinitis have failed to achieve any symptomatic improvement.

Comments on the case

This case tests the ability of the candidate to think about the possible differential diagnoses before commencing the consultation, otherwise important aspects of the history will be missed. Again, it is a typical case where investigations may be normal and a clinical diagnosis is made purely on the history. It is also a typical case of where no obvious immediate cure may be available and this has to be communicated to the patient; she may be expecting an answer to all her symptoms that day. Chronic cough is a symptom that can cause immense impact on the rest of the family and so the candidate must show empathy and have an understanding rapport throughout the consultation.

Case 12 | Diabetic feet

Candidate information

You are the medical SHO in the diabetic clinic. Mr Gordon Wright has been referred to you by his GP.

Please read this letter (it should take no more than 2 min) and then continue with the consultation.

Dear Doctor

Re: Mr Gordon Wright, aged 67

Thank you for seeing this man urgently in clinic. He has a long history of diabetes and, when seen by the local chiropodist last week, a small ulcer over his left fourth toe was seen. I saw him in my surgery today and I found that the toe has turned black. Mr Wright has a long history of a sensory neuropathy and I could not detect any pulses in the left foot.

Current medication: Mixtard 30/70 20 units a.m. and 40 units p.m., simvas-tatin 10 mg o.d., Imdur 60 mg o.d., aspirin 150 mg o.d., amlodipine 5 mg o.d., lisinopril 5 mg o.d. Please advise on diagnosis and management.

Yours sincerely

Dr G. Practitioner

You have 14 min until the patient leaves the room, followed by 1 min for reflection, before the discussion with the examiners. Be prepared to discuss the solutions to the problems posed by the case and how you might reply to the GP's letter.

Patient information

Mr Gordon Wright is a 67-year-old retired salesman. He has had diabetes mellitus for 12 years and has been on insulin for 4 years. Last week, after wearing some new shoes, he noticed an ulcer over the fourth toe on his left foot. He booked an emergency appointment with the chiropodist as he had been advised to do so if this ever happened. The ulcer was dressed and the chiropodist said that he did not need antibiotics as it was very superficial. Today he went back to have it redressed. He had been worried, even before the dressing came off, because the toe had been throbbing all night and he was horrified to see that it had turned black. He was immediately seen by the GP who could not detect any pulses in the left foot. He has had a bilateral sensory neuropathy (characterized by numbness) for 3 years and laser therapy for retinopathy 2 years ago. He was converted to insulin 4 years ago although this was delayed as long as possible because of a phobia of self-injection. Previous history includes a myocardial infarction (MI) in 1992 when he presented with central, crushing chest pain. He remembers being given streptokinase. He made a good recovery but does get occasional angina when walking uphill against a cold wind. He does not suffer from calf claudication. He also has hypertension for which he takes amlodipine and lisinopril. Otherwise, he is reasonably well, ambulant and self-caring. He smokes 5 cigarettes a day and is trying hard to give up. He does not drink and lives with his wife who needs help with washing and dressing as she has severe rheumatoid arthritis. He is obviously concerned about the state of his toe with fears of an imminent amputation and any admission will mean arranging care for his wife. He also believes that delaying the insulin conversion may have caused this.

Examiner information

1 Data gathering in the interview

A good candidate would be able to elicit:
- a detailed history of the events surrounding the gangrenous toe
- a detailed history of the diabetes and especially any past history of microvascular (retinopathy, neuropathy) and macrovascular complications (previous myocardial infarction, absent left foot pulses)
- history of the myocardial infarction and any history suggestive of angina and peripheral vascular disease
- other past medical history and cardiovascular risk factors, e.g. hypertension, hyperlipidaemia, family history of coronary artery disease
- drug and dietetic history, including that of insulin and a diabetic and low fat diet
- smoking history
- social circumstances, especially care for the wife
- concerns of the patient

2 Identification and use of information gathered

The candidate should be able to interpret the history and create a problem list. The objectives for the candidate are to:
- speculate on the contribution of the micro- and macrovascular disease to the ischaemic toe and to his neuropathy
- explain to the patient that he will need an urgent assessment by the vascular surgeons and that management will be jointly shared by the diabetologists and the surgeons
- explain that vascular studies will determine whether he will need surgery to his arteries to improve the blood supply or just local treatment for his toe
- consider whether this patient needs admission or close follow-up in a diabetes foot clinic. Inquire whether arrangements need to be made for his wife's care
- explain the importance of good blood pressure and glycaemic control

- advise on stopping smoking and suggest referral to an appropriate counsellor
- explain that diabetic complications are usually a result of a long period of poor control and are made worse by smoking, but at least reassure him that he has been right in seeking urgent advice for the toe

3 Discussion related to the case

- This gentleman has both macro- and microvascular complications of diabetes. He has type 2 diabetes which is now insulin-treated, and from the history we note that contributory risk factors have been poor glycaemic control, hyperlipidaemia and smoking.
- Approximately 15% of individuals with diabetes mellitus develop a foot ulcer, and a significant subset of those individuals will at some time undergo amputation (14–24% risk with that ulcer or subsequent ulceration). Risk factors for foot ulcers or amputation include: male sex, diabetes > 10 years duration, peripheral neuropathy, abnormal structure of foot (bony abnormalities, callus, thickened nails), peripheral vascular disease, smoking and history of previous ulcer or amputation. Bad glycaemic control is also a risk factor—each 2% increase in the HbA1c increases the risk of a lower extremity ulcer by 1.6 times and the risk of lower extremity amputation by 1.5 times.
- This gentleman was at risk of foot ulceration because of established neuropathy and additionally he probably has macrovascular disease affecting the legs in view of the missing foot pulses, although he does not have a history of intermittent claudication. He will also have a contribution from microvascular disease and superimposed infection is a distinct possibility. The need for inpatient or outpatient treatment will depend on the extent of the ulceration/gangrene and the findings of the vascular surgeons. He may get away without admission as the vascular surgeons can arrange urgent outpatient angiography, and he can be managed in a multidisciplinary foot clinic with an admission for angioplasty or bypass. If this arrangement is not possible, and with the high likelihood of infection and the need

for intravenous antibiotic treatment, the patient ought to be admitted, with arrangements made for the wife. Subcutaneous low molecular weight heparin and a pressure-relieving mattress should be included in the management plan. Activity should be restricted and temporary footwear provided. Intensive control of blood glucose is important. The toe may need amputation but if the arterial supply can be improved it may dry up and autoamputate.

- Ischaemia and neuropathy assessment is a basic need for the patient; both may coexist. Ischaemia is characterized by rest pain, claudication, cold feet, poor pulses with painful ulceration, especially heels, ankles and toes, and sensory neuropathy is usually painless with warm feet and bounding pulses.
- Patient education should emphasize: (a) careful selection of footwear; (b) daily inspection of the feet to detect early signs of poor-fitting footwear or minor trauma; (c) daily foot hygiene to keep the skin clean and moist; (d) avoidance of self-treatment of foot ab-

normalities and high-risk behaviour (e.g. walking barefoot); and (e) prompt consultation with a health-care provider if an abnormality arises.

- Discussion with the examiners may include the incidence of vascular disease in patients with diabetes, the contributing causes for diabetic foot disease and the importance of a multidisciplinary care team in the management of the diabetic foot.

Comments on the case

This case tests the candidate's ability to take a diabetic foot history. The patient, like many other such patients, has several complications as a result of the diabetes, and so it is essential for the candidate to explore deeply into these problems in order to be able to manage the patient optimally.

Case 13 | Difficulty in walking

Candidate information

You are the SHO in a neurology clinic. Mrs Sheila Harrison has been referred to you by her GP.

Please read this letter (it should take no more than 2 min) and then continue with the consultation.

> Dear Doctor
>
> **Re: Mrs Sheila Harrison, aged 63**
>
> Thank you for seeing Mrs Harrison so quickly. She has been complaining of a gradual progression of difficulty in walking for 5 months with some numbness in her feet. She has chest pain and a long-standing cough from her chronic bronchitis. She smokes 40 cigarettes a day. She uses a salbutamol inhaler and needs paracetamol for the pain. Please see and advise.
>
> Yours sincerely
>
> Dr G. Practitioner

You have 14 min until the patient leaves the room, followed by 1 min for reflection, before the discussion with the examiners. Be prepared to discuss the solutions to the problems posed by the case and how you might reply to the GP's letter.

Patient information

Mrs Sheila Harrison is a 63-year-old retired hospital domestic who complains of a gradual, progressive weakness affecting both legs and leading to difficulty in walking over the last 5 months. Her symptoms have deteriorated, particularly in the last 4 weeks. At the onset 5 months ago she remembers tripping over while shopping one day. During the last 6 weeks she has found walking up stairs much harder and indeed has had two falls at home last week. She has global weakness in both legs and finds getting out of a chair difficult without using her arms. She has noticed a progressive loss of sensation, initially in the feet and now up to and around the middle of her chest. The symptoms are constant throughout the day and she has no headache, diplopia, muscle wasting or tremor. She has recently noticed difficulty in micturating and has occasional urinary incontinence (bowel control is presently intact). Her general systemic symptoms include constant dull central chest pain with a band-like radiation bilaterally, which is worse on sneezing, coughing and straining. The pain is worsening and now keeps her awake at night. She has had a productive cough for more than 4 years and this is caused by her chronic bronchitis. She smokes 40 cigarettes a day and has done so for over 40 years. There is no haemoptysis, gastrointestinal or gynaecological symptoms, loss of weight or loss of appetite. There is no past history of diabetes mellitus, spinal injury/trauma, intervertebral disc disease, sciatica, arthritis, neuromuscular disorder (e.g. myasthenia), or any endocrine or metabolic history (e.g. hyperthyroidism,

Cushing's syndrome or electrolyte disturbance). She takes a salbutamol inhaler for her bronchitis and regular paracetamol for her pain. She has had a lot of breakthrough pain in the chest recently. There is no previous history of taking corticosteroids or diuretics and she does not drink alcohol. She has no family history of neuromuscular disorders. She is widowed and lives alone and is naturally worried about her progressive symptoms. She has found that she is relying on her neighbour to do the shopping and now does not go out of the house. She lives in a big four-bedroomed house with stairs and now finds the general maintenance of the house difficult.

Examiner information

1 Data gathering in the interview
A good candidate would be able to elicit:
- how long the symptoms have persisted and whether they are deteriorating
- if there is weakness in both legs and where (distal vs. proximal vs. global)
- if she is having any falls or trips
- if she can get out of a chair without using her arms. Can she walk up stairs?
- if the symptoms are worse towards the end of the day (myasthenia gravis)
- if there are any other neurological symptoms, e.g. headache, diplopia, muscle wasting, sphincter problems, tremor of hands, backache and paraesthesia (if so to what level)
- other respiratory, abdominal and gynaecological symptoms especially suggestive of a neoplasm (primary)
- band-like chest pain worse on coughing, sneezing and straining may suggest a level of spinal cord compression. Is there adequate pain relief?
- a history of diabetes mellitus, spinal injury/trauma, disc disease, sciatica, arthritis, neuromuscular disorder (e.g. myasthenia gravis), metabolic history (e.g. hyperthyroidism, Cushing's syndrome or electrolyte disturbance).
- drug history especially corticosteroids (proximal myopathy), diuretics
- alcohol and smoking history
- the impact of her symptoms on activities of daily living
- the concerns of the patient

2 Identification and use of information gathered
The candidate should be able to interpret the history and create a problem list. The objectives for the candidate are to:
- assemble a list of differential diagnoses
- discuss these possibilities with the patient
- discuss the investigations to be arranged
- consider admission as she lives alone and her social circumstances are deteriorating
- address the concerns of the patient, especially regarding cancer and admitting that you are not sure if the diagnosis is definitely cancer but that this has to be a possibility that needs exploring

3 Discussion related to the case
- This case illustrates how spinal cord compression in the thoracic region may present. Causes of spinal cord compression include neoplastic such as extradural (e.g. metastatic particularly from the lung and breast — although onset is usually more acute), extramedullary such as meningioma, neurofibroma and ependymoma, and intramedullary such as glioma (usually over many years), and ependymoma. This case illustrates that radicular pain at the site of the compression (thoracic band-like pain worse on coughing, straining and sneezing), spastic paraparesis and sensory loss up to the level of the compression are typical in a case such as an extradural meningioma. Other possibilities include vertebral disc protrusion especially in the cervical spine, inflammatory causes such as tuberculous and epidural abscess and, rarely, epidural haemorrhage and haematoma.
- The candidate must have a plan of investigations to relay to the patient. Time wasted on lengthy and random investigations cannot be tolerated. A routine chest X-ray may detect an unsuspected lung cancer, and plain spinal X-ray films may show destruction of a vertebral body, but the investigation of choice is an *urgent* MRI scan.

Comments on the case

This is a case where the symptoms are classic and the candidate really should have an idea of exactly what he or she is dealing with. The patient is obviously anxious that this may be cancer and although the candidate cannot say whether it is or is not, he or she must be seen to share the patient's worry and urgency.

Case 14 | Dizziness and feeling faint

Candidate information

You are the SHO in a care of the elderly clinic. Mrs Edna Richards has been referred to you by her GP.

Please read this letter (it should take no more than 2 min) and then continue with the consultation.

Dear Doctor

Re: Mrs Edna Richards, aged 83

Thank you for seeing Mrs Richards who has complained of several episodes of feeling faint and dizzy over the last few months. On examination, I heard a carotid bruit on the left and I wonder if this may be a reason for her symptoms. She has a past history of hypertension and takes bendrofluazide (bendroflumethiazide) 2.5 mg o.d. She has never smoked. Her BP is 155/88 mmHg. I am concerned that, as she lives alone and has no family, she may harm herself. Please see and advise.

Yours sincerely

Dr G. Practitioner

You have 14 min until the patient leaves the room, followed by 1 min for reflection, before the discussion with the examiners. Be prepared to discuss the solutions to the problems posed by the case and how you might reply to the GP's letter.

Patient information

Mrs Edna Richards is an 83-year-old retired secondary school headmistress who has had several episodes of dizziness and of feeling faint with transient disturbance of consciousness during the last 6 months. These are occurring about once a fortnight and on the last three occasions she has fallen and had some difficulty in getting up again. The symptoms come on suddenly and unexpectedly, usually when she is at home. Once, it occurred when she was hanging up the washing. The dizziness lasts for about 1–2 min. Normally she has to sit down to rest and by 10 min she is back to her normal self. She cannot remember much else about the symptoms. There are no obvious spinning feelings, palpitations, chest pain, dyspnoea, tinnitus, vomiting, headache, weakness or numbness in the arms or legs or urinary incontinence. The symptoms do not occur during micturition nor if she gets up quickly from the chair. Her past medical history includes hypertension for the last 12 years for which she takes bendrofluazide 2.5 mg and the GP is reasonably happy with the blood pressure. She is otherwise fit and well, living on her own (widowed for 3 years) and doing her own shopping and cooking. She has no other family and has never smoked. She does not drink alcohol.

Examiner information

1 Data gathering in the interview

A good candidate would be able to elicit:

- a full description of the symptoms, especially whether the symptoms are a sensation of imbalance or faintness, or does she mean vertigo, e.g. sensation of revolving in space or the surroundings revolving around the patient
- the frequency of the episodes and how long each lasts
- what triggers the dizzy spell, e.g. stooping, standing up quickly from a sitting position or turning her head sharply
- whether the dizzy spells abate spontaneously, e.g. by lying down, or do they lead to unconsciousness
- if there is any associated nausea, vomiting, nystagmus, tinnitus (vertigo)
- if there are any associated palpitations, syncope (cardiac dysrhythmias)
- if there is any associated diplopia, paresis, confusion, dysphasia and numbness (transient ischaemic attacks)
- details regarding the falls, if she has difficulty in getting up or whether she has had any injuries
- drug history, especially antihypertensives, diuretics
- past medical history of diabetes mellitus, ischaemic heart disease, hyperlipidaemia, hypertension
- any obvious blood loss leading to anaemia
- social history, particularly about the house and especially an accident risk assessment, e.g. steepness of stairs, etc.
- impact of the symptoms on the patient

2 Identification and use of information gathered

The candidate should be able to interpret the history and create a problem list. The objectives for the candidate are to:

- understand the exact circumstances surrounding the case and establish whether there is a witness available to give more details of the episodes
- explain the possible causes for her symptoms
- have a plan of investigations
- explain in simple terms that the GP has found a carotid bruit and that this may or may not be related to the symptoms
- explain what a carotid ultrasound involves, stressing that the test is non-invasive

3 Discussion related to the case

- This case tests the candidate's ability to take a detailed history of dizziness and to differentiate the possible causes, such as carotid artery stenosis, carotid sinus hypersensitivity, orthostatic hypotension, cardiac dysrhythmias, transient ischaemic attack, drug-induced and anaemia.
- This scenario suggests carotid sinus hypersensitivity brought about by excessive sensitivity of the carotid sinus, commonly found in the elderly. She describes symptoms when she moves her neck, especially when hanging up the washing.
- Investigations should include routine tests looking for anaemia and disturbed urea and electrolytes as a result of the bendrofluazide, resting ECG, 24-h ECG tape, sitting and standing blood pressure and carotid Doppler ultrasound. Tilt table assessment may be useful in cases of impaired autonomic reflexes as a cause of postural hypotension, particularly in the elderly.
- As she lives alone it would be prudent to admit her for investigations and for an occupational therapy assessment regarding her safety at home; the GP has expressed concern as well.

Comments on the case

This is a typical case where the candidate has a patient who: (a) may not remember too many details of the symptoms; and (b) may use terms such as 'dizziness' to mean something completely different to what the candidate understands. Hence it is vitally important to ask exactly what the patient means by 'dizziness' or feeling 'faint', etc. Do not assume that you and the patient are talking about the same thing! It is important to read the GP's letter carefully to make a judgement about his or her concerns. Do not dismiss these concerns; the GP knows the patient better than you do so you must respect these anxieties.

Case 15 | Double vision

Candidate information

You are the SHO in a general medical clinic. Mr Alfred Lee has been referred to you by his GP.

Please read this letter (it should take no more than 2 min) and then continue with the consultation.

> Dear Doctor
>
> **Re: Mr Alfred Lee, aged 50**
>
> Thank you for seeing Mr Lee who gives a 12-month history of diplopia. He felt this was caused by fatigue when working late but now he finds it difficult to keep his eyes open in the evenings. Routine blood tests including FBC, U/E, LFT, calcium and a chest X-ray are all normal. Please see and advise.
>
> Yours sincerely
>
> Dr G. Practitioner

You have 14 min until the patient leaves the room, followed by 1 min for reflection, before the discussion with the examiners. Be prepared to discuss the solutions to the problems posed by the case and how you might reply to the GP's letter.

Patient information

Mr Lee is a 50-year-old lawyer who has had diplopia for the last 12 months. The diplopia is worse towards the end of the day. He has also noticed recently, when he is at his desk, that when looking up at someone for a prolonged time, his eyelids close. Initially he put all this down to general fatigue which he has had over the last year. The fatigue has become worse over the last 3 months and he finds that walking home from the train station, which includes two flights of steps, in the evenings is particularly arduous; walking to the station in the morning is not such a problem. He has also noticed that he has some weakness in his limbs. When his son asked him to help assemble a set of shelves, he could not hold these up for more than a minute. He has not had any problems with chewing, swallowing, speaking or breathing. He does not have any other cardiovascular, gastrointestinal, hyperthyroid or neurological symptoms, such as headache, loss of consciousness or ataxia. There have been no obvious precipitants causing an acute deterioration of his symptoms. He has always been well with no significant past medical history. There is no past history or family history of autoimmune disorders, such as pernicious anaemia, rheumatoid disease, hyperthyroidism or SLE. He has never smoked and drinks wine occasionally at home. He lives with his wife and his main concerns are the effect of these symptoms on his work. He is particularly worried that this may be motor neurone disease.

Examiner information

1 Data gathering in the interview

A good candidate would be able to elicit:

- details of the diplopia, when and how first noticed (usually early sign of myasthenia), ascertain in which direction the patient sees two of a thing, whether it is worse towards the evenings and whether he can read print (visual acuity). Whether there is associated ptosis and, if so, is it bilateral. Is the ptosis worse after looking upwards for a prolonged time?
- tiredness, weakness and fatigability—whether it is worse after repetitive usage of muscle groups and improves with rest or sleep. Which limbs and which muscle groups, e.g. proximal, distal or all muscle groups feel weak? Seek examples of when he has had particular problems with limb weakness
- weakness of other muscle groups, e.g. facial (myasthenic 'snarl' when attempting to smile), bulbar involvement (difficulty in chewing and swallowing, dysarthria or dysphoria at the end of sentences), respiratory muscle weakness
- other neurological symptoms suggestive of an intracranial lesion, or other systemic symptoms suggestive of a neoplasm (e.g. Lambert–Eaton syndrome secondary to small-cell lung cancer)
- past history of autoimmune disorders (associated with myasthenia gravis), e.g. hyperthyroidism, thyroiditis, SLE, rheumatoid disease and pernicious anaemia
- drug history, e.g. D-penicillamine for rheumatoid arthritis, aminoglycosides in large doses, procainamide
- smoking and alcohol history
- impact of symptoms on family and work
- concerns of the patient

2 Identification and use of information gathered

The candidate should be able to interpret the history and create a problem list. The objectives for the candidate are to:

- explain the possible differential diagnoses to the patient
- have a list of investigations and explain this to the patient
- concede that it is a disabling disorder and will need treatment

- outline the main principles of management
- address the concerns of the family and reassure that this is not motor neurone disease

3 Discussion related to the case

- This scenario illustrates myasthenia gravis (IgG antibodies to acetylcholine receptor (AChR) protein) particularly as the patient describes fatigability when looking up at someone or holding up shelves. He also describes extraocular muscle weakness and diplopia as a result.
- Investigations to confirm diagnosis are important, e.g. anti-AChR radioimmunoassay: 90% positive in generalized myasthenia gravis, 50% in ocular myasthenia and 25% in those in remission. The diagnosis is definite if positive but a negative result does not exclude myasthenia. Edrophonium chloride (Tensilon) 2 mg test dose, then 8 mg IV (an anticholinesterase); highly probable diagnosis if progressive improvement—weakness within 30 s; unequivocal if an immediate and complete improvement in weakness. Repetitive nerve stimulation shows a decrement of muscle-evoked muscle action potential > 15% at 3 Hz.
- The candidate will be expected to discuss other relevant diagnoses. Other conditions that cause weakness of the cranial and/or somatic musculature include drug-induced myasthenia, Lambert–Eaton myasthenic syndrome (LEMS), hyperthyroidism, botulism, intracranial mass lesions (if suspected, e.g. sphenoid ridge meningioma, must have MRI), non-organic cause of apathy and tiredness and progressive external ophthalmoplegia with mitochondrial muscular dystrophy.
- The candidate would also be expected to discuss the importance of a thymoma in the general outcome, the management of myasthenia gravis (oral pyridostigmine) and of myasthenic crises.

Comments on the case

In this case the candidate must ask the patient for examples of his weakness and fatigue to get a feel of the history and to make sure that this is not motor neurone disease which is the patient's foremost worry.

Case 16 | **Dysphagia**

Candidate information

You are the SHO in a gastroenterology clinic. Mr Fred Williams has been referred to you by his GP for an urgent consultation.

Please read this letter (it should take no more than 2 min) and then continue with the consultation.

Dear Doctor

Re: Mr Fred Williams, aged 63

Thank you for seeing Mr Williams who complains of difficulty in swallowing for the last 12 weeks. As a consequence he has lost 2 kg in weight. He is naturally concerned about the possibility of a cancer. In the past he has had arthritis of the right knee for which he takes paracetamol. He has had heartburn for many years for which he takes ranitidine.

Yours sincerely

Dr G. Practitioner

You have 14 min until the patient leaves the room, followed by 1 min for reflection, before the discussion with the examiners. Be prepared to discuss the solutions to the problems posed by the case and how you might reply to the GP's letter.

Patient information

Mr Fred Williams is a 63-year-old former accountant for the city council. He has had difficulty in swallowing for the last 12 weeks. This has gradually progressed from an inability to eat large meals to having to cut up meat into small pieces, and to now finding that these meat pieces intermittently stick in the lower part of the chest and are associated with some pain. He has no pain between meals. He also suffers from heartburn which he has had for many years. He has had two recent episodes of waking up in the middle of the night choking with a feeling of acid in the mouth. There has been a 2-kg loss of weight but no other symptoms of vomiting, haematemesis, loss of appetite, dyspnoea or hoarseness of the voice. He has no neurological symptoms or history of having swallowed any foreign bodies. He has been taking ranitidine which has provided some relief until now. There is no history of taking NSAIDs, although he does take paracetamol for an arthritic knee. He has never smoked and rarely takes alcohol. He lives with his wife. He is concerned he may have cancer.

Examiner information

1 Data gathering in the interview

A good candidate would be able to elicit:
- the duration of the symptoms, whether they are getting

progressively worse (e.g. cancer) or are intermittent (e.g. motility disorder)
- if there is chest pain between meals or any pain on swallowing
- whether solid food (obstructive) and/or liquids

(motility) are equally difficult to swallow (achalasia)

- if the patient can point to where food seems to stick
- any high dysphagia (compression web, pharyngeal pouch, thyroid swelling)
- if swallowing is easier in a different posture
- any associated vomiting, haematemesis, regurgitation, heartburn, weight loss, loss of appetite, hoarseness, dyspnoea, cough, choking or spluttering especially when lying flat (typical in achalasia)
- the past history of reflux oesophagitis with any precipitating and relieving factors
- any neurological symptoms (bulbar palsy)
- history of foreign body ingestion
- drug history, e.g. NSAIDs, potassium (which can cause oesophagitis) or aspirin
- any history of scleroderma (poorly localized dysphagia, skin changes and Raynaud's phenomenon), though the dysphagia may precede the other symptoms
- impact of symptoms and the concerns of the patient

2 Identification and use of information gathered

The candidate should be able to interpret the history and create a problem list. The objectives for the candidate are to:

- develop a list of possible differential diagnoses
- explain the possible causes for the dysphagia, including the impossibility of totally excluding a cancer without an endoscopy
- describe what an endoscopy entails
- address any concerns with regard to the procedure and diagnosis
- arrange follow-up to discuss these results

3 Discussion related to the case

- This case tests the ability of the candidate to develop a list of differential diagnoses: benign oesophageal stric-

ture, reflux oesophagitis, oesophageal tumour (e.g. carcinoma, benign such as leiomyoma) or motility disorder, e.g. achalasia, spasm, scleroderma. Other conditions which need to be considered are drug-induced oesophagitis especially as a result of the NSAIDs, infective oesophagitis (e.g. candida, herpes, cytomegalovirus (CMV)) neuromuscular disorders, e.g. bulbar palsy, pharyngeal disorder e.g. pouch or web, globus hystericus (high dysphagia in the throat that is related to anxiety), foreign body obstruction.

- The candidate should give a list of investigations, such as routine blood tests especially looking for malnutrition and anaemia, chest X-ray looking for signs of pulmonary aspiration, barium swallow and an upper gastrointestinal endoscopy.
- For discussion, the candidate should know what an upper gastrointestinal endoscopy entails with knowledge of the diagnostic and therapeutic uses of this test, knowledge of motility disorders and their presentation and investigations, diagnosing tumours and their management. The candidate must be able to distinguish certain features of the history that may suggest a neoplasm, e.g. unrelenting progressive worsening of symptoms, continuous pain, loss of weight and appetite, and aspiration.

Comments on the case

This is a case where the history of dysphagia must be taken carefully, looking especially for symptoms suggestive of cancer. It cannot be certain if this is a neoplasm and, as concerns will not be alleviated until the results of the endoscopy are known, the candidate must be seen to show a sense of urgency and concern.

Case 17 | Epigastric pain and nausea

Candidate information

You are the SHO in a general medical clinic. Mrs Sarah Thompson has been referred to you by her GP.

Please read this letter (it should take no more than 2 min) and then continue with the consultation.

Dear Doctor

Re: Mrs Sarah Thompson, aged 39

Thank you for seeing this lady who has complained of epigastric pain with nausea on and off for 4 months. I cannot find any abnormalities on abdominal examination. She was prescribed ranitidine for 4 weeks with only intermittent relief of symptoms. Her full blood count, urea and electrolytes and liver function tests were all normal. Her past medical history is unremarkable except that she has had episodes of allergic rhinitis. I wonder if you would consider whether an endoscopy is warranted.

Yours sincerely

Dr G. Practitioner

You have 14 min until the patient leaves the room, followed by 1 min for reflection, before the discussion with the examiners. Be prepared to discuss the solutions to the problems posed by the case and how you might reply to the GP's letter.

Patient information

Mrs Sarah Thompson is a 39-year-old domestic cleaner weighing 82 kg who gives a 4-month history of intermittent epigastric pain and nausea. The symptoms have been progressively increasing in frequency and at present are occurring 4–5 times each week. Each episode is colicky and sharp in nature, lasting between 30 and 60 min and with no obvious radiation to the shoulder or to the back. Alcohol may precipitate the pain. The pain is not worse with particular movements or on deep inspiration and is not relieved by food, belching and defaecation. She had some intermittent relief with antacids and ranitidine but admits to poor compliance. The nausea is related to the pain. She has had 2 days off work in the last 4 months. There is no history of heartburn, vomiting, bloating, haematemesis, change in bowel habit, rectal bleeding, jaundice or loss of weight and appetite. In the past she has had seasonal allergic rhinitis for which she takes a Beconase nasal spray. She also suffers from headaches for which she takes paracetamol. She does not take any NSAIDs. She smokes 15 cigarettes a day and occasionally drinks two glasses of wine during the evening. She lives with her husband and has two children. Her mother died from colonic carcinoma and she is worried that she may have a neoplasm as a cause of her symptoms.

Examiner information

1 Data gathering in the interview

A good candidate would be able to elicit:

- a detailed history of her symptoms, particularly the site of the pain, the timing, character, constant or intermittent, radiation (to the back or the shoulder), precipitating factors (e.g. movement, food, inspiration), relieving factors (e.g. food, belching, antacids, defaecation), timing of the nausea
- any other gastrointestinal symptoms, such as heartburn, dysphagia, vomiting, haematemesis, change in bowel habit, rectal bleeding, jaundice, pale stools, dark urine, loss of weight and appetite, bloating
- a complete drug history, especially NSAIDs, codeine phosphate, coproxamol, aspirin
- her response to ranitidine and possible reasons for the non-compliance—this may be important if further treatment regimens are recommended
- a detailed alcohol and smoking history
- the impact of this pain on her life, e.g. time off work
- her concerns, especially the family history of colon cancer

2 Identification and use of information gathered

The candidate should be able to interpret the history and create a problem list. The objectives for the candidate are to:

- explain the possible diagnoses
- explain how these may be investigated
- aim to address the worsening nature of the symptoms
- determine any possible precipitating factors, especially NSAIDs usage
- discuss the possibility of an endoscopy with an explanation of the procedure
- discuss her concerns about cancer
- reassure the patient that cancer is unlikely without any 'alarm symptoms', especially dysphagia, weight loss and gastrointestinal bleeding

3 Discussion related to the case

- This case is very common in clinical practice and tests the ability of the candidate to differentiate the diagnosis of non-specific dyspepsia from peptic ulcer disease, gallstones and gastrointestinal neoplasia. The candidate must be able to elicit any possible 'alarm symptoms'.
- The candidate should have a plan of investigations. Generally, in young people (<45 years) with dyspepsia and an absence of 'alarm symptoms', gastrointestinal malignancy is highly unlikely. It would be worthwhile to assess the patient's *Helicobacter pylori* status serologically by measuring IgG antibodies. If these are positive then eradication therapy may be instituted. If negative, then a trial of proton-pump inhibition may be tried, ensuring that she takes the drug regularly.
- The candidate should be able to discuss the pros and cons of an upper gastrointestinal endoscopy at this stage, as this task has been requested by the GP. Further investigation, such as an endoscopy, should ideally be reserved for when 'alarm symptoms' develop or when symptoms persist despite a trial of therapy. It is important to review the patient again in clinic to discuss further the need for an endoscopy.
- The candidate should be able to discuss the epidemiology of *H. pylori*, its mechanism of action, clinical features and diagnostic methods (non-invasive vs. invasive). The candidate may be asked to discuss the pros and cons of eradication with or without peptic ulcer disease and their side-effects.

Comments on the case

This is a common case in the outpatient clinic and stresses the importance of taking a detailed history, especially eliciting the symptoms suggestive of neoplasia. The case tests the candidate's ability to explore any concerns the patient may have. The possibility of cancer is always a worry for many of these patients—the referral to a specialist is itself anxiety-provoking and so exploration of these worries followed by reassurance is very useful. It is important to address the issue of an endoscopy as requested by the GP.

Case 18 | Facial swelling

Candidate information

You are the SHO in a general medical clinic. Mrs Lorna Smith has been referred to you by her GP.

Please read this letter (it should take no more than 2 min) and then continue with the consultation.

Dear Doctor

Re: Mrs Lorna Smith, aged 31

Thank you for seeing Mrs Smith who has complained of two episodes of itchy facial swelling in the last 6 weeks. I treated her with chlorpheniramine (chlorphenamine, Piriton) and prednisolone on both occasions but I am at a loss to know the cause. She has no relevant past medical history. Please see and advise.

Yours sincerely

Dr G. Practitioner

You have 14 min until the patient leaves the room, followed by 1 min for reflection, before the discussion with the examiners. Be prepared to discuss the solutions to the problems posed by the case and how you might reply to the GP's letter.

Patient information

Mrs Lorna Smith is a 31-year-old housewife who has had two recent similar episodes, 2 weeks apart, of soft tissue swelling of her face over the last 6 weeks. She is presently asymptomatic. Both episodes developed rapidly over 20 min, with swelling around the eyes, lips and tongue. She had some cutaneous discrete swellings (weals) in both hands that were intensely itchy and erythematous. Her tongue felt numb but there was no laryngeal oedema (no stridor or dyspnoea). On the second occasion her eyes became fully closed causing her distress. On both occasions the GP gave oral chlorpheniramine (Piriton) 4 mg 4-hourly and prednisolone (30 mg o.d.) to treat the urticaria. The symptoms improved within 6 h, but were not fully resolved until after 72 h. Once recovered, there was no lasting rash. There has been no obvious precipitant, such as extreme temperatures, pressure, inhalatory allergens (pollen, moulds, animal dander), and she is normally tolerant of foods such as fresh fruits, shellfish, fish, milk products, chocolate, peanuts or medication such as NSAIDs, aspirin or penicillin. There has been no recent unusual contact sensitivity to metal jewellery or dog/cat hair and saliva. She has no other symptoms such as gastrointestinal symptoms (diarrhoea), respiratory symptoms of dyspnoea, cough or wheeze or other systemic symptoms, e.g. fever, arthralgia, myalgia. She has no other previous history of allergies, asthma, allergic rhinitis, eczema or of recent viral infections. There is no family history of allergy or angio-oedema. She does not take any routine medication and does not smoke or drink alcohol except a glass of beer now and again. She lives with her husband and three young children who are all well. The family is concerned about the swellings and wishes to know the cause and how it can be prevented.

Examiner information

1 Data gathering in the interview

A good candidate would be able to elicit:
- the exact description of the weals on the hands and the facial oedema, and the parts that are affected
- how quickly the urticaria appeared and for how long it persisted
- the response of the symptoms to antihistamines and prednisolone
- any associated symptoms, especially those suggestive of laryngeal oedema (stridor, dyspnoea), or gastrointestinal or systemic disorders (fever, arthralgia, myalgia)
- any obvious precipitating cause, e.g. trauma, local pressure, emotional stress, inhalatory allergen (pollen, animal dander, mould), extreme cold or heat, solar rays, allergic contact substances such as metallic jewellery or dog/cat hair and saliva
- any previous food allergies, e.g. fruit (strawberries), food colouring, shellfish, chocolate, peanuts
- any past history of atopy, eczema, allergic rhinitis, asthma or recent viral illnesses, SLE, thyrotoxicosis or lymphoma which may present with urticaria
- a family history of angio-oedema
- full drug history, especially NSAIDs, aspirin, opiates and penicillins
- alcohol and smoking history
- social history
- occupational history
- the concerns of the family

2 Identification and use of information gathered

The candidate should be able to interpret the history and create a problem list. The objectives for the candidate are to:
- assess fully the past symptoms as she describes them now that she is asymptomatic
- assess fully the possibility of a precipitating allergen
- show empathy and reassure the family that the symptoms are rarely severe and dangerous, but explaining what to do if laryngeal swelling should occur (urgent admisson to hospital if she develops any breathing or swallowing difficulties associated with the facial swelling)
- explain there is no obvious cause for the urticaria and angio-oedema and it is not uncommon for the cause to remain unknown so routine detailed investigations are not justified
- explain that most idiopathic cases may last for a few months before resolving altogether, although occasionally some go on to have chronic urticaria with recurrent episodes
- have a management plan including the avoidance of aspirin and opiates and to consider regular, non-sedating oral antihistamines for prevention, e.g. cetirizine 10 mg o.d. or loratadine 10 mg o.d.

3 Discussion related to the case

- This case tests the ability of the candidate to take an accurate history of urticaria (well-circumscribed erythematous weals) and angio-oedema (localized oedema involving the deeper layers of the skin). It is important to search for an allergic cause although in this case there is no obvious precipitant. If urticaria was caused by a physical stimulus, such as cold, deep pressure, heat and stress, then avoiding such a known cause is the primary treatment. Hereditary angio-oedema is a rare autosomal dominant condition brought about by deficiency of C1-esterase inhibitor with low levels of C2 and C4, presenting with angio-oedema but not urticaria. It may be worthwhile checking the complement levels but further complex immunological tests are probably not justified.
- Management primarily includes reassurance, avoidance of aspirin and opiates which can degranulate mast cells, and the regular use of oral non-sedating antihistamines which should prevent recurrences. It is important to stress to the patient, and in the letter to the GP, that severe angio-oedema with laryngeal swelling (stridor) will need urgent admission to casualty for emergency treatment and observation.
- The examiner may ask for other possibilities, such as contact sensitivity (a vesicular eruption that pro-

gresses to chronic thickening of the skin with continued allergenic exposure), atopic dermatitis (a condition that may present as erythema, oedema, papules, vesiculation and oozing), cutaneous mastocytosis (reddish-brown macules, papules and urticaria with pruritus upon trauma), and systemic mastocytosis (episodic systemic flushing with or without urticaria but no angio-oedema).

Comments on the case

This case highlights the importance of taking a good history in the absence of current symptoms, with particular emphasis on precipitating factors.

Case 19 | Funny turns

Candidate information

You are the medical SHO in a diabetes clinic. Mr Donald Tiverton has been referred to you by his GP.

Please read this letter (it should take no more than 2 min) and then continue with the consultation.

Dear Doctor

Re: Mr Donald Tiverton, aged 69

Thank you for seeing this gentleman ahead of his routine appointment. He has been having episodes of altered consciousness, mainly during the late mornings. He has insulin-controlled diabetes and had a coronary artery by-pass graft (CABG) in November last year. He is currently under investigation for leg pain with suspected peripheral vascular disease. His medications comprise Mixtard insulin b.d., aspirin 75 mg o.d., frusemide (furosemide) 40 mg o.d., lisinopril 10 mg o.d., Bezalip-Mono 400 mg o.d. and nizatidine 150 mg b.d. I am uncertain if these 'funny turns' are caused by hypoglycaemia. Please would you advise.

Yours sincerely

Dr G. Practitioner

You have 14 min until the patient leaves the room, followed by 1 min for reflection, before the discussion with the examiners. Be prepared to discuss the solutions to the problems posed by the case and how you might reply to the GP's letter.

Patient information

Mr Donald Tiverton is a 69-year-old retired market trader who has had diabetes mellitus for 15 years treated with subcutaneous insulin for the last 7 years. He had been reasonably well until the last 2 months when his wife noticed that he was getting drowsier towards noon (before lunch) on most days. According to his wife these episodes seem to start around 11.30 a.m. They come on over about 10 min with a sense of oblivion to what is going on around him and he looks pale, sweaty and he mumbles. He has no limb-shaking or tongue-biting typical of a fit and no collapses typical of dysrhythmias. Symptomatically, during these episodes Mr Tiverton feels light-headed and hungry and sometimes has palpitations. When a blood sugar test was carried out on one occasion, the count was unrecordable. He eventually comes round after a 'Lucozade drink' from his wife. She is adamant that these are hypoglycaemic attacks. Mr Tiverton cannot understand why he may be having frequent hypoglycaemic episodes; his diet has not changed (including the timing) and neither has the insulin dose. Previous to these episodes, his hypoglycaemic attacks would occur approximately once every 3 months, usually after an imbalance between the injected insulin and his diet. His activity has not changed and in fact he rarely does much exercise. His glycaemic control is excellent with home glucose monitoring running mainly between 4 and 8 mmol/L and a recent HbA1c was 6.1%. He takes Mixtard 30/70 human insulin using a pen device, 26 units in the morning and 24 in the evening. His other symptom of note is bilateral leg pain when walking, which is improved by resting, but returns when he restarts walking. The pain starts in the left calf followed by the right one. He is awaiting a review by a vascular surgeon for suspected peripheral vascular disease. Two years ago he had persistent, severe, central chest pain and underwent a CABG for coronary artery disease; unfortunately with a suboptimal result because of early graft failure. Presently his angina is infrequent (treated with sublingual glyceryl trinitrate (GTN) spray) and the cardiothoracic surgeons are not keen to undertake further intervention. His weight is steady. He is under regular follow-up by the ophthalmologist and has not needed retinal laser therapy. His medication includes aspirin 75 mg o.d., lisinopril 10 mg o.d., Bezalip-Mono 400 mg o.d. and nizatidine 150 mg b.d.; he does not take any extra oral hypoglycaemics. He does not drink alcohol and there is no suggestion of him taking extra doses of insulin surreptitiously. They are concerned about the frequent episodes of possible hypoglycaemia and his wife is worried that she cannot leave him alone at home.

Examiner information

1 Data gathering in the interview
A good candidate would be able to elicit:
- details of the nature of these 'funny turns', i.e. frequency, timing (e.g. before lunch), any symptoms of hypoglycaemia (e.g. palpitations, aura, hunger, blurred vision, light-headedness, sweating) and any association with posture or movement
- whether any blood glucose testing was carried out during these episodes
- the possibility of unawareness and any episodes of unconsciousness
- symptoms suggestive of other possible causes of altered consciousness, e.g. epilepsy, dysrhythmia, postural hypotension, vasovagal syncope, transient ischaemic attacks (TIAs)
- insulin regimen, usual level of control (home glucose monitoring or recent HbA1c)
- if a record of home glucose monitoring is kept and if the patient has it with him
- injection technique and any 'lumps'
- diet, use of snacks, timing of meals in relation to insulin doses
- patient's usual pattern of activity and any deviations from it related to these episodes
- macro- and microvascular complications of diabetes, especially in view of his coronary artery disease and peripheral vascular disease
- drug history, e.g. beta-blockers
- smoking and alcohol history
- suggestions of factitious overdosing of insulin and/or usage of oral hypoglycaemics
- symptoms suggestive of other causes of hypoglycaemia, e.g. endocrine (hypopituitarism, Addison's disease), tumours (sarcomas) and hepatic disease
- fears and concerns of the patient and his wife

2 Identification and use of information gathered
The candidate should be able to interpret the history and create a problem list. The objectives for the candidate are to:
- consider the differential diagnoses for these episodes
- establish whether the episodes are a fault of the insulin regimen or unusual activity or due to an imbalance with his diet
- appreciate the macro- and microvascular complications of diabetes mellitus, giving a differential diagnosis for the leg pain including peripheral vascular disease, neuropathy, nerve entrapment or spinal problems
- provide a management plan (as suggested below) with reassurance

3 Discussion related to the case
- Hypoglycaemia occurs most commonly as a result of very tight treatment of patients with diabetes mellitus. However, a number of other disorders including in-

sulinoma (although not in this case), large mesenchymal tumours, end-stage organ failure, alcoholism, endocrine deficiencies, postprandial reactive hypoglycaemic conditions and inherited metabolic disorders are also associated with hypoglycaemia. Hypoglycaemia is sometimes defined as a plasma glucose level <2.5 mmol/L. However, the glucose thresholds for hypoglycemia-induced symptoms and physiological responses vary widely depending on the clinical setting. Therefore, Whipple's triad provides an important framework for making the diagnosis of hypoglycaemia: (a) symptoms consistent with hypoglycaemia; (b) a low plasma glucose concentration; and (c) relief of symptoms after the plasma glucose level is raised.

- Hypoglycaemia is a common problem and may result from an imbalance between injected insulin and a patient's normal diet, activity and basal insulin requirements. Before meals are the most hazardous times. Irregular eating habits (e.g. shift work) or exertion and excessive alcohol intake may precipitate an attack. However, changing absorption of insulin (which may be the case here) may also be the cause. It is therefore necessary to take an accurate account of diet including snacks and insulin dosage and timing history.

- Hypoglycaemia unawareness (occurs in some longstanding diabetics, sometimes with coincident non-selective beta-blockers) refers to loss of the warning symptoms of hypoglycaemia, which normally alert individuals to the presence of hypoglycaemia and prompt them to eat in order to abort the episode. This issue must be addressed during the history taking. Some patients who have previously been treated with animal insulins complain of reduced awareness of hypoglycaemia when changed to human insulin.

- Management of hypoglycaemic attacks includes patient education, frequent self-monitoring of blood glucose, realistic glycaemic goals and ongoing professional support. Appropriate adjustments to medications, diet and lifestyle should be recommended. Non-selective beta-blockers may attenuate the recognition of hypoglycaemia and they impair glycogenolysis; a relatively selective beta-1 antagonist (e.g. metoprolol or atenolol) is preferable if a beta-blocker is indicated. Management also includes strict avoidance of hypoglycaemia, possibly a change of insulin regimen (e.g. insulin q.d.s., use of new rapidly acting insulin analogues) or, in the case of patients previously on animal insulins (who may have insulin antibodies), converting back to a porcine or bovine insulin. Lifestyle factors and diet may need adjusting.

Comments on the case

This patient with diabetes has recently developed episodes of hypoglycaemia before lunch. He has a number of macrovascular complications. Although the 'funny turns' are not difficult to elaborate, the history is very suggestive of hypoglycaemic attacks and importance should be placed on why these episodes have developed.

Case 20 | Haemoptysis

Candidate information

You are the SHO in a respiratory clinic. Mr Gordon Bell has been referred to you by his GP.

Please read this letter (it should take no more than 2 min) and then continue with the consultation.

Dear Doctor

Re: Mr Gordon Bell, aged 75

Thank you for seeing this man who has had two episodes of haemoptysis during the last 3 weeks. He has a long history of COPD for which he takes beclomethasone, ipratropium, salmeterol and salbutamol inhalers. He has been a chronic smoker for many years. A chest X-ray performed last week is reported as normal but I am concerned that we may be missing a neoplasm.

Yours sincerely

Dr G. Practitioner

You have 14 min until the patient leaves the room, followed by 1 min for reflection, before the discussion with the examiners. Be prepared to discuss the solutions to the problems posed by the case and how you might reply to the GP's letter.

Patient information

Mr Gordon Bell is a 75-year-old man who has had two episodes of haemoptysis in the last 3 weeks. Both occurred while at home in the morning, about 2 weeks apart. The haemoptysis was fresh blood with mucoid phlegm, and about a spoonful in volume. He has never had any previous episodes of haemoptysis. He has had COPD for many years. This manifests as breathlessness on exertion especially on an incline, and he has to stop twice when walking up a flight of stairs. He has no chest pains, ankle swelling, palpitations or loss of weight or appetite. There is no previous history of a deep vein thrombosis, pulmonary embolism, bleeding disorders or tuberculosis. Apart from the inhalers he takes no other medication and no anticoagulants. He has been a chronic 20 cigarettes a day smoker since the age of 14 years and has worked as a plumber all his life. He has been exposed to asbestos during his work with pipe insulation. He lives with his wife in a terraced house and she does most of the household chores. The patient is concerned that he may have lung cancer.

Examiner information

1 Data gathering in the interview

A good candidate would be able to elicit:

- when the haemoptysis was first noticed and whether he has coughed up blood before
- whether the haemoptysis occurs daily or has he had it only once

- the volume of haemoptysis, e.g. eggcupful or spoonful
- whether the haemoptysis is fresh red blood; discoloured brown or mixed in with sputum (colour of sputum, mucoid vs. purulent)
- any other associated symptoms, such as pleuritic chest pain, dyspnoea, fever, syncope, palpitations, or leg swelling suggestive of a deep vein thrombosis
- an idea of his exercise ability, i.e. stairs, distance on the flat or on an incline
- any past history of cardiac, pulmonary (e.g. COPD, childhood pneumonia, tuberculosis) or bleeding disorders
- drug history, including anticoagulants
- smoking history
- occupational history, especially asbestos exposure
- family history of tuberculosis
- daily living abilities
- the concerns of the patient, particularly regarding the possibility of lung cancer

2 Identification and use of information gathered

The candidate should be able to interpret the history and create a problem list. The objectives for the candidate are to:
- explain the possible differential diagnoses; although the chest X-ray was normal one still has to consider the potential chance of lung cancer
- give a list of investigations
- explain that the patient needs a bronchoscopy and give a description of the procedure
- share a sense of concern with some arrangement for a follow-up appointment to discuss the results

3 Discussion related to the case

- This case tests the ability of the candidate to create a list of differential diagnoses for haemoptysis. Although this patient has a normal chest X-ray, lung cancer is still the main diagnosis to rule out. A chest X-ray does not necessarily exclude a small bronchial neoplasm. Haemoptysis is also common in patients with COPD, especially during exacerbations. A history of increased sputum volume and purulence with dyspnoea may

point to this. Other possibilities include bronchiectasis, pulmonary embolism, infective causes such as tuberculosis and pneumonia, and mitral stenosis.
- Investigations should include FBC, U/E, LFT and calcium, ECG, spirometry and oxygen saturation on air. These should also help to decide if the patient would be able to tolerate a bronchoscopy. If the bronchoscopy is normal then the next step would be a CT scan of the thorax though this may be ideally done before any invasive procedures. A ventilation–perfusion scan may be necessary if pulmonary embolization is suspected.
- The candidate is expected to be aware of the bronchoscopy procedure, the use of sedation and the diagnostic and therapeutic scope of this procedure. The examiners expect the candidate to know the different histological types of lung cancer, the manifestations of lung cancer (direct/metastatic spread and non-metastatic extrapulmonary manifestations), investigations and treatment, i.e. surgical (including contraindications), radiotherapy, chemotherapy and palliative care.

Comments on the case

This case tests the ability of the candidate to take a history giving particular attention to the possibility of cancer. Most patients in these situations want to know if it is cancer or not, so avoiding the matter altogether will do the patient no favours. Although the chest X-ray is normal, the candidate must be able to convey to the patient that this may not rule out the possibility completely and hence it would be wise for the patient to have a bronchoscopy. Most doctors, in the authors' experience, have found that patients are quite keen to undergo such a test for the purposes of reassurance. This case also raises the issue of smoking cessation, although it is usually best to address this at a later date.

Case 21 | Headache

Candidate information

You are the SHO in a neurology clinic. Mrs Sarah Wittington has been referred to you by her GP.

Please read this letter (it should take no more than 2 min) and then continue with the consultation.

> Dear Doctor
>
> **Re: Mrs Sarah Wittington, aged 45**
>
> I would appreciate your help with this pleasant housewife who has had migrainous headaches on-and-off for 3 years. They usually occur around the left side of her head with occasional vomiting. I have tried paracetamol, codeine and sumatriptan without much success. I am now struggling to control her symptoms. She is normally fit and well but does suffer from bouts of depression for which she takes paroxetine 50 mg o.d. I could not find any obvious neurological deficits on examining her.
>
> Yours sincerely
>
> Dr G. Practitioner

You have 14 min until the patient leaves the room, followed by 1 min for reflection, before the discussion with the examiners. Be prepared to discuss the solutions to the problems posed by the case and how you might reply to the GP's letter.

Patient information

Mrs Sarah Wittington is a 45-year-old housewife who has been complaining of episodes of facial pain for the last 3 years. The pain usually begins around the left eye (always the left side), is excruciating in nature and increases in intensity over about 30 min. It may last for up to 2 h, usually occurring at night time and with a strange feeling of heaviness on that side of the face with nasal stuffiness. There is no radiation and there are no obvious precipitating factors. These episodes usually keep her awake and tend to occur around once or twice a day for a fortnight and then there are none for about 6–8 months. There has been little relief from painkillers and sumatriptan. She does get another pain that is different from the facial pain. This is a headache with a feeling of a tight band throughout the whole head, throbbing in nature, lasting for around 2–4 h, with no radiation, usually exacerbated by bouts of depression and normally relieved by paracetamol. She has had these headaches for a number of years but it is the facial pain that causes the most trouble. There are no precipitating factors such as straining, coughing or sneezing nor do they occur on wakening. There is no history of any previous head trauma or seizures. There are no other symptoms of drowsiness, confusion, weakness, ataxia, photophobia, neck stiffness, visual changes or fever. She has had no problems with the teeth, sinuses or ears, or any previous herpetic neuralgia, temporomandibular arthritis or temporal arteritis. She has had depression for 6 years, first presenting as low mood and difficulty in sleeping. She has been on paroxetine 50 mg o.d. during this time. Family rows and worry about the children usually aggravate the depression. She has no other relevant past medical history. Apart from the painkillers and paroxetine, she is on no other medication. She rarely drinks alcohol and smokes 5 cigarettes a day. She is divorced and has brought up two teenage children single-handedly. Her concerns are that the facial pain is causing the depression to worsen and she is desperate for help.

Examiner information

1 Data gathering in the interview

A good candidate would be able to elicit:
- that two types of pain are present: facial and headache
- confirm how long the pains have been a problem and if they come on suddenly; how long are the longest pain-free periods; when was the last attack
- ask for a description of where each pain is located
- whether the headaches radiate anywhere, e.g. back of head and neck
- if the pains are constant or intermittent and whether they are deteriorating
- if they are worse at any particular time of the day, e.g. on wakening. Does the pain wake her up and does it ever change sides
- how long the pains last for
- any particular triggers, e.g. coughing, straining, exertion, stress at work, particular foods, bright lights
- any associated drowsiness, confusion, nausea, vomiting, weakness, ataxia, photophobia, neck stiffness, visual changes or fever
- when differentiating facial pain — ask about problems with teeth, sinuses, ears, and elicit any history of herpetic neuralgia, temporomandibular arthritis or temporal arteritis
- any suggestions of depression, anxiety and, if so, how they present
- any recent history of head trauma or seizures
- drug and alcohol history — ask in detail the response to painkillers and 5-hydroxytryptamine ($5HT_1$) agonists
- a past history of hypertension
- a detailed social history with attention to work and family dynamics
- any concerns she may have and what she thinks the headaches are caused by

2 Identification and use of information gathered

The candidate should be able to interpret the history and create a problem list. The objectives for the candidate are to:
- identify and explain the presence of two different pains
- describe the possible causes of these pains
- reassure that it is very unlikely that there is a neoplastic reason for her pains and that there are unlikely to be any serious consequences
- have a management plan, i.e. prevention strategy for the facial pain

3 Discussion related to the case

- This case tests the ability of the candidate to assemble two lists of differential diagnoses. The facial pain described here is typical of cluster headaches (although more common in males) but other causes of facial pain to be aware of are diseases of the teeth, sinuses, ears and throat, temporal arteritis, postherpetic neuralgia, trigeminal neuralgia, temporomandibular arthritis and glaucoma. The headache she describes sounds like a tension headache exacerbated by depression. Other alternatives include migraine and raised intracranial pressure. If migraine is suspected, the history should also include any prodromal symptoms (classical migraine) with visual symptoms of flashing lights and blind patches together with associated gastrointestinal (nausea and vomiting) and cerebral symptoms and signs, such as numbness and weakness of limbs.
- Treatment usually involves reassurance and explanation with particular emphasis on the very remote chance of a neoplasm, particularly in the absence of symptoms and signs such as weakness or par-

aesthesia. If such symptoms and signs were present, a CT scan of the head may need to be considered.

- With regard to managing the cluster headaches, prevention is important and in some patients beta-blockers or lithium (400–1200 mg daily) has been shown to be useful. Managing the attacks is difficult and painkillers are normally ineffective. Meanwhile, the tension headaches are normally managed adequately with paracetamol (if not, add codeine).

Comments on the case

This case highlights the importance of keeping an open mind after reading the GP's correspondence, i.e. do not assume this is migraine. There are two different types of pain and the candidate must be seen to take a full history of both pains—otherwise it will be impossible to diagnose correctly and manage both symptoms.

Case 22 | **Hoarse voice**

Candidate information

You are the SHO in a general medical clinic. Mrs Kathy O'Donnell has been referred to you by her GP.

Please read this letter (it should take no more than 2 min) and then continue with the consultation.

Dear Doctor

Re: Mrs Kathy O'Donnell, aged 49

Thank you for seeing this lady who has complained of a hoarse voice for 6 months. She smokes 15 cigarettes a day and, after a bout of winter bronchitis 2 years ago, she was started on beclomethasone and salbutamol inhalers. She is also known to have oesophageal reflux for which she takes a maintenance dose of lansoprazole. She has no other past medical history and takes no other medication. Please see and advise.

Yours sincerely

Dr G. Practitioner

You have 14 min until the patient leaves the room, followed by 1 min for reflection, before the discussion with the examiners. Be prepared to discuss the solutions to the problems posed by the case and how you might reply to the GP's letter.

Patient information

Mrs Kathy O'Donnell, aged 49 years, is a Dubliner living in the UK. She works as a barmaid at the local Irish centre. Six months ago she noticed she was becoming a little 'croaky' and 4 weeks later her voice had reached the present degree of hoarseness, remaining unchanged with no particular association with a time of day. She has never had bouts of hoarseness before. She had a lower respiratory tract infection two winters ago manifesting as purulent sputum, wheeze and one episode of haemoptysis (blood mixed in with the sputum) lasting for 1 day. A chest X-ray at that time was normal. Since then she continues to have a slight cough with mucoid sputum at night time and a wheeze in the morning. She was also started on beclomethasone inhaler 200 μg, two inhalations twice a day and salbutamol as needed (usually taken at the same time as the beclomethasone). However, she does admit to having used the inhalers up to four times a day most days of the week for the last 4 weeks. She does not use a volumatic nor gargle after the beclomethasone inhalations. She did not have a hoarse voice when she first started using the inhalers. She still suffers from heartburn, particularly at night time, and she now props herself up with three pillows. She commonly wakes up at night with an acid taste in the mouth. She has had no haemoptysis, chest pain, dyspnoea, dysphagia, loss of weight or noticed any enlarged lymph glands in her neck. She has had no recent coryzal illnesses or sore throat, and no past history of hypothyroidism or exposure to environmental hazards such as coal fires. She lives with her husband who has been insisting that she should have sought advice about the voice earlier. She has been working at the Irish centre for 16 years and admits that she needs a clear booming voice during work; there have been times when she is unable to make herself heard. She has always been a heavy smoker since the age of 12 and currently smokes 15 cigarettes a day. She does tend to have about three measures of gin per day during her work.

Examiner information

1 Data gathering in the interview

A good candidate would be able to elicit:

- how long she has noticed the hoarse voice. Has she had a hoarse voice before?
- how the hoarseness started. Was it after a bout of viral laryngitis? Has the hoarseness plateaued or is it still worsening?
- if the hoarse voice coincided with starting the beclomethasone inhaler
- if she uses a volumatic with the beclomethasone and gargles afterwards. Has she been using the inhalers excessively?
- if she has been overusing her voice
- any associated sore throats and upper respiratory tract coryzal illnesses
- any associated dyspnoea, cough, sputum, haemoptysis, chest pain, heartburn — if so, is it worse at night, does she prop herself up at night time?
- any associated dysphagia with aspiration
- any associated symptoms suggestive of hypothyroidism
- recent inhalational history, e.g. exposure to fire/smoke
- drug history
- smoking history
- occupational history — whether she needs a loud voice at work. What does she use her voice for, e.g. announcements, etc.?
- her concerns and the impact of the hoarseness on her work and family life
- if she would be receptive to smoking cessation advice

2 Identification and use of information gathered

The candidate should be able to interpret the history and create a problem list. The objectives for the candidate are to:

- assemble the possible differential diagnoses
- explain the possible causes of the hoarse voice
- explain and describe a plan of investigations
- arrange follow-up soon to discuss any results

3 Discussion related to the case

- The hoarseness of the voice in this case could be the result of a number of possibilities: chronic laryngitis secondary to corticosteroid inhaler or gastro-oesophageal acid reflux disease or even overuse, laryngeal polyp, laryngeal carcinoma, vocal cord paralysis secondary to lung cancer or, rarely, hypothyroidism.
- Investigations in this case would be first a chest X-ray to rule out a bronchial neoplasm with left recurrent nerve palsy, routine blood tests and, most importantly, asking an ENT surgeon to have a look at the vocal cords with a laryngoscope.
- If there are no vocal cord lesions, e.g. polyps or evidence of candida, but only inflammation, this may suggest acid reflux as the cause and this will need to be addressed appropriately. Evidence of candida would suggest that the beclomethasone is the cause. This should be addressed by advising the patient to take the beclomethasone less often, using a volumatic that would prevent the aerosol impacting on the pharynx and larynx, and gargling after inhalation.

Comments on the case

This is a common case and highlights the importance of taking all the details of inhaler usage with particular timing to the onset of hoarseness. The candidate must ascertain the impact of the symptoms on her work.

Case 23 | Hypercalcaemia

Candidate information

You are the medical SHO in a general medical clinic. Mrs Freda Davidson has been referred to you by her GP.

Please read this letter (it should take no more than 2 min) and then continue with the consultation.

Dear Doctor

Re: Mrs Freda Davidson, aged 53

Thank you for seeing Mrs Davidson who, after a routine blood test, was found to have a calcium of 2.84 mmol/L and an albumin of 39 g/L. She has a past history of peptic ulcer disease 10 years ago and takes fluoxetine for depression. Please see and advise.

Yours sincerely

Dr G. Practitioner

You have 14 min until the patient leaves the room, followed by 1 min for reflection, before the discussion with the examiners. Be prepared to discuss the solutions to the problems posed by the case and how you might reply to the GP's letter.

Patient information

Mrs Davidson is a 53-year-old housewife who has been found to have hypercalcaemia on routine testing by the GP. She is normally well although she has bouts of tiredness which she puts down to not being able to sleep at night. She has no obvious gastrointestinal symptoms apart from a poor appetite and a tendency towards constipation if she is not careful with her diet. She has a history of depression for the last 4 years after the death of her mother. Presently she feels low in mood with some loss of self-esteem. She is on fluoxetine for this. Ten years ago she presented to hospital with dyspepsia and an upper gastrointestinal endoscopy revealed a duodenal ulcer. This was treated with antacids but she does occasionally have dyspeptic symptoms, particularly after a spicy meal. She has no bony pains, nor any past history of renal stones. She lives with her husband and generally leads a fairly active life running the household, doing the shopping and cleaning. She does not smoke or drink and she takes no other medication. There is no family history of hypercalcaemia. She is on a normal diet with no real excessive intake of dairy products. Mrs Davidson is not quite sure why she has been referred to the specialist.

Examiner information

1 Data gathering in the interview

A good candidate would be able to elicit:

- the history of the symptoms relevant to hypercalcaemia, e.g. tiredness, malaise, depression, abdominal pain (e.g. from a peptic ulcer), constipation, urinary symptoms and renal colic from stones, bony pain, etc.
- symptoms suggestive of respiratory disorders (e.g. sarcoidosis), gastrointestinal disorders (e.g. peptic ulcer), endocrine disorders (e.g. hyperparathyroidism, thyrotoxicosis), malignancy (bony secondaries from breast and lung, lymphoma, myeloma)
- history of the depression
- drug history (i.e. any vitamin D analogues, thiazides, lithium)
- family history (hypocalciuric hypercalcaemia)
- immobility
- concerns of the patient

2 Identification and use of information gathered

The candidate should be able to interpret the history and create a problem list. The objectives for the candidate are to:

- take a history relevant to hypercalcaemia
- determine any specific cause for the hypercalcaemia
- ascertain the history of the peptic ulcer and the depression and to think about a possible link between these and the hypercalcaemia (hyperparathyroidism)
- explain the biochemical findings to the patient
- have a plan of further investigations and management

3 Discussion related to the case

- Hypercalcaemia can be caused by: (a) excessive parathyroid hormone secretion (primary, tertiary or ectopic, lithium and hypocalciuric hypercalcaemia); (b) excessive vitamin D-related (vitamin D intoxication, sarcoidosis and other granulomatous diseases); (c) malignancy-related (breast, lung, haematological), but unlikely if asymptomatic; (d) high bone turnover (immobility); (e) drugs (thiazides, vitamin D analogues); and (f) endocrine (hyperthyroidism).
- Primary hyperparathyroidism is the most common cause of hypercalcaemia discovered by chance. Hypercalcaemia from any cause can result in fatigue, depression, mental confusion, anorexia, nausea, vomiting, constipation, peptic ulcer (particularly in patients with renal calcification), short Q-T interval on the electrocardiogram and, in some patients, cardiac dysrhythmias. There is a variable relation between the severity of the hypercalcaemia and the symptoms. Generally, symptoms are more common at calcium levels >2.9 mmol/L but some patients, even at this level, are asymptomatic. When the calcium level is >3.2 mmol/L calcification in the kidneys, skin, vessels, lungs, heart and stomach can occur and renal insufficiency may develop, particularly if the blood phosphate levels are normal or elevated as a result of impaired renal function. Severe hypercalcaemia, usually 3.7–4.5 mmol/L, can be a medical emergency as coma and cardiac arrest can occur. Hypercalcaemia in an adult who is apparently asymptomatic is usually a result of primary hyperparathyroidism. In malignancy-associated hypercalcaemia it is the malignancy that brings the patient to the physician and the hypercalcaemia is discovered during the routine investigations. Investigations include serum calcium, phosphate and parathyroid hormone levels. Parathyroid hormone values are elevated in >90% of parathyroid-related causes of hypercalcaemia, are undetectable or low in malignancy-related hypercalcaemia, and undetectable or normal in vitamin D-related and high-bone-turnover causes of hypercalcaemia.
- Therapy for primary hyperparathyroidism is primarily surgical, particularly in those with stones, bony involvement, calcium levels above 2.9 mmol/L or a previous episode of severe acute hypercalcaemia. Patients with primary hyperparathyroidism often get used to chronic fatigue that is dramatically improved after parathyroidectomy.
- The candidate will be expected to discuss preoperative localization investigations, especially the role of MRI, radioisotope subtraction scanning and the management of acute hypercalcaemia.

Comments on the case

This case presents with an abnormal biochemical finding and the candidate will be expected to tailor the history towards finding a cause and recognizing that previous medical illnesses may be related.

Case 24 | Hyperlipidaemia

Candidate information

You are the medical SHO in the diabetic clinic. The GP has written a note about this patient whom you are about to see for his annual review.

Please read this letter (it should take no more than 2 min) and then continue with the consultation.

Dear Doctor

Re: Mr David Palmer, aged 54

Please would you advise on the treatment of this gentleman's hyperlipi-daemia. He is a known diabetic and his cholesterol level was 7.0 mmol/L 6 months ago. I started him on a statin and after 3 months his cholesterol fell to 5.4 mmol/L with a HDL cholesterol of 1.5 mmol/L and a raised triglyceride (fasting) level of 4.14 mmol/L. At this recent visit, I also found proteinuria on dipsticking. He is overweight and dietary advice has been unsuccessful. His medication is currently Actrapid insulin t.d.s., Insulatard insulin noct, metformin, atorvastatin, perindopril and aspirin.

Yours sincerely

Dr G. Practitioner

You have 14 min until the patient leaves the room, followed by 1 min for reflection, before the discussion with the examiners. Be prepared to discuss the solutions to the problems posed by the case and how you might reply to the GP's letter.

Patient information

Mr David Palmer is a 54-year-old ex-taxi driver who was found to have a raised cholesterol (7 mmol/L) 6 months ago after a routine visit to the GP's diabetic surgery. He was started on atorvastatin and a repeat test 3 months later showed the cholesterol to have dropped to 5.4 mmol/L. He is reasonably well in himself and is self-caring. He has had diabetes mellitus for 8 years for which he takes insulin four times daily by NovoPen (Actrapid 12 units t.d.s. before meals and Insulatard 18 units at night). He developed diabetic eye problems for which he has had laser treatment to both eyes 2 years ago; eye disease was the reason for him giving up work. He also has had numbness of both feet and was found to have proteinuria on dipsticking 3 months ago by the GP. He has a history of hypertension for 8 years for which he initially took bendrofluazide. However, 4 years ago he had an episode of gout and the thiazide was changed to an ACE inhibitor (perindopril). He does not have a history of ischaemic heart disease but his father died of an MI when he was young. Despite dietary advice from the practice nurse, he is struggling to keep his weight down (he is presently 92 kg) and he does not want to increase his insulin dose any further as he worries that this may increase his weight. He does not think he eats excessively. He has three meals a day; breakfast includes cereal and buttered toast, followed by lunch which usually consists of salad and buttered sandwiches and in the evening a cooked meal usually pork with potatoes and vegetables. When he increases his insulin, he does notice his appetite increases as well and he has a tendency to have snacks between meals with resulting weight gain. Home monitoring of glucose reveals levels between 8 and 13. Other medications include metformin 500 mg t.d.s. and aspirin 75 mg o.d. He smokes 5 cigarettes a day and is trying to cut down. He used to smoke 20 a day but, as he does not work, stopping altogether has been difficult. He does not undertake any exercise. He drinks on average 3 pints of beer a day and lives with his wife and three grown-up children. He does not seem too concerned about the hyperlipidaemia as he is not symptomatic from this, but he is slightly concerned about the urine protein finding.

Examiner information

1 Data gathering in the interview

A good candidate would be able to elicit:
- the details of the hyperlipidaemia (some patients will know the exact lipid values)
- cardiovascular history — suggestive of ischaemic heart disease and of peripheral vascular disease
- a full diabetic history, including micro- and macrovascular complications. Treatment of diabetes
- history of hypertension
- smoking history
- family history of ischaemic heart disease
- alcohol, a full dietary and exercise history
- concerns of the patient

2 Identification and use of information gathered

The candidate should be able to interpret the history and create a problem list. The objectives for the candidate are to:
- ascertain the cardiovascular risk factors in this patient
- explain the importance of minimizing these risk factors by improving glycaemic control and hence the need for reducing weight and alcohol intake, increasing insulin, stopping smoking, keeping blood pressure and lipids stringently under control and improving daily life activities, e.g. more exercise, weight control, etc.
- explain that total calorie intake (alcohol and dietary fat) is excessive and this must be reduced. Also explain that increasing insulin increases food intake and hence the weight gain
- explain the possible significance of the proteinuria finding and the need for doing further tests, i.e. 24-h urine protein collection

- address any concerns, particularly the balance between the increase in insulin dose and the possible weight gain

3 Discussion related to the case
- This patient has numerous cardiovascular risk factors which need to be addressed. The patient has hyperlipidaemia although with a relatively good HDL level, hypertension, diabetes mellitus, a bad family history and he also smokes and drinks.
- The cardiovascular risk in patients with type 2 diabetes without a history of MI is said to be equivalent to that of a non-diabetic patient who has had an MI. Instead of defining treatment cut-off levels for hypercholesterolaemia, the use of cardiovascular risk profiles ought to be favoured. Previous recommendations have been for the treatment of elevated blood pressure with a cardiovascular risk of >15% over 10 years and treatment of elevated cholesterol with a cardiovascular risk of >30% over 10 years. However, these cut-off levels were believed to be mainly financially driven and recommendations for the treatment of cholesterol with cardiovascular risks of >20% are becoming acceptable. The traditional risk calculations, however, will not apply in this case as the patient has established proteinuria which increases the risk a further 2–3 times. Many physicians would treat as for secondary prevention in these cases. With respect to proteinuria and hypertension, the current debate is whether treatment should be with an ACE inhibitor, an angiotensin-II receptor antagonist or both.
- As well as improving glycaemic control, general management should include further advice on diet, especially reducing fat intake, alcohol, weight and increasing exercise; considering increasing the dosage of atorvastatin, adding a fibrate and considering the

use of fast-acting insulins (Humalog and Novonorm) as these possibly help with weight control as there is no need for snacks.

- Discussion with examiners may include the increased risk of side-effects of statin plus fibrate combinations (gemfibrozil and cerivastatin combination led to the withdrawal of the latter) and combined use of thiazides and beta-blockers may adversely affect the lipid profile. The candidate will be expected to know the up-to-date guidelines for hyperlipidaemia management.

Comments on the case

This is a complicated case and tests the ability of the candidate to assess the many possible risk factors rather than purely focusing on the hyperlipidaemia.

Case 25 | Jaundice

Candidate information

You are the SHO in a gastroenterology clinic. Mr Brian Jones has been referred to you by his GP.

Please read this letter (it should take no more than 2 min) and then continue with the consultation.

> Dear Doctor
>
> **Re: Mr Brian Jones, aged 56**
>
> Thank you for seeing this solicitor who has complained of jaundice with right hypochondrial pain, malaise and nausea for the last 4 days. He has had arthritis of his hip since breaking his femur in a road traffic accident 16 years ago. For this he takes co-codamol. Please see and advise.
>
> Yours sincerely
>
> Dr G. Practitioner

You have 14 min until the patient leaves the room, followed by 1 min for reflection, before the discussion with the examiners. Be prepared to discuss the solutions to the problems posed by the case and how you might reply to the GP's letter.

Patient information

Mr Brian Jones is a 56-year-old solicitor, working in the city centre, who complains of a sudden onset of jaundice 4 days ago with right hypochondrial pain. The jaundice has progressed during these 4 days but there are no pale stools and only slight discoloration of the urine. The pain is a dull, constant ache and is worse on deep inspiration. There is also malaise, nausea with loss of appetite and a loss of weight of 2 kg. He has no abdominal swelling, haematemesis, melaena, vomiting, pruritus, fever, peripheral oedema or altered sleep pattern. Past medical history includes a road traffic accident as a pedestrian 16 years ago, when he broke the neck of his femur. Despite repair, he has suffered from subsequent arthritic pain for which he takes co-codamol regularly. This pain is sometimes severe enough to affect his sleep and cause depression. Occasionally, he has taken more than the prescribed dose of co-codamol but has not taken any overdoses. He says he drinks 'socially' but more detailed questioning reveals that he has been a heavy consumer for 12 years, drinking two bottles of wine a day, particularly after work with clients. He does admit to drinking heavily during 'working lunches' as well. He does not drink beer but has some spirits at home in the evening, usually two measures of whisky. He does not drink in the morning nor does he suffer from any early morning withdrawal tremor. He believes he had some units of blood at the time of his fractured hip but no recent transfusions. There has been no recent travel abroad nor are there any obvious HIV risk factors. There is no past history of autoimmune illnesses. He was divorced 6 years ago and he lives alone. He has had one conviction for drink-driving 3 years ago.

Examiner information

1 Data gathering in the interview

A good candidate would be able to elicit:

- when the patient first noticed the jaundice, whether it is gradually deepening and if the skin and sclerae are yellow
- any previous episodes of jaundice and any family history of jaundice
- associated pruritus, discoloured stools or urine (implying biliary obstruction)
- any abdominal pain and its nature. Causes of painful jaundice include alcoholic, infective, drug-induced, Wilson's disease, hepatitis, biliary colic, pancreatitis, cholecystitis, metastatic and Budd–Chiari syndrome
- or painless, e.g. haemolysis (hyperbilirubinaemia, Gilbert's syndrome), pancreatic or biliary malignancy and hepatic cirrhosis (e.g. related to alcohol), haemochromatosis (associated with arthritis), primary biliary cirrhosis (itching and malaise)
- any associated symptoms, including nausea/vomiting, haematemesis, fatigue, malaise, fever, loss of appetite, weight loss, rash, arthritis, peripheral oedema, abdominal swelling, confusion/altered sleeping pattern (encephalopathy)
- any respiratory or cardiac symptoms
- full alcohol history, including drinking at work — CAGE questionnaire, driving offences, psychological and social problems as a consequence
- any relevant past medical history, e.g. liver and gallstone disorders, malignancy, recent anaesthesia (especially halothane), blood transfusions, history of other autoimmune disorders (e.g. coeliac, diabetes, hypothyroidism, etc.) important for primary biliary cirrhosis and autoimmune hepatitis
- full drug history, including antibiotics, paracetamol (any overdoses in an attempt to relieve arthritic pain) and antirheumatic drugs
- any risk factors for viral hepatitis, e.g. hepatitis A (travel abroad, shellfish consumption), hepatitis B and C (intravenous drug abuse, tattoos, sexual)
- other risk factors for hepatitis, such as blood transfusion, contact with environmental sources (e.g. leptospirosis)

- any concerns the patient may have, especially with regard to the possibility of cirrhosis or cancer
- any psychological difficulties which may be associated with the high alcohol consumption, especially depression, and also gain an appreciation of the impact the current illness may have on his work

2 Identification and use of information gathered

The candidate should be able to interpret the history and create a problem list. The objectives for the candidate are to:

- create a list of differential diagnoses
- ascertain any risk factors for hepatitis
- have a plan for investigations
- be able to approach the patient about the high alcohol consumption with regard to encouraging abstinence and offering help, especially counselling
- arrange a follow-up appointment to discuss the results of investigations

3 Discussion related to the case

- This case tests the ability of the candidate to develop a list of differential diagnoses for jaundice (painful vs. non-painful) and to ask appropriate questions to decide with which particular diagnosis the case fits best. The most likely diagnosis is alcoholic hepatitis. However, questioning should reflect the possibility of other diagnoses, such as obstructive jaundice (e.g. gallstones), viral hepatitis and liver metastases.
- The candidate's plan of initial investigations should include FBC, U/E, LFT, GGT, a clotting screen, glucose, viral hepatitis screen, CMV antibodies, autoimmune antibodies (antimitochondrial antibodies), alpha-fetoprotein and, most importantly, an abdominal ultrasound.
- For discussion, the candidate will need to know the causes of jaundice and cirrhosis, the pathological changes of alcoholic liver disease, the consequences of the alcohol dependency syndrome (physical, psychological and social), management of liver failure and complications of portal hypertension.
- A common discussion topic is management of the alcoholic patient with regard to recognition and

counselling. The CAGE questionnaire has been developed to aid the identification of alcohol abuse and a detection rate of up to 70% has been claimed in those who say yes to two or more of the following four questions.

(1) Have you ever felt you ought to Cut down your drinking?

(2) Have people Annoyed you by criticizing your drinking?

(3) Have you ever felt bad or Guilty about your drinking?

(4) Have you ever had a drink first thing in the morning to steady your nerves or to get rid of a hangover (Eye opener)?

Comments on the case

This case typifies the common scenario of a patient underestimating the quantity of alcohol he consumes. The candidate must not just assume 'social drinking' equates to 1 pint per evening; the candidate's and the patient's definition of a 'social drinker' may have no concordance. The candidate must be prepared to burrow further into the alcohol history, with recognition of the possible psychological and social consequences.

Case 26 | Joint pains

Candidate information

You are the SHO in a rheumatology clinic. Mrs Margaret Rees has been referred to you by her GP.

Please read this letter (it should take no more than 2 min) and then continue with the consultation.

> Dear Doctor
>
> **Re: Mrs Margaret Rees, aged 35**
>
> Thank you for seeing Mrs Rees who has complained of painful, swollen joints in her hands during the past 5 weeks. This is associated with tiredness, particularly in the mornings. She is finding that her symptoms are interfering with her work and she has now taken the last 2 weeks off as sick leave. She presently takes co-codamol and she is intolerant of NSAIDs as they exacerbate her oesophageal reflux. Please see and advise.
>
> Yours sincerely
>
> Dr G. Practitioner

You have 14 min until the patient leaves the room, followed by 1 min for reflection, before the discussion with the examiners. Be prepared to discuss the solutions to the problems posed by the case and how you might reply to the GP's letter.

Patient information

Mrs Margaret Rees is a 35-year-old right-handed lady who works behind the counter at the local Lloyds TSB bank. Over the last 5 weeks she has complained of a gradual onset of swollen, painful joints in the proximal interphalangeal (PIP) and metacarpophalangeal (MCP) distribution of both hands (initially the right). This is associated with stiffness, particularly in the mornings, which improves with usage of the hands, and generalized tiredness that may on occasions persist throughout the day. Her pain, swelling and stiffness are worse in the right hand than the left. The only other joint affected is the right shoulder. There are no obvious precipitating factors but gentle activity may improve the stiffness. There are no associated skin rashes, nodules, nail changes, sensory loss or radiation of the pain in the hands. Other general symptoms of the respiratory, neurological or ophthalmic systems are absent. There have been no acute attacks of swelling. Her symptoms are particularly affecting her ability to write and type which are essential for work and because of this and the tiredness she has taken the last 2 weeks off work. This is particularly upsetting as she never takes time off work and she is worried that she may be made redundant. Another disability she has noticed is with buttoning up her blouses. She is taking co-codamol without a great deal of relief. She also takes a maintenance dose of lansoprazole for oesophageal reflux and because of this she is intolerant to NSAIDs. There is no other past history of arthritis, autoimmune disorders, recent infections or trauma. Her mother suffered with osteoarthrosis when in her seventies. She does not smoke or drink alcohol. She lives with her husband and two children who are very supportive. She is naturally anxious as to whether this may be rheumatoid arthritis and, if so, about any potential long-term disability.

Examiner information

1 Data gathering in the interview

A good candidate would be able to elicit:
- which joints in the hands are affected
- if other joints are affected, e.g. wrists, shoulders, neck, back, hips, knees, feet, etc.
- how long the swelling has been present for, if there are any acute attacks of swelling and, if so, how often and what precipitates an attack
- whether the swelling affects both hands at the same time (symmetrical arthropathy)
- any associated pain with radiation, morning stiffness, skin rash, nodules, sensory loss
- other general symptoms related to systemic rheumatological disorders, e.g. fatigue, malaise, fever, eye changes, respiratory, neurological
- history of the oesophageal reflux and inability to tolerate NSAIDs
- detailed occupational history, with any history of repetitive strain injuries or trauma
- any disability, e.g. dressing, writing, using cutlery, socially and at work, e.g. typing
- any past medical history, e.g. connective tissue disease, vasculitis, autoimmune disorders, infections, gastrointestinal disorders (cirrhosis, peptic ulcer), skin disorders, e.g. psoriasis
- any family history of rheumatoid arthritis
- drug history, e.g. thiazides precipitating gout, procainamide or hydralazine causing lupus erythematosus and ask if the patient is intolerant of NSAIDs as this may determine certain pharmacological therapy regimens
- smoking and alcohol history
- concerns of the patient (social and work)

2 Identification and use of information gathered

The candidate should be able to interpret the history and create a problem list. The objectives for the candidate are to:
- explain the possible diagnoses

- express that the diagnosis may be rheumatoid arthritis but it is impossible to comment at this stage on long-term prognosis
- show full understanding, with empathy, about the restriction on her daily activities
- describe in detail the necessary tests to be performed
- illustrate that you would like to admit her to carry out these tests and to start therapy once the diagnosis is made
- attempt to reassure her that alternative treatments other than NSAIDs are available for rheumatoid arthritis
- endeavour to address any other concerns she may have

3 Discussion related to the case

- This case tests the candidate's ability to take a detailed joint history and to consider the primary diagnosis of rheumatoid arthritis, with particular relevance to the systemic symptoms. Other possible diagnoses to be considered are other seronegative arthropathies, such as psoriasis or Reiter's syndrome, both of which may present with asymmetrical distal interphalangeal joint arthropathy. Nodal osteoarthrosis rarely presents under the age of 50 years.
- The candidate should consider admission with a plan of investigations; FBC, serology (rheumatoid factor which is present in approximately 70% of cases), X-rays of the affected joints and aspiration of a joint if an effusion is present with culture for bacteria. Further imaging of the joints (e.g. MRI scan) may be required, especially if the neck is involved. Physiotherapy input may also be considered.
- The candidate would be expected to have a detailed knowledge of the systemic effects of rheumatoid arthritis, its immunopathology, the role of disease-modifying antirheumatic drugs and their potential side-effects and the development of the new anticytokine therapies, such as anti TNF-alpha monoclonal antibody.

Comments on the case

This case highlights the importance of taking a detailed 'impact of symptoms' history. The history is typical for rheumatoid arthritis but extra marks will be awarded if the candidate can visualize the patient in the social setting with the burden of her illness on work and family life. This case will also test the ability of the candidate to address the anxieties and concerns that the patient may have.

Case 27 | Loin pain

Candidate information

You are the medical SHO in an endocrine clinic and about to see this patient for his annual review. The GP has sent a letter with the patient.

Please read this letter (it should take no more than 2 min) and then continue with the consultation.

> Dear Doctor
>
> **Re: Mr Ronald Tweedle, aged 76**
>
> Thank you for seeing Mr Tweedle whom you see for acromegaly on an annual basis. He has been complaining of recurrent left-sided loin pain which has been getting gradually worse over the last 3 weeks. He was treated for a urinary tract infection (UTI) with trimethoprim but his pain has not resolved. Please see and advise.
>
> Yours sincerely
>
> Dr G. Practitioner

You have 14 min until the patient leaves the room, followed by 1 min for reflection, before the discussion with the examiners. Be prepared to discuss the solutions to the problems posed by the case and how you might reply to the GP's letter.

Patient information

Mr Ronald Tweedle, a 76-year-old gentleman, presents with a 3-week history of left-sided loin pain. The pain may come on at any time of the day; it is usually severe, sharp and intermittent and may last up to 2 h. Sometimes the pain radiates anteriorly but there is no dysuria or haematuria. He has had these pains now on two separate occasions. The GP made a home visit on each instance and gave Voltarol, which resulted in some relief, and trimethoprim to cover any infection. He has a previous history of a staghorn calculus in the right kidney which was surgically removed 12 years ago. He has been otherwise well in himself and only suffers symptomatically from prostatism which manifests as postmicturition dribbling with poor stream. He is on finasteride for this. He also has a previous history of acromegaly 20 years ago which was treated surgically and he is under regular yearly follow-up in the endocrine clinic. He has some residual peripheral visual field loss, but the acromegaly is inactive at the moment. A recent CT scan of the head showed no recurrence of the tumour. He has a past history of sick sinus syndrome presenting as dizziness and bradycardia for which a pacemaker was inserted 8 years ago. He takes ramipril for hypertension. He lives alone in a ground floor flat. He is self-caring and he does not smoke or drink. He is concerned about the possibility of recurring renal stones.

Examiner information

1 Data gathering in the interview

A good candidate would be able to elicit:

- a complete history of the pain, i.e. frequency, position, radiation, nature, relieving/exacerbating factors (e.g. alcohol, drinking large quantities of fluids), associated dysuria, haematuria, history of prostatism
- previous history of renal stones, presence of hypercalcaemia at the time
- history of acromegaly and particularly ascertaining the activity, i.e. worsening visual field defects, sweating, headaches, etc. Other symptoms, e.g. change in appearance, increased size of hands, ring tightening, deep/hollow voice, tiredness, impotence or poor libido
- history of other features resulting from acromegaly, e.g. hypertension, heart failure, arthropathy, carpal tunnel syndrome, diabetes mellitus, galactorrhoea, goitre
- when the pacemaker was inserted and what type—this would be a contraindication for MRI scanning
- other drug history
- social history
- concerns of the patient

2 Identification and use of information gathered

The candidate should be able to interpret the history and create a problem list. The objectives for the candidate are to:

- ascertain that the history does sound like renal stones and correctly establish the previous history of renal calculi
- link the acromegaly with the renal calculi and the cardiovascular disease
- provide a plan of action for the patient

3 Discussion related to the case

- Differential diagnoses in this case would be renal stones, pyelonephritis and prostatic obstruction predisposing to hydronephrosis.
- Investigations would include blood tests for calcium and U/E, midstream urine (MSU), a plain abdominal X-ray and an intravenous urogram.
- Long-term sequelae of acromegaly potentially include the deficiency of other pituitary hormones; visual loss caused by compression of the optic nerve; impaired glucose tolerance and diabetes; hypertension; renal stones as a result of increased urinary excretion of calcium; increased risk of gastric and colonic neoplasms; skeletal problems such as kyphosis, scoliosis and accelerated osteoarthrosis; cardiac problems including accelerated atherosclerosis and cardiomyopathy; overgrowth of soft tissues which may not entirely resolve after treatment including a goitre and nerve entrapment syndromes such as carpal tunnel syndrome. Skin changes in acromegaly include acral bony overgrowth (frontal bossing), soft tissue swelling (nose, lips, hands and feet), excessive sweating and hypertrichosis.

> **Comments on the case**
>
> This is quite a typical case where the past medical history is 'retrospectively' interlinked and hence it is vitally important not to dismiss past illnesses but to speculate on any possible connection with the present symptoms.

Case 28 | Loss of weight

Candidate information

You are the SHO in a general medical clinic. Mrs Marlene Llewellyn has been referred to you by her GP.

Please read this letter (it should take no more than 2 min) and then continue with the consultation.

> Dear Doctor
>
> **Re: Mrs Marlene Llewellyn, aged 40**
>
> Thank you for seeing Mrs Llewellyn who has complained of a 5-kg loss of weight over the last 6 months. Her appetite is good but she has noticed an increasing frequency of bowel actions during the last few weeks. She has a past history of anxiety for which she takes zopiclone. A recent FBC, U/E, LFT and chest X-ray are all normal. Please see and advise.
>
> Yours sincerely
>
> Dr G. Practitioner

You have 14 min until the patient leaves the room, followed by 1 min for reflection, before the discussion with the examiners. Be prepared to discuss the solutions to the problems posed by the case and how you might reply to the GP's letter.

Patient information

Mrs Llewellyn is a 40-year-old housewife who has complained of a 5-kg loss of weight over the last 6 months from 54 to 49 kg. She has always been thin. She first noticed the weight loss when her clothes started to feel looser and the children were saying that she looked much thinner than before. She eats well and there has been no loss of appetite. Her diet is non-vegetarian with fresh fruit and cereals in the morning, followed by a sandwich at lunch and usually a cooked meal with meat and potatoes in the evening. She does no physical exercise apart from her daily living activities. There has been no purposeful dieting and no abuse of laxatives or diuretics. She has no other bowel symptoms apart from occasional loose stools recently but no steatorrhoea. Normally she goes once a day but in the last few weeks it has been up to three times a day. There is no constipation, rectal bleeding, nausea/vomiting, vaginal bleeding, cough, sputum or haemoptysis. Her past medical history includes an anxiety neurosis for which she takes zopiclone. She continues to feel 'on edge' most days with occasional tremors and palpitations during the anxious episodes, which are usually triggered by family rows. Recently she has noticed that she is not sleeping well with early morning wakening. She has smoked 10 cigarettes a day since the age of 16 and does admit to smoking more when she is anxious. She does not drink alcohol but her husband drinks heavily and this exacerbates her worries. She lives in a three-bedroom semidetached house in a deprived area with her husband and two children. She has always been a housewife. She cannot understand why she is losing weight despite an unchanged diet.

Examiner information

1 Data gathering in the interview

A good candidate would be able to elicit:
- if the patient feels her clothes are looser, whether she is looking thinner and if friends/family have noticed any change
- how much weight she has lost. Take a dietary history with assessment of intake and any change in appetite
- if the weight loss is intentional, e.g. dieting, exercise, laxatives/diuretics
- previous history of weight loss
- previous body weight
- associated gastrointestinal symptoms, e.g. dysphagia, abdominal pain, nausea/vomiting, gastrointestinal bleeding, altered bowel habit, steatorrhoea
- endocrine symptoms, e.g. thyrotoxicosis (tremors, increased appetite, diarrhoea, palpitations, eye symptoms), adrenal insufficiency (weakness, dizziness, excessive sweating)
- other cardiovascular and respiratory symptoms
- drug history, especially diet pills, laxatives, amphetamines
- symptoms suggestive of anxiety and depression
- social history, recent separation or job loss/change
- alcohol and smoking history (smoking reduces appetite)
- other past medical history, e.g. gastrointestinal disorders, emphysema, neoplasia, diabetes mellitus
- the patient's concerns regarding the weight loss

2 Identification and use of information gathered

The candidate should be able to interpret the history and create a problem list. The objectives for the candidate are to:
- create a list of differential diagnoses
- plan a list of investigations
- convey these to the patient with explanations
- educate her on the hazards of smoking
- arrange quick follow-up with reweighing and to discuss the results of investigations

3 Discussion related to the case

- This case tests the ability of the candidate to decide if the loss of weight is non-gastrointestinal, e.g. thyrotoxicosis or anxiety/depression, or gastrointestinal, e.g. primary neoplasm, malabsorption (coeliac disease, Crohn's disease), poor dietary intake as a result of alcoholism or functional dyspepsia/peptic ulcer. Do not forget the possibility of concurrent disease.
- Investigations including FBC, U/E, TFT, LFT, GGT, glucose, chest X-ray and, if these are all normal, one may consider looking specifically for gastrointestinal causes.
- If all investigations are normal, observation of her weight with a daily food diary over a few weeks/months may be necessary.
- The diagnosis here is between an anxiety neurosis and thyrotoxicosis though coeliac disease must be excluded. The anxiety neurosis may well be exacerbated by thyrotoxicosis and it is not uncommon for patients to be labelled 'anxious' only to be subsequently found that they are thyrotoxic. The candidate will be expected to describe the systemic effects of thyrotoxicosis, the complications (e.g. crises) and treatment (antithyroxine synthesis drugs vs. radioactive iodine).

> **Comments on the case**
>
> This is a common general medical case of 'weight loss ?cause'. Do not assume the weight loss is psychological or gastrointestinal. The clues are in the history and the candidate must have made a mental note of all the possible causes before the consultation in order to tailor the history along the lines of that list. If you feel the case may be thyrotoxicosis, then you can really concentrate specifically on the long list of possible symptoms to gain extra marks. Again, you must have a plan of investigations on hand and be prepared to reply to the patient's query, 'Have I got cancer?'

Case 29 | Lower gastrointestinal haemorrhage

Candidate information

You are the SHO in the gastroenterology clinic. Mr John Davies has been referred to you by his GP.

Please read this letter (it should take no more than 2 min) and then continue with the consultation.

> Dear Doctor
>
> **Re: Mr John Davies, aged 53**
>
> Thank you for seeing Mr Davies so quickly. He has complained of rectal bleeding for the last 3 weeks without any loss of weight. His past medical history includes osteoarthritis of both knees and haemorrhoids. He takes diclofenac only. I am concerned that he may have a neoplasm. Please see and advise.
>
> Yours sincerely
>
> Dr G. Practitioner

You have 14 min until the patient leaves the room, followed by 1 min for reflection, before the discussion with the examiners. Be prepared to discuss the solutions to the problems posed by the case and how you might reply to the GP's letter.

Patient information

Mr John Davies is a 53-year-old car mechanic who, one morning 3 weeks ago, noticed dark red blood mixed in with his stools at the bottom of the toilet pan. He thought at first that this was from his haemorrhoids but these normally present intermittently with bright red blood on the toilet paper and not mixed in with the stools. The blood is present every day and he passes stools regularly once a day. There has been no change in his bowel habit, and he has had no haematemesis, loss of weight, abdominal pain, diarrhoea, vomiting, jaundice, hypochondrial tenderness or malaise. He does not suffer from urgency, tenesmus or pain on passing stools. He has not noticed any lumps protruding through his anus. He has had haemorrhoids for many years and the last time he noticed any blood from these was 3 months ago. The new symptom is definitely different. There is no other history of bleeding disorders, other gastrointestinal history or of food poisoning. He takes diclofenac for his arthritis but does not suffer from NSAID-induced dyspepsia. There is no other relevant drug history, e.g. iron or bismuth. There is no family history of polyps or colonic carcinoma. He does not drink or smoke. He lives with his wife and both lead active lifestyles. Mr Davies is naturally concerned that this may be cancer.

Examiner information

1 Data gathering in the interview

A good candidate would be able to elicit:

- if he had passed blood rectally before and, if so, the nature and frequency of this
- the description of the present blood in the stools, e.g. fresh red blood, dark red or black, mixed with stool, on the surface of the stool or on the toilet paper only. How much blood and mucus is present
- any associated diarrhoea or any nocturnal diarrhoea (sometimes seen in ulcerative colitis)
- how often he passes bloody stools in a day
- any change in bowel habit
- if he has abdominal pain, urgency or tenesmus when passing stools
- any straining, constipation, anal pain (fissure), rectal lumps/masses
- any weight loss and, if so, over how long a period
- any associated symptoms, such as loss of appetite, nausea, vomiting, haematemesis, abdominal mass, fatigue and tiredness, bleeding elsewhere
- other previous gastrointestinal history, haemorrhoids, bleeding disorders, food poisoning
- drug history, especially NSAIDs, anticoagulants, iron and bismuth (black stool not red)
- alcohol history
- family history of gastrointestinal neoplasia, polyps
- any obvious concerns regarding cancer

2 Identification and use of information gathered

The candidate should be able to interpret the history and create a problem list. The objectives for the candidate are to:

- decide clearly the difference between the previous rectal bleeding and the present symptom
- explain that cancer cannot be totally excluded unless the proper investigations are carried out
- explain what these investigations are and describe what is involved with a sigmoidoscopy, double-contrast barium enema and, if needed for confirmation of doubtful lesions, a colonoscopy including the description of preoperative sedation, biopsies and retaining of tissue for histology

3 Discussion related to the case

- The case tests the ability of the candidate to compare the present history with the past symptoms and to judge if these are from the same aetiology or not. The history of the previous haemorrhoids is clearly different to the present symptom. The most worrying differential diagnosis includes a lower gastrointestinal neoplasm, the history of which can sometimes point to the possible site of the cancer, e.g. altered bowel habit with or without abdominal pain is common in descending colonic lesions, rectal and sigmoid carcinomas tend to present with bleeding commonly mixed in with stools whereas caecal lesions may just present with an iron-deficiency anaemia and no other obvious bowel symptom. Other possibilities include colonic and/or rectal polyps which may intermittently bleed, particularly the larger ones; colitis such as ulcerative colitis, although diarrhoea is more common with bleeding; diverticular bleeding which can occasionally be massive and can be detected on double-contrast barium enema as pouches of mucosa extruding through the muscular wall. Haemorrhoids and anal fissures present with fresh bleeding with pain on defaecation (particularly with the fissures). Angiodysplasia may also be a cause of lower gastrointestinal bleeding. The candidate should have a plan of investigations including FBC, routine biochemistry, flexible sigmoidoscopy, double contrast barium enema (good preparation essential) and colonoscopy to confirm the presence of a suspicious lesion.
- The candidate will be expected to discuss the importance of neoplastic polyps with regard to transformation to carcinoma, genetics of colonic carcinoma, use of faecal occult blood testing, screening and prevention, and treatment (surgical and chemotherapy).

Comments on the case

This case is an important one to stress the value of collating details of the previous haemorrhoid history and comparing this to the present history. The candidate will get extra marks if he or she makes it obvious to the examiner that the line of questioning is conforming to this thought processes while searching for the possible site of the lesion.

Case 30 | Macrocytic anaemia

Candidate information

You are the SHO in a general medical clinic. Mr Arthur Evans has been referred to you by his GP.

Please read this letter (it should take no more than 2 min) and then continue with the consultation.

Dear Doctor

Re: Mr Arthur Evans, aged 84

Thank you for seeing Mr Evans who was noticed to be pale by his carers. He has been in the residential home for 2 years since the death of his wife. He is normally mobile with a stick. A full blood count shows: Hb 6.3 g/dL, white cell count (WCC) 5.8 × 10^9/L, platelets 213 × 10^9/L and mean cell volume (MCV) 112 fl. He does not normally complain of any symptoms but the carer has noticed a decline in activity levels over the last year. He also has arthritis of the right hip for which he takes paracetamol.

Yours sincerely

Dr G. Practitioner

You have 14 min until the patient leaves the room, followed by 1 min for reflection, before the discussion with the examiners. Be prepared to discuss the solutions to the problems posed by the case and how you might reply to the GP's letter.

Patient information

Mr Evans is an 84-year-old retired machine operator who does not complain of any symptoms but recently has been noticed to be very pale by the residential home carers. He has been in the home for 2 years since the death of his wife. Normally he is mobile with a stick, has no obvious symptoms of dementia, is self-caring and takes an active role in the daily activities at the home. However, over the last year his activity has reduced with increasing tiredness, particularly towards the end of the afternoon, and there has been a tendency to retire to bed early in the evening. Closer questioning reveals that he has lost about 4 kg in weight, his appetite has diminished over the last few months and he has mentioned to the carer that he has a sore mouth. He does not complain of vomiting, dysphagia, abdominal pain, diarrhoea or gastrointestinal bleeding. There are no cardiovascular, respiratory, hypothyroid or neurological symptoms such as limb weakness or numbness. His past medical history includes arthritis of the right hip which does restrict his movement and for which he needs a stick. He has never been referred to an orthopaedic surgeon. He has no past history of liver disorders, alcohol problems, autoimmune disorders such as Graves' disease, myxoedema, thyroiditis, idiopathic adrenocortical insufficiency, vitiligo, or hypoparathyroidism, or of any gastrointestinal disorders or previous operations. There is no family history of any of the abovementioned autoimmune conditions. He eats a normal diet supplied by the home which includes meat, vegetables and fruit. His only medication is paracetamol. He used to smoke 5 cigarettes a day until 12 years ago and he does not drink alcohol. Although he does not have any concerns about his condition, Mr Evans is aware that the residential home staff have expressed their concern about the pallor.

Examiner information

1 Data gathering in the interview

A good candidate would be able to elicit:

- how the patient has deteriorated with regard to activity at the home
- a description of any tiredness, dyspnoea, weight loss or poor appetite
- his premorbid state, especially mobility, self-caring abilities and dementia
- a full gastrointestinal history, especially loss of weight—how much? Suggestions of small bowel disease, e.g. steatorrhoea (ileal disease, bacterial overgrowth), jaundice, a sore tongue (glossitis) in pernicious anaemia
- a dietary history—?vegan
- full systemic history to identify heart failure, vitamin B_{12} deficiency-related subacute combined degeneration (any paraesthesia), autoimmune disease
- past medical history, especially of gastrointestinal surgery (gastrectomy, ileal resection), gastrointestinal disease (coeliac disease, Crohn's disease, bacterial overgrowth, tropical sprue), malignancy, renal dialysis (folate)
- full drug history, especially antifolate drugs such as phenytoin, methotrexate, trimethoprim
- family history of autoimmune disorders, including pernicious anaemia
- alcohol history (folate deficiency)
- fish tapeworm (very rare)
- the concerns of the patient and his carers

2 Identification and use of information gathered

The candidate should be able to interpret the history and create a problem list. The objectives for the candidate are to:

- assemble a list of the possible causes of the macrocytic anaemia
- have a plan of investigations
- explain to the patient that he has an anaemia and that

the symptoms of weight loss, poor appetite and tiredness are most likely to be related to this
- address any concerns that he, the carers and the GP may have
- arrange follow-up

3 Discussion related to the case

- The main problem is the macrocytic anaemia and the consultation needs to address finding a cause for this, i.e. megaloblastic vs. non-megaloblastic.
- This case tests the candidate's ability to assimilate a list of differential diagnoses from the information given by the GP and to take an appropriate history. Essentially, this patient describes an insidious illness manifesting with tiredness, loss of weight and appetite and with a sore mouth suggesting a glossitis; these point to a diagnosis of pernicious anaemia.
- Causes of macrocytic anaemia are megaloblastic (bone marrow contains erythroblasts with delayed nuclear maturation) such as vitamin B_{12} or folate deficiency, or non-megaloblastic, e.g. hypothyroidism, alcohol excess, liver disease, reticulocytosis or drug-induced. An MCV of over 110 fl is more suggestive of megaloblastic than non-megaloblastic anaemia. Pernicious anaemia is common in the elderly and is characterized by atrophy of the gastric mucosa with consequent failure of intrinsic factor production leading to vitamin B_{12} malabsorption.
- Investigations should include vitamin B_{12} and folate levels (values less than 100 ng/L and 4 μg/L, respectively, are highly suggestive of vitamin B_{12} and folate deficiencies, respectively), LFT looking for a raised bilirubin, parietal cell antibodies (present in 90% of patients) and intrinsic factor antibodies (found in 50% of patients but is specific for pernicious anaemia) and, if there are any doubts, a bone marrow examination. A Schilling test may be performed to delineate the cause of vitamin B_{12} deficiency, i.e. pernicious anaemia, or terminal ileal disease or bacterial overgrowth. Further small bowel investigations are only relevant if small bowel disease is suspected.

- Treatment of vitamin B_{12} deficiency is with hydroxo-cobalamin 1000 μg intramuscularly to a total of 5 mg over 3 weeks and then 1000 μg intramuscularly every 3 months for life. If any gastrointestinal symptoms persist then endoscopy should be considered as gastric carcinoma has twice the normal incidence in those with pernicious anaemia than in the normal population.

Comments on the case

This case tests the ability of the candidate to evaluate the results given in the letter. This is a typical case where the candidate must know the causes of a macrocytic anaemia. If not, the history taking will be insufficient to score points.

Case 31 | Neck lump

Candidate information

You are the SHO in a general medical clinic. Mr Abdul Hussein has been referred to you by his GP.

Please read this letter (it should take no more than 2 min) and then continue with the consultation.

Dear Doctor

Re: Mr Abdul Hussein, aged 41

Thank you for seeing Mr Hussein who presents with a firm nodule on the right side of his neck of 3 months' duration. He seems otherwise well and a recent chest X-ray was reported as normal. There is no tuberculosis in the family and he has no significant past medical history apart from *Plasmodium vivax* malaria 2 years ago. Please see and advise.

Yours sincerely

Dr G. Practitioner

You have 14 min until the patient leaves the room, followed by 1 min for reflection, before the discussion with the examiners. Be prepared to discuss the solutions to the problems posed by the case and how you might reply to the GP's letter.

Patient information

Mr Hussein is a 41-year-old Bangladeshi who came to the UK 4 years ago. Since then he has worked as a waiter but back in Bangladesh he was a shop assistant. The nodule was first noticed 3 months ago when he was washing. It is situated on the right side of the neck, is firm and has not changed in size. He thinks he has also felt another lump on the right side but towards the back of the neck. The lumps are not tender. There have been no symptoms of cough, sputum, haemoptysis, fever, malaise, pruritus, diarrhoea, weight loss or rash. He feels tired but puts this down to working late nights. There has been no recent history of a sore throat or tonsillitis. There is no family history of tuberculosis, including the family back in Bangladesh. He smokes up to 10 cigarettes a day, does not drink alcohol and lives with his wife and three children who are all fit and well.

Examiner information

1 Data gathering in the interview

A good candidate would be able to elicit:
- where the glands are and if he has noticed any other glands
- when the gland was first noticed and how
- if the gland is increasing or fluctuating in size
- if the gland is hard or soft, non-tender or tender
- if he has a history of tuberculosis or recurrent sore throat or tonsillitis
- any past history of head and neck cancer

- if there has been any recent family history of sore throats, viral illnesses or tuberculosis
- other associated symptoms of cough, sputum, haemoptysis, fever, fatigue, pruritus, malaise, diarrhoea, weight loss, rash or eye problems (sarcoidosis)
- occupational history and contacts at work
- family history and well-being of present family
- smoking history
- concerns of the patient

2 Identification and use of information gathered

The candidate should be able to interpret the history and create a problem list. The objectives for the candidate are to:

- develop a list of differential diagnoses (the most likely diagnosis in this case is tuberculous lymphadenitis)
- discuss the possibility of tuberculosis with the patient
- arrange investigations
- discuss the need for a fine-needle aspiration and, if a dry tap, excision biopsy for cytology and microscopy and culture for acid–alcohol fast bacilli (surgical referral)
- have an idea about the family members with regard to possible contact tracing if tuberculous lymphadenitis is confirmed
- reassure the patient that in the absence of an abnormal chest X-ray and respiratory symptoms the patient's chance of being infectious is very low

3 Discussion related to the case

- This case tests the candidate's ability to determine the probable cause of an enlarged lymph node. The possible diagnoses are: (a) tuberculous lymphadenitis — most likely in this case despite a normal chest X-ray; (b) metastatic lymph node from a head and neck neoplasm; (c) non-specific viral — doubtful in the absence of a sore throat and persistence of the nodule for 3 months — or infectious mononucleosis or CMV; (d) lymphoproliferative disorder — watch out for weight loss and fever; (e) sarcoidosis — watch out for eye and joint symptoms; and (f) HIV lymphadenopathy — a never-to-be-forgotten contender. Tuberculous lymphadenitis is a common presentation of *Mycobacteria*, particularly in patients from South Asia, and not necessarily associated with an abnormal chest X-ray. The patient may be feeling well but, despite this, full investigation including a fine needle or excision biopsy is imperative to make a firm diagnosis.
- Mantoux test may be considered but is not confirmatory and the investigation of choice is a biopsy looking for *Mycobacteria* bacilli and caseating granulomas. Commonly, the fine-needle aspirate is non-yielding and a complete excision biopsy by the surgeon is necessary. Tell the surgeon to send part of the node to microbiology in normal saline and not formalin; the histology sample can be sent in formalin. A raised ACE level in the presence of non-caseating granulomas would support sarcoidosis but the chest X-ray is commonly abnormal. An abnormal chest X-ray, such as hilar lymphadenopathy, with fever and loss of weight, may indicate a lymphoproliferative disorder.
- The candidate may be asked about the other presentations of tuberculosis, treatment of tuberculosis including the side-effects, multidrug resistance, length of treatment, contact tracing and prevention.

Comments on the case

This is a common case and tests the candidate's ability to make decisions. The node has been present for 3 months and hence a biopsy is warranted.

Case 32 | Painful shins

Candidate information

You are the SHO in a general medical clinic. Mrs Doreen Fredericks has been referred to you by her GP.

Please read this letter (it should take no more than 2 min) and then continue with the consultation.

Dear Doctor

Re: Mrs Doreen Fredericks, aged 43

Thank you for seeing Mrs Fredericks who has developed painful, red, raised lesions on her shins for the last 2 weeks and which have been accompanied by malaise. She is otherwise well although I treated her with a course of amoxicillin 1 month ago for a bout of bronchitis. She smokes 15 cigarettes a day.

Your sincerely

Dr G. Practitioner

You have 14 min until the patient leaves the room, followed by 1 min for reflection, before the discussion with the examiners. Be prepared to discuss the solutions to the problems posed by the case and how you might reply to the GP's letter.

Patient information

Mrs Fredericks is a 43-year-old healthcare assistant who works at a residential home. She has had painful, red, raised lesions on both shins for the last 2 weeks. She has felt unwell with malaise and has been off work for the last week. She does not have a fever, arthralgia, loss of weight, any eye complaints, sore throats, bowel symptoms or other skin rashes. One month ago, she had a bout of bronchitis manifesting as cough and purulent sputum for which she had a 7-day course of amoxicillin. She has had a persistent cough with occasional mucoid sputum for the last 6 months but her GP has suggested that this is most likely a result of her smoking; she smokes 15 cigarettes a day. She has an unremarkable past medical history and takes no medication apart from the oral contraceptive pill. She lives with her husband and two teenage children who are all well. She has not been abroad for over 15 years.

Examiner information

1 Data gathering in the interview
A good candidate would be able to elicit:
- the features of the skin lesions: site, shape, size, colour, raised or flat, painful or painless, any deterioration or improvement, relieving or aggravating factors
- other systemic symptoms, e.g. malaise, fever, arthralgia, loss of weight, cough, sputum, haemoptysis or gastrointestinal symptoms
- other symptoms particularly suggestive of sarcoidosis,

streptococcal infection, tuberculosis or inflammatory bowel disease
- the details of the recent bout of bronchitis
- any recent history suggestive of infection, e.g. fungal, atypical organisms
- the history of the recent course of antibiotics
- other drug history, especially the oral contraceptive pill
- any travel abroad and any exposure to atypical organisms and tropical infectious agents
- the impact of the painful skin lesions on her life and work
- the concerns of the patient

2 Identification and use of information gathered

The candidate should be able to interpret the history and create a problem list. The objectives for the candidate are to:
- confirm a history suggestive of erythema nodosum
- explore the possible aetiology from the history
- explain the possible diagnosis to the patient
- detail the investigations to be carried out

3 Discussion related to the case

- Erythema nodosum presents as painful, tender, dusky blue-red nodules, commonly over the lower limbs or shins which may fade over a couple of weeks leaving a bruised appearance. It is common in young adults, particularly females, and can be associated with arthralgia, malaise and fever. Inflammation occurs in the dermis and the subcutaneous layer (panniculitis).
- Streptococcal infections and sarcoidosis (accompanied with bilateral hilar lymphadenopathy) are the most common causes in adults. In children, erythema nodosum is most commonly caused by upper respiratory tract infections, especially from streptococci. Less common causes, except in endemic areas, include tuberculosis, mycoplasma, leprosy, coccidioidomycosis, histoplasmosis, psittacosis, lymphogranuloma venereum and ulcerative colitis. The condition can also be a reaction to drugs (sulphonamides, iodides, bromides, oral contraceptives). In some cases, no cause may be found.
- Investigations should include a chest X-ray, erythrocyte sedimentation rate (ESR), ACE level, throat swab if streptococcal sore throat is suspected and a search for an infective organism, e.g. mycoplasma serology, sputum for *Mycobacterium*.
- Treatment is symptomatic, with NSAIDs and bedrest. Oral steroids are sometimes necessary and stopping the oral contraceptive pill may need to be considered in this case.

Comments on the case

This case tests the candidate's ability to develop a list of differential diagnoses and to tailor the history towards finding a cause for her symptoms. The history of the cough must be detailed to determine if the patient is describing possible sarcoidosis or tuberculosis. It is possible that no cause will be found.

Case 33 | **Painful shoulders**

Candidate information

You are the SHO in the general medical clinic. Mr Alfred Swindon has been referred to you by his GP.

Please read this letter (it should take no more than 2 min) and then continue with the consultation.

Dear Doctor

Re: Mr Alfred Swindon, aged 71

Thank you for seeing Mr Swindon who has been suffering for the last 4 weeks with painful shoulders and a stiff neck. I have treated him with diclofenac but with no success. I am worried that he may have cervical myelopathy. Please see and advise.

Your sincerely

Dr G. Practitioner

You have 14 min until the patient leaves the room, followed by 1 min for reflection, before the discussion with the examiners. Be prepared to discuss the solutions to the problems posed by the case and how you might reply to the GP's letter.

Patient information

Mr Alfred Swindon is a 71-year-old retired shopkeeper who has been suffering from painful, stiff shoulders and neck for the last 4 weeks. These symptoms appeared suddenly and are worse in the mornings, lasting up to 2–3 h. He does not have any stiffness or pain in the lumbar spine or hips. Other associated features include tiredness, fever, weight loss and a feeling of low mood. He does not have any weakness of his limbs and no restriction of head movements once the stiffness of the neck is relieved. He is otherwise well and has no respiratory, cardiovascular or gastrointestinal symptoms. He does not have any other neurological symptoms such as dizziness, blurred vision, tinnitus, headache, scalp tenderness, claudication of the jaw or tender temporal or occipital arteries. He is on no medication and used to smoke 10 cigarettes a day up to 30 years ago. He has an occasional glass of wine in the evenings and lives with his wife.

Examiner information

1 Data gathering in the interview

A good candidate would be able to elicit:
- the history of the painful, stiff shoulders and neck (suggesting polymyalgia rheumatica) including time of onset, the limbs affected, any variation of severity during the day, the duration of symptoms and any proximal muscle weakness (polymyositis if proximal pain is present or myopathy if pain and stiffness are absent)
- any associated systemic features, e.g. tiredness, fever, weight loss or depression
- any suggestion of giant cell arteritis, e.g. painless loss of

vision, severe headache, tenderness of the scalp, jaw claudication when eating, tenderness over the temporal and/or occipital arteries
- any other neurological symptoms
- symptoms suggestive of rheumatoid arthritis, e.g. symmetrical arthropathy in both hands, etc.
- any symptoms suggestive of cervical myelopathy, e.g. head movement restriction, pain along the distribution of the dermatomes in the arms, wasting of the small muscles of the hand
- symptoms suggestive of hypothyroidism
- past medical history
- drug history
- the impact of the illness on the patient

2 Identification and use of information gathered

The candidate should be able to interpret the history and create a problem list. The objectives for the candidate are to:
- identify the symptoms clearly and to differentiate the three main possibilities: polymyalgia rheumatica, polymyositis and myopathy
- detail a list of investigations
- explain the possible cause for his symptoms and outline a management plan

3 Discussion related to the case

- The prevalence, aetiology and pathogenesis of polymyalgia rheumatica (PMR) are unknown. In some patients the disorder is a manifestation of underlying temporal arteritis. Most patients are not at any significant risk from the complications of temporal arteritis but should be warned of the possibility and should immediately report such symptoms as headache, visual disturbance and jaw pain on chewing. PMR usually occurs in patients over 60 years old and the female : male ratio is 2 : 1.
- Onset may be acute or subacute. PMR is characterized by severe pain and stiffness of the neck, pectoral and pelvic girdles, morning stiffness, stiffness after inactivity and systemic complaints such as malaise, fever, depression and weight loss (cachectic PMR may mimic cancer). There is no selective muscle weakness

or evidence of muscle disease on electromyography (EMG) or biopsy. A normochromic normocytic anaemia may be present. In most patients, the ESR is dramatically elevated, often >100 mm/h. C-reactive protein levels are usually elevated and may be a more sensitive marker of disease activity in certain patients.
- PMR is distinguished from rheumatoid arthritis by the usual absence of small joint synovitis (although some joint swelling may be present), erosive or destructive disease, rheumatoid factor or rheumatoid nodules. PMR is differentiated from polymyositis by finding normal muscle enzymes, EMG and muscle biopsy and by the prominence of pain over weakness. Hypothyroidism can present as myalgia with abnormal thyroid function tests and an elevated creatine kinase. PMR is differentiated from myeloma by the absence of a monoclonal gammopathy and from fibromyalgia by the systemic features and the elevated ESR.
- Corticosteroids produce a reduction in the symptoms within 48 h of starting treatment. This should reduce the risk of developing giant cell arteritis. NSAIDs are less effective and should be avoided. PMR usually responds dramatically to prednisolone initiated at around 15 mg o.d. If temporal arteritis is suspected, treatment should be started immediately with 60 mg o.d. to prevent blindness. As the symptoms subside, corticosteroids are tapered to the lowest effective dose, regardless of the ESR. Some patients are able to discontinue corticosteroids within 2 years whereas others require small amounts for years. Prevention of corticosteroid-induced bone loss using bisphosphonates should also be considered.

Comments on the case

This case tests the candidate's ability to clearly ascertain the history of painful, stiff shoulders and to differentiate the diagnosis of polymyalgia rheumatica from polymyositis and myopathy. The GP wondered if the patient had cervical myelopathy but the candidate should be able to rule this out by taking a comprehensive history.

Case 34 | Palpitations

Candidate information

You are the SHO in a cardiology clinic. Mr Colin Jeffreys has been referred to you by his GP.

Please read this letter (it should take no more than 2 min) and then continue with the consultation.

Dear Doctor

Re: Mr Colin Jeffreys, aged 78

Thank you for seeing Mr Jeffreys who is normally a fit and healthy man. However, he had an attack of palpitations and dizziness while on the golf course 2 weeks ago. I would be grateful if you could rule out any serious cardiac disease. He takes salbutamol for mild, late-onset asthma. He also had a transient ischaemic attack 5 years ago and he takes aspirin for this. He was in sinus rhythm today and his BP was 130/68 mmHg. His recent FBC, U/E and TFT were all normal. Please see and advise.

Yours sincerely

Dr G. Practitioner

You have 14 min until the patient leaves the room, followed by 1 min for reflection, before the discussion with the examiners. Be prepared to discuss the solutions to the problems posed by the case and how you might reply to the GP's letter.

Patient information

Mr Colin Jeffreys is a 78-year-old retired city councillor who had one episode of palpitations 2 weeks ago when teeing off at the local golf course. The palpitations came on suddenly, lasted for around 5 min and then abruptly disappeared. He remembers that the palpitations were rapid and regular with no missed beats, and there was a feeling of heaviness in his chest, with dyspnoea and faintness and he felt extremely ill. Once back home he felt exhausted for the rest of the day. He visited the GP the next day at which point the referral to the cardiology clinic was made. Currently he feels fine, with no obvious irregular heartbeats. He has had no more chest pain, dyspnoea or any symptoms of hyperthyroidism (such as anxiety, tremor, loss of weight or increased appetite). There were no previous episodes of palpitations or chest pains and he has no symptoms suggestive of an anxiety–depressive neurosis. His asthma is stable with no nocturnal symptoms and he only uses his salbutamol inhaler once a day (he does not have a tremor or any other side-effects from the inhaler). He does not take any other inhalers such as long-acting beta-2 agonists. He had a transient ischaemic attack 5 years ago which presented as weakness of his right hand but this subsided after 1 h. He had no palpitations then. He was started on aspirin and has had no similar events since. There is no past history of ischaemic heart disease, hypertension, diabetes mellitus or hypercholesterolaemia. He stopped smoking 23 years ago, when he used to smoke 10 cigarettes a day. He has a glass of sherry in the evenings but no more. He does not drink tea or coffee and takes no other drugs. He lives alone in a three-bedroomed house and has no family. His main concerns are that his GP has told him to stop playing golf until investigations have revealed a cause for his recent illness.

Examiner information

1 Data gathering in the interview
A good candidate would be able to elicit:
- how long ago the palpitations occurred and what the patient was doing at the time
- any previous history of palpitations
- if they started and stopped abruptly (supraventricular tachycardia) and how long they lasted for
- how fast did the heart race — ask the patient to tap it out on the desk
- did the patient take his own pulse at the time of the palpitation? If so, how fast was the pulse rate and was the pulse regular or irregular. If the patient did not take his own pulse, did he feel any thumping in his chest. If so, how fast and how regular was the thumping. Was there a missed beat and, if so, did the next one feel heavier
- whether he currently has any palpitations or irregular heartbeats
- any other associated symptoms, such as chest pain, dyspnoea, faintness, anxiety, tremor, recent loss of weight or increased appetite (hyperthyroidism)
- drug history, e.g. sympathomimetics or salbutamol tablets. How often does he use the salbutamol inhaler? Does he also use a beta-2 long-acting agonist inhaler?
- details of alcohol, caffeine (often an increased consumption initiates an attack) and tobacco consumption. Has he taken other illicit drugs or herbal remedies
- details of the TIA. Did he have a rhythm problem (e.g. atrial fibrillation) at that time
- any previous history of heart disease, hypertension, thyroid disorders
- any symptoms of anxiety and depressive disorders
- address any concerns that the patient may have

2 Identification and use of information gathered
The candidate should be able to interpret the history and create a problem list. The objectives for the candidate are to:
- explain the possible differential diagnoses
- arrange a set of investigations

- assure him that all tests will be carried out as soon as possible

3 Discussion related to the case
- This case tests the ability of the candidate to: (a) decide if the palpitations are related to ischaemic heart disease or resulting from a non-cardiac cause (other causes of palpitations in the clinic situation, particularly in young people, are caffeine/tobacco-induced, anxiety disorder and, occasionally, thyrotoxicosis); and (b) decide if the palpitations were regular (supraventricular tachycardia, SVT, atrial fibrillation, AF 2 : 1 block) or irregular (AF, variable block).
- The most likely cause of the palpitations in this case is related to ischaemic heart disease and sinoatrial disease and investigations would be tailored towards this (GP has said TFTs are normal). This would include glucose, cholesterol, resting ECG, chest X-ray, echocardiogram and a 24-h ECG.
- The examiners will expect the candidate to be able to discuss: (a) the management of paroxysmal atrial fibrillation including issues of anticoagulation; and (b) the acute management of narrow complex and broad complex dysrhythmias.

Comments on the case

This is a typical case where the patient is currently asymptomatic and the emphasis is on taking a detailed history to work out exactly what rhythm the palpitations characterize — a 24-h ECG will probably show *'sinus rhythm with a few ventricular ectopics'*.
Tapping out the palpitations is a good way of determining rate, rhythm and mode of onset and offset. Do not expect the patient to have measured his own pulse when he felt ill.

Case 35 | **Personality change**

Candidate information

You are the medical SHO in a liver clinic. Mr Matthew Hayward has been referred to you by his GP. He is accompanied by his wife.

Please read this letter (it should take no more than 2 min) and then continue with the consultation.

Dear Doctor

Re: Mr Matthew Hayward, aged 42

Thank you for seeing Mr Hayward earlier than usual. You see him regularly for Wilson's disease of the liver. Over the last 4 weeks he has been irritable with bouts of anger directed towards his wife for no obvious reason together with odd sleeping patterns. Compared to the previous investigations, his liver function tests, clotting indices and the albumin levels have deteriorated. Please see and advise.

Yours sincerely

Dr G. Practitioner

You have 14 min until the patient leaves the room, followed by 1 min for reflection, before the discussion with the examiners. Be prepared to discuss the solutions to the problems posed by the case and how you might reply to the GP's letter.

Patient information

Mr Hayward, a 42-year-old unemployed man, first presented 7 years ago with a tremor and abnormal liver function tests. Further investigations confirmed Wilson's disease and slit lamp examination of the eyes showed Kayser–Fleischer rings. Since then he has been reasonably well although his tremor has persisted. He was initially started on penicillamine but developed a rash and fever and was switched over to trientine. Over the last 4 weeks his wife has noticed him to be more irritable, with poor concentration, confusion, bursts of temper and sleeping during the day but not at night. These symptoms are variable with good and bad days. She has not noticed him to be obviously jaundiced but he has been complaining of tiredness and nausea with a poor appetite. There have been no convulsions, loss of weight, constipation, or any obvious abdominal swelling suggestive of ascites and no gastrointestinal bleeding. His diet has not changed, although he is probably not eating as much, nor is he on any other medication. There is no history of taking benzodiazepines or any illicit drugs which may cause hepatic damage. He does drink alcohol, usually about 6 pints of beer during the week but there has been no sudden increase in alcohol consumption. His compliance to trientine has been patchy as a result of occasional drug-induced nausea. He does not smoke and has not been abroad recently.

There are no other risk factors for concomitant viral hepatitic infections. Mrs Hayward is particularly concerned about the personality changes as his current behaviour is certainly out of character.

Examiner information

1 Data gathering in the interview

A good candidate would be able to elicit:

- the history of the Wilson's disease: presentation (neurological, hepatic and eye), diagnosis (serum and urinary copper with caeruloplasmin and liver biopsy), treatment, treatment changes, side-effects to treatment
- present history of behavioural and psychiatric changes and the effect of this on his wife, e.g. personality, mood, tempers, sleep pattern, poor concentration, irritation, confusion, disorientation, slurred speech, self care
- other liver disease symptoms, e.g. jaundice, ascites, ankle swelling, bruising, itching, urine changes, weight loss, convulsions, nausea and vomiting
- factors suggesting reasons for possible precipitation of portosystemic encephalopathy, e.g. high protein diet/poor nutrition, gastrointestinal haemorrhages, alcohol, constipation, infection (peritonitis), drug-induced (e.g. benzodiazepines or illicit drugs), development of hepatocellular carcinoma, or worsening cirrhosis. Other causes include electrolyte imbalance, e.g. hypokalaemia or hyponatraemia (?diuretic usage)
- any suggestions of additional hepatic disease to the Wilson's disease, e.g. viral hepatitis
- poor compliance to medication and, if so, why
- social and psychological impact on the family

2 Identification and use of information gathered

The candidate should be able to interpret the history and create a problem list. The objectives for the candidate are to:

- obtain a history of the Wilson's disease
- obtain a history of the present symptoms suggestive of portosystemic encephalopathy
- determine possible triggers for the encephalopathy, especially poor drug compliance
- provide a plan of investigations and management, including admission to hospital
- explain the possible causes for the deterioration

3 Discussion related to the case

- Portosystemic encephalopathy refers to a chronic neuropsychiatric syndrome secondary to liver cirrhosis presenting as a fluctuating disorder of personality, intellect, mood and reversal of normal sleep pattern. Other features include nausea, vomiting and weakness. The most important factors in the pathogenesis are severe hepatocellular dysfunction and/or intra- and extrahepatic shunting of portal venous blood into the systemic circulation so that the liver is largely bypassed. As a result of these processes, various toxic substances absorbed from the intestine are not detoxified by the liver and lead to metabolic abnormalities in the central nervous system (CNS).
- Factors precipitating portosystemic encephalopathy include those mentioned above. Signs include a coarse flapping tremor, constructional apraxia and decreased mental function. Investigations include routine biochemistry, clotting and haematology and an EEG which will show triphasic slow waves.
- A number of conditions can mimic the clinical features of hepatic encephalopathy. These include acute alcohol intoxication, sedative overdose, delirium tremens, Wernicke's encephalopathy, Korsakoff's psychosis, subdural haematoma, meningitis and hypoglycaemia. Other metabolic encephalopathies must also be considered, especially in patients with alcoholic cirrhosis.
- Basic management includes identification and removal of the precipitant, protein restriction and intestinal purgation with lactulose (aiming for increased frequency of motions, at least four a day).
- The neurological manifestations of Wilson's disease include both resting and intention tremors, spasticity, rigidity, chorea, drooling, dysphagia and dysarthria. Psychiatric disturbances are present in most patients with neurological symptoms. Schizophrenia, manic-depressive psychoses and the classic neuroses may occur, but the most common disturbances are bizarre behavioural patterns that defy classification. Improvement in the psychiatric state can occur with pharmacological reduction of the copper excess, but psychotherapy may be required.
- Treatment of Wilson's disease consists of removing and detoxifying the deposits of copper as rapidly as possible and must be instituted once the diagnosis is secure, whether the patient is ill or asymptomatic. Penicillamine is administered orally in an initial

dosage of 1 g daily in single or divided doses at least 30 min before and 2 h after eating (maintenance dosage). Because penicillamine has an antipyridoxine effect, 25 mg/day of pyridoxine is also given. Sensitivity to penicillamine develops early in nearly 10% of patients. White blood cell and platelet counts should be assessed and urinalysis performed several times during the first month of treatment. Penicillamine should be discontinued and replaced by trientine if rash, fever, leucopenia, thrombocytopenia, lymphadenopathy or proteinuria develops or if neurological worsening accompanies the institution of penicillamine and persists for a week or more. Treatment must be continued for life. Trientine is not recommended as long-term therapy. It is possible to restart penicillamine after a period of cessation. The symptoms may not recur if oral prednisolone is given before restarting penicillamine. Inadequate treatment, or interruption of therapy, can be fatal or cause irreversible relapse. Zinc acetate is a useful adjunct for maintenance therapy of Wilson's disease. Because zinc is essentially non-toxic and the other two agents do have toxic side-effects, zinc may indeed turn out to become the preferred maintenance therapy for Wilson's disease. It must not be given with penicillamine or trientine as both these agents chelate zinc. The beneficial effect of zinc results from it blocking the intestinal absorption of copper. It accomplishes this by inducing intestinal cell metallothionein, which binds copper and prevents its transfer into the blood. As intestinal cells slough the copper contained in these cells is eliminated in the stool. Thus, the end result is reduced intestinal absorption of copper.

Comments on the case

This case tests the ability of the candidate to establish the diagnosis of porto-systemic encephalopathy and to detect a precipitant for it. In this case compliance to taking drugs is an important factor.

Case 36 | Pins and needles

Candidate information

You are the SHO in a neurology clinic. Mr Leonard Willis has been referred to you by his GP.

Please read this letter (it should take no more than 2 min) and then continue with the consultation.

Dear Doctor

Re: Mr Leonard Willis, aged 64

Thank you for seeing Mr Willis who still works part-time as a gardener. He gives a 2-month history of pins and needles in both hands. He has a past history of hypercholesterolaemia for which he takes simvastatin 20 mg a day. His last cholesterol level was 4. 8 mmol/L. Other previous history includes an inguinal hernia repair 14 years ago. He also takes aspirin 75 mg o.d. His BM glucose in the practice was 5.0.

Yours sincerely

Dr G. Practitioner

You have 14 min until the patient leaves the room, followed by 1 min for reflection, before the discussion with the examiners. Be prepared to discuss the solutions to the problems posed by the case and how you might reply to the GP's letter.

Patient information

Mr Willis is a 64-year-old part-time gardener who has been complaining for the last 2 months of pins and needles with pain, tingling and numbness in both hands. He is right-handed and the pain first appeared in that hand which was soon followed by pain in the left hand. The symptoms are worse particularly in the thumb, index and middle finger but it does sometimes affect the whole hand. The symptoms are now occurring at night time causing sleep disruption. Shaking the hands sometimes helps, but in the mornings his hands feel clumsy and swollen although later in the day the symptoms are better. He does not have similar symptoms in the feet or arms nor does he complain of any burning sensation in the feet. There are no other neurological symptoms such as weakness in the limbs, tremor, headache, blurred vision, muscle wasting, dysphasia or dysphagia. He has no other respiratory, cardiovascular or abdominal symptoms. His past history includes hypercholesterolaemia (cholesterol 8.0 mmol/L) for which he takes simvastatin 20 mg o.d. and an inguinal hernia repair 14 years ago. The latest cholesterol measurement last year was 4.8 mmol/L. He has no history of ischaemic heart disease, cerebrovascular disease, peripheral vascular disease, diabetes mellitus, trauma or renal disease. He has never smoked and only drinks one bottle of beer a day at home. He has a normal diet and does not take any medication except for aspirin and simvastatin. He works with another gardener, usually doing weekly contract jobs. He noticed that during one job last week, where he had to use a stone cutter to take down an old coal shed, his symptoms immediately returned and persisted for much longer during that day and night. He has not suffered from any cuts or injuries to his hands during his work. He lives with his wife and his main concerns are that his job is being affected by the symptoms.

Examiner information

1 Data gathering in the interview

A good candidate would be able to elicit:

- the duration of the symptoms and whether they are deteriorating
- if the patient is left- or right-handed
- which hand had the symptoms first and which part of the hand is affected, including which fingers. Are the feet also affected
- what are the exact symptoms, e.g. pain, burning sensation, numbness, weakness, clumsiness, feeling of heaviness or tingling
- other neurological symptoms, especially weakness, paraesthesia, tremor or muscle wasting
- other cardiovascular, respiratory and abdominal symptoms, looking for the possibility of cancer, vascular disease or diabetes mellitus
- any previous trauma
- full drug history, including enquiry about drugs which may cause peripheral neuropathy, especially isoniazid and nitrofurantoin
- full alcohol history
- dietary history (vitamin B_1, B_6 and B_{12} deficiencies)
- metabolic history, especially osmotic symptoms suggestive of diabetes mellitus, renal failure, thyrotoxicosis
- positive hereditary history of neuropathies, such as hereditary motor and sensory neuropathy
- causes of carpal tunnel syndrome, e.g. obesity, arthritis, previous fractures of wrists, repetitive strain injury, e.g. vibrating tools (stone cutter), hypothyroidism, acromegaly, pregnancy
- address any concerns that the patient has

2 Identification and use of information gathered

The candidate should be able to interpret the history and create a problem list. The objectives for the candidate are to:

- assimilate a list of differential diagnoses
- explain these diagnoses to the patient
- have a plan of investigations
- arrange follow-up to discuss the investigations

3 Discussion related to the case

- This case tests the ability of the candidate to differentiate carpal tunnel syndrome from peripheral neuropathy and explore the possible underlying cause.
- The case presents with the typical features of carpal tunnel syndrome which tend to affect mainly the dominant hand. In this case the vibrating tool exacerbated the symptoms. For diagnosis and confirmation, nerve conduction studies should be performed which will show a reduced or absent median sensory nerve action potential (SNAP) from the index finger and prolongation of the latency. EMG may show denervation of the abductor pollicis brevis.
- Treatment may include night time splints, local steroid injections (temporary relief) and, if necessary, surgical decompression.
- The examiners would expect the candidate to be able to discuss the differential diagnoses for a peripheral neuropathy.

Comments on the case

This case again demonstrates the importance of taking a detailed history in order to provide the probable diagnosis and distinguish this entrapment neuropathy from a peripheral neuropathy.

Case 37 | Polyuria

Candidate information

You are the SHO in a general medical clinic. Mrs Janet Abrahams has been referred to you by her GP.

Please read this letter (it should take no more than 2 min) and then continue with the consultation.

Dear Doctor

Re: Mrs Janet Abrahams, aged 42

Mrs Abrahams gives a 2-week history of polyuria, feeling unwell and being generally tired. Four months ago she had a bout of 'flu followed by acute bronchitis. The cough has persisted despite three courses of antibiotics. Her recent blood glucose test performed at the clinic was 5.8. A chest X-ray is reported as showing 'numerous pulmonary infiltrates and bilateral hilar lymphadenopathy. Please refer to a physician.' Please see and advise.

Yours sincerely

Dr G. Practitioner

You have 14 min until the patient leaves the room, followed by 1 min for reflection, before the discussion with the examiners. Be prepared to discuss the solutions to the problems posed by the case and how you might reply to the GP's letter.

Patient information

Mrs Janet Abrahams is a 42-year-old accountant who presents with a 2-week history of polyuria and thirst. The symptoms came on suddenly over 2 days and she now passes copious amounts of urine daily (volume exceeds 4 L), including during the night. She says she has to pass urine about every 15 min and it is very dilute. In response to this she is having to drink an equivalent amount of liquid (especially cold fluids) during the day. Associated with this is a cough which first presented 4 months ago after a bout of 'flu. Despite three courses of antibiotics, the cough persists and is non-productive with no wheeze, sputum or haemoptysis. She feels tired with generalized aches in her body. She has no chest pains, feelings of faintness, palpitations, gastrointestinal, arthritic or eye symptoms. She has not noticed a change in her periods, or her weight. The past medical history includes an appendicectomy when she was 6 years old but no recent head trauma or neurosurgery. Currently, she takes no medication and she finished her last course of antibiotics 6 weeks ago. She has never taken corticosteroids. She does not smoke or drink alcohol. She has no psychiatric history. There is no family history of note, such as diabetes mellitus or asthma. She lives with her husband and two children who are all well. She has now stopped working as it was impossible to do her work with the polydipsia and polyuria. She is obviously concerned about her symptoms.

Examiner information

1 Data gathering in the interview

A good candidate would be able to elicit:

- a chronological history of the events
- the polyuria and polydipsia; the onset, volume of urine passed, frequency of micturition (day and night) and volume of fluid intake (type of fluids, e.g. cold drinks), colour of urine
- appetite, weight, cough history (dry or with sputum and/or haemoptysis, worse in the mornings with wheeze), any associated heartburn and sinusitis. Precipitating factors such as common household allergens
- other general symptoms which may suggest a cause for the polyuria: diabetes mellitus (osmotic); cranial diabetes insipidus; tumours (primary craniopharyngioma, ependymoma, hypothalamic pituitary glioma, lung and breast metastases); infections (tuberculosis, meningitis, cerebral abscess); infiltrations (sarcoidosis, Langerhan's cell histiocytosis); postsurgical (transfrontal or transphenoidal); postradiotherapy; vascular (haemorrhage or thrombosis, aneurysm) or head trauma; nephrogenic diabetes insipidus, e.g. drug-induced (lithium, glibenclamide), metabolic (hypokalaemia, hypercalcaemia), familial; renal tubular acidosis
- symptoms suggestive of pituitary dysfunction, e.g. galactorrhoea, amenorrhoea, hypogonadism, visual field defects, hypothyroidism, hypoadrenalism
- psychiatric history (compulsive water drinking)
- full drug history
- relevant past history, e.g. head trauma, head neurosurgery
- smoking and alcohol history
- impact of symptoms on family and work
- the concerns of the patient

2 Identification and use of information gathered

The candidate should be able to interpret the history and create a problem list. The objectives for the candidate are to:

- have a complete list of possible differential diagnoses
- explain the chest X-ray findings and to suggest the possibility of sarcoidosis as the cause for the patient's symptoms
- explain what sarcoidosis is
- explain the need to admit for further investigations
- explain the investigations in detail

3 Discussion related to the case

- This case tests the ability of the candidate to explore the possible causes of polyuria and polydipsia. The differential diagnoses are stated above. The most likely cause is sarcoidosis either through its pituitary infiltration or due to the associated hypercalcaemia.
- Initial investigations are biochemistry including osmolalities of blood and urine, serum calcium, ACE, MRI scan of the head and bronchoscopy with a transbronchial biopsy to confirm a tissue diagnosis of non-caseating granuloma. In this case there is no need to carry out water-restricting investigations.
- The diagnosis of cranial diabetes insipidus may be made on early morning paired plasma and urine osmolalities but if these are normal a water deprivation test will need to be undertaken. The principle of this test is to withhold fluids while monitoring plasma and urinary osmolalities. If the patient loses more than 3% of the total body weight on hourly measurements during the test and the serum osmolality is >300 mOsm/kg it should be stopped and a dose of desmopressin given and the patient allowed to drink. Otherwise, monitoring is continued by plasma and urinary osmolalities for 8 h, then desmopressin is given and the patient allowed to drink. A normal response is for the plasma osmolality to remain within the normal range (280–295 mOsm/kg) and the urine:plasma (U:P) osmolality ratio to rise to >2.0.
- In pituitary diabetes insipidus the urine osmolality fails to rise appropriately and the urine volume remains inappropriately high in spite of a rising plasma osmolality. Plasma osmolality rises to >295 mOsm/kg and the U:P ratio remains <2.0 with urine concentration increasing normally after administration of desmopressin.
- Treatment should include the intranasal synthetic vasopressin analogue desmopressin (DDVAP) 10–20 µg o.d. or b.d. or orally 100–200 µg t.d.s. The patient should start on high dose corticosteroids, e.g. prednisolone 40 mg o.d. for the sarcoidosis and tailed down slowly. She should be offered bisphosphonates as well because of the long-term steroids.

Comments on the case

This case highlights the importance of the information given by the GP to enable the candidate to direct the history taking and establish the precise cause of polyuria and polydipsia.

Case 38 | Pruritus

Candidate information

You are the SHO in a general medical outpatient clinic. Mrs Shirley Baxter has been referred to you by her GP.

Please read this letter (it should take no more than 2 min) and then continue with the consultation.

Dear Doctor

Re: Mrs Shirley Baxter, aged 52

Thank you for seeing Mrs Baxter who has been complaining of generalized pruritus and increasing fatigue for the last 6 months. I have tried her with lubricant bath oils, initially with some soothing effect, but now her itch is worse and keeps her awake at night. She is normally fit and well and I enclose the following routine blood results. She takes no regular medication. Please see and advise.

Haemoglobin 11.3 g/dL, white cell count 6.8×10^9/L, platelets 354×10^9/L, sodium 139 mmol/L, potassium 4.1 mmol/L, urea 3.9 mmol/L, creatinine 74 mmol/L, bilirubin 12 µmol/L, alanine transaminase (ALT) 29 U/L, alkaline phosphatase 290 U/L, albumin 39 g/L, glucose 5.1 mmol/L.

Yours sincerely

Dr G. Practitioner

You have 14 min until the patient leaves the room, followed by 1 min for reflection, before the discussion with the examiners. Be prepared to discuss the solutions to the problems posed by the case and how you might reply to the GP's letter.

Patient information

Mrs Baxter is a 52-year-old school secretary who has been normally fit and well without any time off work for ill-health. However, over the last 6 months she has been complaining of a persistent generalized pruritus. She has tried various bath oils with some initial soothing effect but the itch has now worsened. She finds that the pruritus keeps her awake at night and she has scratched herself to such an extent that her skin is raw and bleeding. Associated with this is a recent feeling of generalized tiredness and she is finding it hard to concentrate at work. There are no other symptoms of loss of weight or appetite, or of cardiovascular, pulmonary or gastrointestinal origin including jaundice, bowel habit alteration, haematemesis or *per rectum* (PR) bleeding or any thyroid or neurological symptoms. No rashes have been seen and her skin looks quite normal except for the scratch marks. There has been no occupational exposure to fibreglass or to pruritus-provoking recreational or domestic agents. The past medical history includes a Colles' fracture when she was 8 years old. She does not suffer from anxiety or depression. She takes only paracetamol for occasional headaches and no herbal remedies. She lives with her husband and has three grown-up children. Her husband is well with no similar itching. She has not been in close contact with anyone else. She does not smoke and only drinks three glasses of wine per week. Her main concerns are about the possible cause for the pruritus and her poor sleeping.

Examiner information

1 Data gathering in the interview

A good candidate would be able to elicit:
- the timing of the pruritus, and whether this is persistent or intermittent, improving or deteriorating, and the extent and severity of her scratching
- which part of her body has the pruritus, which part of her body started first and whether her eyes itch
- any relieving factors (e.g. bath oils) or provoking factors (e.g. stress, depression, drugs, certain foods)
- whether the pruritus affects sleep and work
- whether there are any associated skin rashes, pruritus ani and/or vulvae
- living conditions and contact history, e.g. anyone with scabies
- occupational exposure, e.g. fibreglass
- systemic symptoms, e.g. tiredness, jaundice (primary biliary cirrhosis, haemochromatosis), fever, weight loss (malignancy, especially lymphoma), osmotic symptoms (diabetes mellitus), thyroid symptoms (hypo or hyper), history of chronic renal failure, history of HIV
- drug history, including herbal remedies
- any new recreational and domestic agents, e.g. skin creams, biological washing powders
- psychiatric illness, especially anxiety and depression
- alcohol and smoking history
- impact of the pruritus on her and her family

2 Identification and use of information gathered

The candidate should be able to interpret the history and create a problem list. The objectives for the candidate are to:
- develop a list of differential diagnoses
- explain the possibilities to the patient
- show that one blood test was slightly abnormal (alkaline phosphatase) and to explain that one cause could be related to the liver
- plan and explain the investigations to be arranged, particularly concentrating on primary biliary cirrhosis

- address the problem of the pruritus with general advice such as avoiding soaps but to tell her that follow-up will be arranged soon with results of further tests

3 Discussion related to the case

- This case tests the ability of the candidate to work out the possible systemic causes of pruritus. The raised alkaline phosphatase possibly suggests primary biliary cirrhosis which can present with pruritis before the appearance of any jaundice. Other possibilities include diabetes mellitus, hypo- or hyperthyroidism, chronic renal failure, haemochromatosis, polycythaemia, HIV infection or internal malignancy such as a lymphoma. However, topical causes (e.g. washing-up liquid, drug-induced) and psychological histories are still very important.
- Other tests not performed as yet include thyroid function, lipids, iron studies, autoantibody screen (mitochondrial M2). If autoantibodies are positive then the next step would be an ultrasound of the liver and a liver biopsy.
- The candidate would be expected to discuss the management of pruritus (usually difficult) using cholestyramine (4 g sachet t.d.s.) and ursodeoxycholate (10–15 mg/kg/day in 2–4 divided doses) in improving liver enzymes and pruritus, the prognosis and the role of liver transplantation.

Comments on the case

This case also tests the candidate's ability to read the GP's letter carefully. The finding of an abnormal alkaline phosphatase level should enable the candidate to structure his or her history taking without forgetting the possibilities of other systemic medical and topical causes. The candidate must not forget to ask about other recreational and domestic skin contacts.

Case 39 | Purpuric rash

Candidate information

You are the SHO in a haematology clinic. Mrs Christine Bunch has been referred to you by her GP for an urgent assessment.

Please read this letter (it should take no more than 2 min) and then continue with the consultation.

Dear Doctor

Re: Mrs Christine Bunch, aged 36

Thank you for seeing urgently this lady who has presented with a 4-day history of a purpuric rash. I cannot detect any obvious bleeding. Her FBC is as follows: haemoglobin 11.1 g/dL, white cell count 8.4×10^9/L, neutrophils 6.7×10^9/L and platelets 20×10^9/L. She is normally fit and well and takes no medication. Please see and advise.

Yours sincerely

Dr G. Practitioner

You have 14 min until the patient leaves the room, followed by 1 min for reflection, before the discussion with the examiners. Be prepared to discuss the solutions to the problems posed by the case and how you might reply to the GP's letter.

Patient information

Mrs Christine Bunch is normally a fit and well 36-year-old lady who works in a florist shop and presents with a 4-day history of a gradual onset of a purpuric, non-blanching rash which started in both hands but now covers both arms and legs. The purpuric spots are flat, bright red, well circumscribed and vary in size with larger lesions seen particularly on the arms. She feels generally quite well although she has always had a tendency to bruise easily. There is no associated epistaxis, bleeding gums, haematuria, lymphadenopathy, fever, weight loss, abdominal pain, arthritic pain or vaginal bleeding. Her last menstrual period (LMP) was 2 weeks ago and her periods do tend to be heavy. There is no recent history of a viral illness or any previous history of purpuric rashes, lymphoproliferative disorders or coagulopathies. She has not taken any medication such as anticoagulants, steroids or antibiotics. Her diet is satisfactory, with fresh fruit and vegetables and there has been no recent history of trauma or blood transfusions. She has no HIV risk factors and lives with her husband and one son who are both well. She does not smoke or drink. She is obviously concerned about the rash.

Examiner information

1 Data gathering in the interview

A good candidate would be able to elicit:

- how long the purpura has been present for and if it has occurred before
- the distribution of the rash
- a description: size, shape, colour, circumscribed, raised, itchy, blanching
- associated symptoms, such as epistaxis, bleeding gums, haematuria, fever, weight loss (?evidence of leukaemia or secondary malignancy), abdominal pain, arthritic pain and vaginal bleeding and menstrual blood loss
- if she has noticed any lymphadenopathy
- relevant past medical history of lymphoproliferative disorders, liver disease or recent viral infections (Epstein–Barr virus (EBV), toxoplasmosis, CMV)
- family history of bleeding and coagulopathies or collagen disorders, e.g. Ehlers–Danlos syndrome, or connective tissue disorders such as SLE
- drug history, especially anticoagulants, steroids, sulphonamides, chloramphenicol
- dietary history, especially vitamin C-containing fruit and vegetables
- recent trauma, head injury or blood transfusions
- the concerns of the patient

2 Identification and use of information gathered

The candidate should be able to interpret the history and create a problem list. The objectives for the candidate are to:

- formulate a list of differential diagnoses
- explain the possibilities to the patient
- explain it would be best to admit for assessment
- have a plan of investigations and include an explanation of the bone marrow biopsy
- explain you may have to treat with steroids and explain their side-effects

3 Discussion related to the case

- This case typically describes idiopathic thrombocytopenic purpura (ITP) in a young female. She does not have any active bleeding. The other possibilities for consideration are: bone marrow failure (e.g. leukaemia, infiltration by secondary malignancy); coagulation deficiency (e.g. thrombotic thrombocy-topenic purpura, disseminated intravascular coagulation, haemolytic uraemic syndrome); drug-induced (e.g. sulphonamides, chloramphenicol, steroids); infection (e.g. EBV, CMV and toxoplasmosis); and others such as Henoch–Schönlein purpura.
- Most adults with ITP have symptoms that persist for many years and it is then referred to as chronic ITP. Women aged 20–40 years are most commonly affected and outnumber men by a ratio of 3 : 1. They may present with an abrupt fall in the platelet count with bleeding similar to that of patients with acute ITP. Usually, they have a prior history of easy bruising or menorrhagia. These patients have an autoimmune disorder with antibodies directed against target antigens on the glycoprotein IIb–IIIa or glycoprotein Ib–IX complex.
- The only blood count abnormality is the thrombocytopenia. Bone marrow examination reveals normal or increased numbers of megakaryocytes. Platelet antibodies can be looked for but are not reliably specific. Antinuclear antibody testing is useful in looking for SLE. Patients with splenic enlargement and atypical lymphocytes should have EBV serology and HIV should not be overlooked in high-risk patients.
- Treatment is aimed at reducing platelet antibodies with corticosteroids. Haemorrhage in patients can be controlled usually with corticosteroids but, in rare cases, the patients may require temporary phagocytic blockade with intravenous immunoglobulin (IVIG). Although IVIG is an effective form of therapy, it is quite expensive and should be reserved for patients with severe thrombocytopenia and bleeding, and for those who have not responded to other measures. Emergency splenectomy is usually reserved for patients with acute or chronic ITP who are desperately ill and have not responded to any medical measures designed to improve haemostasis.
- The candidate will be expected to discuss the differential diagnoses of purpura, the investigations and the treatment of ITP.

Comments on the case

This case is an important 'describe the rash' history. For all rashes the candidate should have a set list of questions to ask: distribution, colour, size, shape, surface, itch, etc.

Case 40 | Pyrexia

Candidate information

You are the SHO in a general medical clinic. Mr Mark Hamilton has been referred to you by his GP.

Please read this letter (it should take no more than 2 min) and then continue with the consultation.

Dear Doctor

Re: Mr Mark Hamilton, aged 35

I would be grateful if you could see this man who works for British Petroleum and, after a business trip to Nairobi 4 weeks ago, has developed a fever. An FBC, U/E, LFT, malarial screen and chest X-ray have all been normal. He has no relevant past medical history. Please see and advise.

Yours sincerely

Dr G. Practitioner

You have 14 min until the patient leaves the room, followed by 1 min for reflection, before the discussion with the examiners. Be prepared to discuss the solutions to the problems posed by the case and how you might reply to the GP's letter.

Patient information

Mr Mark Hamilton is a 35-year-old previously fit gentleman who works for British Petroleum overseeing their investment in Africa. He attended a 1-week business meeting in Nairobi 4 weeks ago. While he was there he felt reasonably well and was staying in a four-star hotel. However, 3 days after coming back he started to feel tired and feverish, particularly at night. He was sweaty but did not drench the bed sheets. He has not measured his temperature but his wife tells him he feels as if he is 'burning'. The temperature comes and goes for around 12 h. He has had a slight cough but he puts this down to smoking. He also has had one bout of loose stools. He has lost 1 kg of weight as a consequence of a reduced appetite. There are no symptoms of sputum, haemoptysis, shortness of breath, abdominal pain, headaches, weakness of the arms/legs or lymph nodes. His past medical history is unremarkable. While he was in Africa he went sightseeing and does admit to being bitten by mosquitoes on one particular day. He took proguanil daily for malaria chemoprophylaxis throughout his trip but stopped these when he arrived back in the UK. He is intolerant to mefloquine (strange dreams) and chloroquine (sickness). In Nairobi he had no bouts of food poisoning nor did he eat uncooked food served at street cafés. There is no family history of tuberculosis or any contact with known cases. Other recent trips include one to Lagos (4 months ago) and one to Cape Town (2 months ago); he was well throughout both these trips. He is heterosexual, never had contact with prostitutes and has never injected drugs. He smokes 15 cigarettes a day, and drinks about 1 pint of beer a day. He lives with his wife and has no children. His wife is a teacher who works with young children. She does admit to having felt slightly coryzal recently.

Examiner information

1 Data gathering in the interview

A good candidate would be able to elicit:

- when he came back from Nairobi, how long he was out there for and whether the fever coincided with the trip. Whether he had other trips abroad and, if so, whether he was well during these
- if he has measured his temperature. If so, how high does it go and is it constant or intermittent. Does the fever ever disappear. How often does it peak
- other symptoms, e.g. rigors, loss of weight, poor appetite, chills, fatigue, pain, respiratory, cardiovascular, gastrointestinal, neurological (headache, neck stiffness), night sweats, lymphadenopathy, joint pains and rashes
- if there is any relevant past medical history, e.g. infections (malaria, pneumonia, tuberculosis) or recent surgery or trauma, neoplasia, connective tissue disorders or liver disorders
- drug history, especially malaria chemoprophylaxis and compliance (ideally 1 week before, during the trip and for 4 weeks after arriving back in the UK), previous immunosuppressives, e.g. corticosteroids, antibiotic therapy
- assess HIV risk, especially contact with prostitutes
- contact history, especially family (viral illness, sore throat)
- alcohol history
- the concerns of the patient

2 Identification and use of information gathered

The candidate should be able to interpret the history and create a problem list. The objectives for the candidate are to:

- assemble a list of differential diagnoses
- explain that the cause of the temperature is uncertain
- explain the possibilities
- highlight a list of investigations to be carried out

3 Discussion related to the case

- This case describes a pyrexia of unknown origin lasting

for 3 weeks or more. The possible diagnoses are vast and include: (a) infective, e.g. malaria, tuberculosis, pyogenic abscess, urinary, biliary, joint, subacute bacterial endocarditis (SBE), viral (EBV, CMV) and others (Q fever, toxoplasmosis, brucellosis); (b) cancer, e.g. lymphoproliferative (lymphoma, leukaemia), renal cell carcinoma, hepatocellular carcinoma; (c) immunogenic, e.g. drug-induced, connective tissue and autoimmune (e.g. SLE, rheumatoid), sarcoidosis; (d) miscellaneous, e.g. inflammatory bowel disease (IBD), thyrotoxicosis; (e) factitious; and (f) unknown causes.

- The possibilities in this case include malaria (proguanil is inadequate for total chloroquine-resistant *Plasmodium falciparum* and he did not take the full chemoprophylaxis for 4 weeks after returning to the UK), tuberculosis (cough, loss of weight, tiredness, night time fever), non-specific viral illness, and always think of HIV infection.

- Investigations include repeating the earlier tests in case something new turns up, especially the malaria screen, blood cultures, repeat chest X-ray, full respiratory pathogen screen which includes viral, *Chlamydia*, *Coxiella* and *Legionella*, sputum, if any, for alcohol–acid fast bacilli and consider giving him a thermometer with a chart and reviewing him again shortly with the chart and blood results. Even if a malarial screen has been normal, it is worth repeating the screen a few more times. Bone marrow aspiration (likely to show the malarial parasites) may have to be considered if none of the investigations points to a diagnosis.

- In order to determine tolerance and to establish habit, prophylaxis should be started 1 week before travel and continued for at least 4 weeks after returning. For Sub-Saharan Africa, where chloroquine resistance is widespread, recommendations include mefloquine 250 mg once weekly or, in the presence of intolerance, chloroquine 300 mg once weekly and proguanil hydrochloride 200 mg o.d.

Comments on the case

This example typifies a case where the diagnosis is not known—it never may be! Unless a detailed history is taken, the investigator will not be able to focus his or her pattern of investigations. Do not be afraid to ask about contact with prostitutes, particularly of those visiting parts of Central and East Africa. Individuals may always conceal such activity and hence one must be vigilant for HIV infection, especially if odd symptoms such as sore throats caused by oral thrush (in the absence of antibiotics and corticosteroids) and lymphadenopathy are present.

Case 41 | **Renal colic and haematuria**

Candidate information

You are the SHO in a general medical clinic. Mr Dennis Bingley has been referred to you by his GP.

Please read this letter (it should take no more than 2 min) and then continue with the consultation.

Dear Doctor

Re: Mr Dennis Bingley, aged 78

Thank you for seeing Mr Bingley who had an episode of left-sided renal colic accompanied by macroscopic haematuria 3 weeks ago. His past medical history is unremarkable except that he has atrial fibrillation for which he takes digoxin 125 μg o.d. and aspirin 75 mg o.d.

Your sincerely

Dr G. Practitioner

You have 14 min until the patient leaves the room, followed by 1 min for reflection, before the discussion with the examiners. Be prepared to discuss the solutions to the problems posed by the case and how you might reply to the GP's letter.

Patient information

Mr Dennis Bingley is a 78-year-old retired gardener. Three weeks ago he developed a severe, sharp, colicky, left-sided pain in the renal area, which lasted for 3 h and was accompanied with macroscopic haematuria. The pain radiated down to his suprapubic area and it was relieved by an intramuscular injection of diclofenac given by his GP. The macroscopic haematuria appeared soon after the onset of the renal colic and was visible throughout the stream. He does not remember passing any stones in his urine. Since this episode he has had no more episodes of renal colic and haematuria. He has suffered with prostatism for many years with symptoms of poor initiation, poor stream and postmicturition dribbling but has no dysuria. He had never noticed any blood in the urine until this recent episode. He was diagnosed as having atrial fibrillation by the GP 5 years ago for which he takes digoxin 125 μg and aspirin 75 mg o.d. He does not take warfarin. He has no respiratory, cardiovascular or abdominal symptoms. He does not complain of any loss of weight or appetite. He does not have diabetes mellitus, any coagulation problems or a previous history of kidney stones. He has not suffered any recent trauma. He lives alone and leads an active life, undertaking his own shopping and house cleaning. He stopped smoking 25 years ago and does not drink alcohol. His GP has told him that he may have kidney stones but he is concerned that he may have cancer.

Examiner information

1 Data gathering in the interview

A good candidate would be able to elicit:

- the history of the renal colic, including the site of the pain, severity, nature, time span, radiation, any relieving factors and any aggravating factors
- the history of the haematuria, including if it was frank blood or diluted by urine and whether the haematuria was visible throughout the stream (suggests that the site of the haemorrhage is the bladder or above), at the beginning of micturition with the urine clearing towards the end of the stream (suggestive of bleeding from the urethra) or at the end of micturition (suggestive of bleeding from the bladder base or prostate)
- whether any stones or gravel were passed in the urine
- other urinary symptoms, such as dysuria, poor stream, postmicturition dribbling
- any past episodes of haematuria and prostatism
- any past history of renal stones or renal disorders
- any history of hypercalcaemia, coagulation disorders or recent trauma to the back
- any medication, including anticoagulants
- any family history of renal disorders, e.g. cystic disease
- other respiratory (cough, sputum, fever, haemoptysis), cardiovascular (palpitations, chest pains) or gastrointestinal (change in bowel habit, *per rectum* bleeding) symptoms
- history of smoking and alcohol
- any known allergies, e.g. contrast medium
- the impact of the illness on the patient and his concerns

2 Identification and use of information gathered

The candidate should be able to interpret the history and create a problem list. The objectives for the candidate are to:

- develop a list of differential diagnoses
- explain the possible causes for his symptoms
- arrange relevant investigations
- address his concerns and particularly his worry of a possible cancer

3 Discussion related to the case

- Haematuria (blood in the urine) can produce red to brown discoloration depending on the amount of blood present and the acidity of the urine. Slight haematuria may cause no discoloration and may be detected only by microscopy or chemical analysis. Haematuria without pain is usually caused by renal, vesical or prostatic disease. In the absence of red blood cell casts, which usually indicate glomerulonephritis, silent haematuria may be caused by a bladder or a kidney malignancy. Such tumours usually bleed intermittently and should not be dismissed if the bleeding stops spontaneously. Intermittent, recurrent haematuria may also occur in IgA nephropathy. Other causes of asymptomatic haematuria include calculi, polycystic disease, renal cysts, sickle cell disease, hydronephrosis and benign prostatic hyperplasia. Haematuria accompanied by excruciating pain (renal colic), as in this case, suggests the passage of a ureteral calculus or a blood clot from renal bleeding. Haematuria with dysuria is also associated with bladder infections or stones.

- The presence of one or more red blood cells per cubic millimetre in an unspun urine sample results in a positive dipstix test for blood and this is abnormal. The test is sometimes too sensitive, giving false positive results in normal individuals. A positive dipstick test should always be followed up by a microscopy of the urine sample to confirm the presence of red cells and so exclude haemoglobinuria or myoglobulinuria which may also give false positive dipstick tests. Microscopy may also demonstrate red cell casts which indicate bleeding from the kidney, particularly in glomerulonephritis.

- Bleeding may come from anywhere within the urinary tract and other investigations include urine cytology, plain abdominal X-ray, ultrasound of the renal tract and intravenous urography. These results will determine any further investigations, e.g. cystoscopy, abdominal CT scan, etc.

- Common causes of bleeding from the kidney include stones, cysts (single or multiple), trauma, carcinoma, glomerulonephritis, tuberculosis, papillary necrosis, infarction, tubulo-interstitial nephritis and coagulation defects.

> **Comments on the case**
>
> This case tests the candidate's ability to obtain a thorough history of haematuria and renal colic. The candidate will be expected to discuss a management plan with the patient and to address his concerns about cancer.

Case 42 | Tiredness

Candidate information

You are the SHO in a general medical clinic. Mr Steven Waugh has been referred to you by his GP.

Please read this letter (it should take no more than 2 min) and then continue with the consultation.

Dear Doctor

Re: Mr Steven Waugh, aged 48

Thank you for seeing this pleasant man who works for the city council as a personnel manager. He complains of tiredness during the day for the last year. At work his colleagues regularly find him asleep at his desk and 5 weeks ago he fell asleep at the wheel of his car, driving off the motorway onto the embankment. Past medical history includes hypertension for which he takes atenolol 50 mg o.d. and he is overweight at 110 kg. Recent FBC, U/E and thyroid function tests have all been normal.

Yours sincerely

Dr G. Practitioner

You have 14 min until the patient leaves the room, followed by 1 min for reflection, before the discussion with the examiners. Be prepared to discuss the solutions to the problems posed by the case and how you might reply to the GP's letter.

Patient information

Mr Waugh is a 48-year-old man who works for the city council as a personnel manager. He gives a 1-year history of falling asleep at his desk during the day. This may happen up to five times per day and particularly during the afternoon. He has an all-day desk job with very little activity or exercise throughout the day. His colleagues have found him asleep at his desk on so many occasions that he is currently at the receiving end of numerous taunts. He does not sleep well at night and feels tired and exhausted from the time he wakes up in the morning. He has always been a heavy snorer and occasionally his wife has noticed him stopping breathing; this induces his wife to shake him to arouse him and this is then followed by a grunting noise. Unfortunately, the snoring has recently been so bad that his wife now sleeps in a separate room. When he is not at work, e.g. at weekends, falling asleep in front of the television has been a common occurrence but more worrying was the recent car accident. Falling asleep at the wheel of the car and swerving from lane to lane, particularly on the motorway, has been a problem for a number of years, but this is the first time he has had an accident. No alcohol was found when the police breathalysed him. Other symptoms of note are nocturia (three times a night) and occasional morning headaches but there is no obvious dyspnoea, chest pain, cough, sputum or ankle swelling. He has been hypertensive for 10 years and takes atenolol. He has always been overweight and wears a size 18 collar. He does no physical exercise and drinks three cans of lager at home in the evening. He does not smoke. The snoring is obviously causing marital strife (with reduced sexual activity) and problems at work and he is desperate for help.

Examiner information

1 Data gathering in the interview

A good candidate would be able to elicit:
- how long the lethargy has been present and whether it is deteriorating or disabling
- an idea of which daily routine activities are impinged upon by the symptoms
- if the fatigue is worse with activity and better during rest (myasthenia)
- symptoms suggestive of obstructive sleep apnoea, such as apnoeic episodes during sleep, feeling of poor sleep quality, daytime somnolence (falling asleep at work, in front of the television and while driving), loud snoring, nocturia, restlessness at night, morning headaches and reduced libido. Ask for the size of neck collar and weight
- other possible physical symptoms suggestive of an endocrine disorder, especially hypothyroidism, cardiac failure, respiratory disease, renal failure and limb weakness
- past medical history of neoplasm, viral illnesses, thyroid disorder or surgery, diabetes mellitus or a psychiatric illness
- psychological symptoms, e.g. stress/anxiety, depression, poor sleep pattern, marital strife
- occupational history
- social history
- smoking and alcohol history, particularly in the evening which may exacerbate sleep apnoea
- drug history (legal and illegal), especially anxiolytics and benzodiazepines which aggravate sleep apnoea
- the concerns of the patient

2 Identification and use of information gathered

The candidate should be able to interpret the history and create a problem list. The objectives for the candidate are to:
- decide which diagnosis fits best
- relay the possible differential diagnoses, although in this case the likelihood is obstructive sleep apnoea (OSA)

- explain what OSA is (without jargon)
- explain that you would like to arrange a sleep study and what this entails
- explain that if the findings of the sleep study are suggestive of OSA then nasal continuous positive airway pressure (CPAP) may be considered
- counsel him on the alcohol intake, explaining that drinking in the evening may exacerbate symptoms, and discuss the strategies for losing weight which can improve symptoms

3 Discussion related to the case

- The case tests the ability of the candidate to take a detailed history about a common but vague symptom, and to differentiate the possible causes of tiredness such as OSA (in this case), endocrine disorders, anaemia, postviral illness, heart failure, metabolic or anxiety/depression (with poor sleep quality).
- The candidate should undertake FBC, U/E, LFT, calcium and thyroid function tests if not already carried out. For sleep apnoea, the Epworth sleepiness scale (a questionnaire) is useful to determine the likelihood of OSA. A score of over 11 out of 24 is suggestive but not totally indicative of OSA. The scale asks the likelihood of falling asleep when: (a) sitting and reading; (b) watching television; (c) sitting in a place of activity (work); (d) passenger in a car for 1 h; (e) lying down to rest in the afternoon; (f) sitting and talking to someone; (g) sitting quietly after lunch (without alcohol); and (h) sitting in the car when stopped. A sleep study (polysomnography) is performed; sleep laboratories differ in ways of performing such studies but most perform pulse oximetry (looking for hypoxic episodes), heart rate variability monitoring (which reflect arousals during sleep) with videoing, EEG traces and a microphone to detect levels of snoring during the night. Other departments may include recording of thoracoabdominal movements to detect any paradox (excessive movements as a consequence of upper airway obstruction).
- The candidate should be able to discuss the use of nasal CPAP, the impact of OSA, especially with regard to road traffic accidents, and discuss other causes of tiredness, especially postviral illnesses.

Comments on the case

Tiredness and lethargy are common complaints but the candidate must be aware of not falling into the automatic assumption that there may be no organic explanation. A detailed history must be taken, considering all the possibilities, especially as OSA can be treated.

Case 43 | Tremor

Candidate information

You are the SHO in a neurology clinic. Mr Walter Matthews has been referred to you by his GP.

Please read this letter (it should take no more than 2 min) and then continue with the consultation.

> Dear Doctor
>
> **Re: Mr Walter Matthews, aged 73**
>
> Thank you for seeing Mr Matthews who works as a part-time bookkeeper at the local church-run library. He is usually fit and well but recently complains of having developed shaking of his hands and is dropping books at work. He is worried that he may have Parkinson's disease. He takes aspirin for a previous TIA which he had 6 years ago. Please see and advise.
>
> Yours sincerely
>
> Dr G. Practitioner

You have 14 min until the patient leaves the room, followed by 1 min for reflection, before the discussion with the examiners. Be prepared to discuss the solutions to the problems posed by the case and how you might reply to the GP's letter.

Patient information

Mr Walter Matthews is a 73-year-old generally fit and well gentleman, who continues to work as a part-time bookkeeper at the local church-run library. Over the last 8 months he has noticed shaking of his hands. These shakes are worse when he is engaged in an activity rather than when he is resting. His wife has now noticed that when he is making the tea, he cannot steadily pass a cup over without some spillage into the saucer. At work, he is finding that putting books back on to the higher shelves is slightly awkward and that he often drops them. His shakes do not seem to be deteriorating and there are no other symptoms such as paraesthesia, tingling, coldness, restlessness, rigidity and immobility, slowness of movements, inability to roll over in bed, dribbling of saliva, loss of memory or attention, or any psychological changes. There are no particular exacerbating or relieving factors. He has no other neurological symptoms such as headache or limb weakness and no cardiovascular, respiratory, thyrotoxic or abdominal symptoms. His past medical history includes one episode of a TIA 6 years ago when he presented to his GP with a 1-h history of weakness of the left leg which returned to full strength. He has taken aspirin 75 mg o.d. since then. He takes no other medication. He and his wife are self-caring, generally fit and active, taking part in weekly church activities. He has never smoked and he does not drink alcohol. He lives in a three-bedroomed house and the toilet is upstairs. His main concerns are the possibility of Parkinson's disease.

Examiner information

1 Data gathering in the interview

A good candidate would be able to elicit:

- the time of onset of the tremor and whether it is slowly or quickly progressive
- whether the tremor is confined to the arms or hands or both. Which hand/arm is worse
- whether the patient is left- or right-handed
- whether the tremor is worse at rest (Parkinson's disease) or on sustained posture (benign essential tremor) or fleeting, purposeless, restless and fidgety (chorea) or intentional (cerebellar)
- examples of difficulty, such as bringing a glass of fluid to his mouth, passing a teacup and saucer to his wife, etc.
- any associated tremor of the head (titubation) (in benign essential tremor) or blepharospasm (seen also with Parkinson's disease)
- any symptoms suggestive of Parkinson's disease, such as paraesthesia, tingling, coldness, restlessness, rigidity and immobility, slowness of movements, inability to roll over in bed, dribbling of saliva, loss of memory or attention, or psychological changes
- other neurological symptoms, especially weakness and numbness of limbs, headaches, blurring of vision, dysphasia and dysphagia
- other respiratory (e.g. cough from aspiration), abdominal (e.g. constipation in Parkinson's disease) and cardiovascular (postural hypotension in Parkinson's disease) symptoms
- history of the TIA
- drug medication (e.g. phenothiazines)
- assessment of any anxiety
- history suggestive of thyrotoxicosis
- alcohol history—does alcohol relieve the tremor
- the impact of the disease on the family

2 Identification and use of information gathered

The candidate should be able to interpret the history and create a problem list. The objectives for the candidate are to:

- assemble a list of differential diagnoses for tremor
- reassure the patient that the tremor is a benign essential tremor but that this is persistent and may progress slowly
- reassure the patient that he does not have Parkinson's disease
- explain that treatment is limited but beta-blockers may be tried
- address any other concerns that the patient may have

3 Discussion related to the case

- This case allows the candidate to explore the causes of a tremor. This case typically describes a benign essential tremor (frequency about 5–8 Hz) during sustained posture and persisting or worsening during action. This is not a Parkinsonian tremor as the other classic features of this disease (resting tremor, rigidity and bradykinesia) are absent. Other possibilities include a physiological tremor exacerbated by anxiety but this is a small-amplitude tremor and rapid (about 8–12 Hz), best seen in the outstretched hands, absent at rest and attenuated through voluntary movements, cerebellar (on reaching a target), alcohol and drug-induced such as those causing Parkinsonism (neuroleptics), and beta-agonist inhalers such as salbutamol, salmeterol and eformoterol.
- Management is purely reassurance but, if symptoms continue to be troublesome, beta-blockers can be considered.
- The candidate will be expected to discuss in depth the causes of Parkinsonism, the features and the treatment of Parkinson's disease from a multidisciplinary perspective.

Comments on the case

This case demonstrates how, by taking a detailed history and asking when the symptoms are worse (at rest or during action), one can come to the diagnosis and relieve the patient's anxieties by ruling out Parkinson's disease.

Case 44 | Visual disturbances

Candidate information

You are the SHO in a diabetic clinic. Mr Norman Baron has been referred to you by his GP.

Please read this letter (it should take no more than 2 min) and then continue with the consultation.

Dear Doctor

Re: Mr Norman Baron, aged 84

Thank you for seeing this gentleman urgently. He complains of episodes of 'zig-zag' vision lasting for up to an hour. He has previously suffered from migraines but he says these current episodes are different. He takes Mixtard insulin for his diabetes and his last HbA1c was 8.9%. He is on long-acting nifedipine for hypertension. His past history includes a myocardial infarction (7 years ago) and a cerebrovascular accident (CVA) (5 years ago) when he was found to have a right carotid artery stenosis. He also takes aspirin and his blood pressure today was 130/72 mmHg. Please advise on diagnosis and management.

Yours sincerely

Dr G. Practitioner

You have 14 min until the patient leaves the room, followed by 1 min for reflection, before the discussion with the examiners. Be prepared to discuss the solutions to the problems posed by the case and how you might reply to the GP's letter.

Patient information

Mr Baron is an 84-year-old widowed gentleman with diabetes mellitus who has experienced occasional episodes of disturbed vision over the last 8 weeks—sometimes zigzag, sometimes blurred, with difficulty in reading newspaper print which can become shimmery. These may last for up to an hour and they usually resolve spontaneously. There are no triggers and they may come on at any time of the day. There are no associated headaches, loss of consciousness, limb weakness, pain, swelling, redness or any movement problems of the eyes. There is no history of a head injury. His diabetes (first diagnosed 9 years ago) was initially treated with tablets but after an MI 2 years later, coupled with poor glycaemic control, he was changed over to insulin. At present he takes Mixtard 30/70 human insulin 16 units a.m. and 12 units p.m. using a pen device. He has no problems with administering the insulin and his blood sugars are usually stable between 8 and 10. He does not suffer from hypoglycaemic attacks although every few weeks he does have a blood glucose reading of around 3 and any associated blurred vision recovers after a sugary drink. He has never had any retinal laser therapy. Other past medical history includes a CVA 5 years ago presenting as weakness in the left arm from which he made a full recovery, and hypertension for which he takes long-acting nifedipine. At the time of his CVA a 50% right carotid artery stenosis was detected but was not operated on. He has had migraine-like headaches but these do not cause any visual problems, only a headache and sickness. He lives alone and is self-caring, mobile and manages to collect his own pension and carry out his own shopping. He used to smoke 35 years ago and does not drink alcohol at present. His only other medication is aspirin o.d. He is worried about losing his sight and is unsure if these symptoms are related to the diabetes.

Examiner information

1 Data gathering in the interview

A good candidate would be able to elicit:
- if the problem relates to one or both eyes and to which particular area of the visual field
- the exact presentation of the visual symptoms in detail: clouding (cataracts); painless visual field loss (glaucoma — as opposed to closed-angle glaucoma presenting with a painful red eye); painless bilateral loss of visual acuity — can he read newspaper print? (macular degeneration); blindness from vitreous haemorrhage and retinal detachment (in diabetes mellitus); progressive night time blindness (retinitis pigmentosa)
- details of the episodes, including frequency, length of symptoms, whether sudden onset and sudden resolution
- if the episodes of visual disturbance occur at any particular time of the day or are caused by any particular movement or activity
- details of previous eye problems, retinal screening history and any cataract surgery
- details of the diabetes mellitus and its treatment
- details of the previous stroke, MI and cholesterol levels
- smoking and drinking history
- social history, driving history
- the effect of symptoms on daily activities
- concerns and worries the patient may have

2 Identification and use of information gathered

The candidate should be able to interpret the history and create a problem list. The objectives for the candidate are to:
- differentiate the possible causes for the patient's visual problems: retinal problems (e.g. macular oedema or retinal detachment), migraine, TIAs, postural hypotension or hypoglycaemia, and explain these possibilities
- consider either paroxysmal atrial fibrillation and/or carotid stenosis/emboli as a cause of TIAs. Hypoglycaemia must be excluded as a cause
- recommend that an ophthalmological opinion should be sought, unless an alternative diagnosis is obvious

3 Discussion related to the case
- Further investigation relevant to the differential diagnoses should be considered; urgent retinal screening/eye hospital referral considered for full retinal examination.
- Postural blood pressure should be measured.
- Further investigations may include CT scan of the head, carotid Doppler, ECG recording (for atrial fibrillation) and a 24-h ECG recording.
- The appearance of neovascularization in response to retinal hypoxia is the hallmark of proliferative diabetic retinopathy. These newly formed vessels may appear at the optic nerve and/or macula and rupture easily leading to vitreous haemorrhage, fibrosis and, ultimately, retinal detachment. Not all individuals with non-proliferative retinopathy develop proliferative retinopathy, but the more severe the non-proliferative disease, the greater the chance of evolution to proliferative retinopathy within 5 years. This creates a clear opportunity for early detection and treatment of diabetic retinopathy. In contrast, clinically significant macular oedema may appear when only non-proliferative retinopathy is present. Fluorescein angiography is often useful to detect macular oedema which is associated with a 25% chance of moderate visual loss over the next 3 years.
- Duration of diabetes mellitus and degree of glycaemic control are the best predictors of the development of retinopathy. Non-proliferative retinopathy is found in almost all individuals who have had diabetes for >20 years (25% incidence with 5 years, and 80% incidence with 15 years of type 1 diabetes mellitus).
- Efforts should be made to establish safe control, e.g. diabetes and hypertension, rather than trying to meet targets that may produce sudden effects such as hypo-

glycaemia or postural hypotension. The choice of the best antihypertensive agents is debatable, calcium channel antagonists and low-dose thiazides have been shown to prevent CVA in this age group but for diabetic patients ACE inhibitors should also be considered.

- New onset of migraine would be unusual at this age, whereas the risk of retinal problems from either diabetes or macular degeneration is greater.

Comments on the case

This case demonstrates an elderly gentleman with episodes of disturbed vision, possibly a result of macular disease or early retinal detachment. The candidate must not forget to ascertain the effect of these symptoms on his daily life. Other causes must be considered and a sense of investigative urgency must be displayed.

Case 45 | Vomiting

Candidate information

You are the SHO in a respiratory clinic. Mr Azhar Khan has been referred to you by his TB health visitor.

Please read this letter (it should take no more than 2 min) and then continue with the consultation.

Dear Doctor

Re: Mr Azhar Khan, aged 24

I have asked Mr Khan to come back to clinic today because of his vomiting. He was started on Rifinah 300 two tablets o.d., pyrazinamide 2 g o.d. and ethambutol 800 mg o.d. 2 weeks ago for pulmonary tuberculosis. I have asked him to stop all his tablets until review. Please see and advise.

Yours sincerely

Mrs TB Health Visitor

You have 14 min until the patient leaves the room, followed by 1 min for reflection, before the discussion with the examiners. Be prepared to discuss the solutions to the problems posed by the case and how you might reply to the health visitor's letter.

Patient information

Mr Azhar Khan is a 24-year-old man born in the UK but of Pakistani origin. He works in Burger King as a food preparer. He first presented to his GP 6 weeks ago with cough, sputum, loss of weight and feeling generally unwell with a fever. Despite a course of oral amoxicillin, his symptoms persisted and a chest X-ray, arranged 3 weeks after the first presentation, showed right upper lobe shadowing typical of *Mycobacteria tuberculosis*. A subsequent sputum sample confirmed the diagnosis on microscopy, making him smear-positive. He was started on quadruple therapy 2 weeks ago in the chest clinic: Rifinah 300 two tablets, pyrazinamide 2 g and ethambutol 800 mg, all once a day 30 min before breakfast. He is 54 kg and the dosage is correct for this weight. Within 5 days he developed nausea and vomiting after taking the tablets. He would be vomiting up to three times in the morning and the nausea would persist into the afternoon. His appetite has decreased and he has not gained any weight. He has some epigastric tenderness, but no jaundice or right hypochondrial pain. There have been no other symptoms such as diarrhoea, dysphagia, abdominal distension, haematemesis, PR bleeding, skin reactions, peripheral neuropathy or visual disturbances suggestive of retrobulbar neuritis. There are no symptoms suggestive of labyrinthine, endocrine or metabolic disorders. Despite trying to persevere with the medication, his nausea and vomiting continued and the TB health visitor advised him to stop the medication, believing that his symptoms were drug-induced. Within 2 days of stopping therapy, his symptoms have improved. LFTs on his first visit to the chest clinic were normal. His cough and sputum persist. Contact tracing has revealed no new cases in his close contacts and, as there were no unusually susceptible individuals such as children or immunocompromised individuals working with Mr Khan at the Burger King, it was felt that contact tracing should not be carried out here. He has not returned to work since the microscopic confirmation of the *Mycobacteria*. He has no past medical history of gastrointestinal disorders such as oesophageal reflux, dyspepsia, pancreatitis or previous gastrointestinal surgery. He has no previous or present psychiatric history and he does not take any other medication such as antidepressants, opioids, antibiotics or dextropropoxyphene. He lives with his parents and two younger sisters. He does not drink alcohol or smoke. There is no family history of tuberculosis here in the UK or Pakistan. He has only visited Pakistan once when he was 7 years old. He is obviously concerned that his respiratory symptoms have not improved and he has lost confidence in the medication.

Examiner information

1 Data gathering in the interview

A good candidate would be able to elicit:

- chronological events of the symptoms in relation to the medication and explore their temporal relationship
- frequency of vomiting and nausea and for how long this persists during the day. When not vomiting does the nausea persist and if there is any relation to meals
- other gastrointestinal symptoms, e.g. acid regurgitation, dysphagia, abdominal pain, dyspepsia, bloating, fullness, intestinal obstruction (distension, pain, constipation, borborygmi), diarrhoea, haematemesis and melaena
- any suggestions of hepatitis (jaundice, biliary pain, itching, dark urine)
- other side-effects of tuberculosis therapy, especially skin reactions, visual disturbances, peripheral neuropathy (isoniazid). Patient would have noticed an orange discoloration of the urine as a result of the Rifinah
- other precipitating factors
- systemic symptoms, e.g. weakness, malaise, weight loss, loss of appetite
- symptoms suggestive of endocrine, metabolic or labyrinth disorders
- past history of gastrointestinal disorders, e.g. reflux oesophagitis, pancreatitis or endocrine disorders and of gastrointestinal surgery
- psychiatric history (e.g. eating disorders, anxiety), alcohol history and family history of tuberculosis

- full drug history, including antituberculous therapy (correct dosage related to the weight of the patient), overdosing, and antidepressants, opioids, antibiotics, dextropropoxyphene
- the contact tracing history and work history, especially contacts there and how long he has been off work
- impact of illness on the patient and his family and his concerns

2 Identification and use of information gathered

The candidate should be able to interpret the history and create a problem list. The objectives for the candidate are to:

- identify quite clearly whether the nausea and vomiting are drug-induced or not, and to relay this to the patient
- have a list of investigations (e.g. LFT)
- explain the importance of taking medication for pulmonary tuberculosis (6 months) in order to reinforce the importance of compliance
- explain it is not known which medication is causing the symptoms and that admission on to the ward with gradual introduction individually of medication at low dosage is needed and this may allow gradual tolerance
- explain that it would be unwise to return to work at this stage until he has had at least 2 weeks of therapy at full dosage without any side-effects and with improvement in the respiratory symptoms. Emphasize that he is still infectious
- address any other concerns and attempt to reverse any loss of confidence in the treatment

- complete a 'yellow' adverse drug reaction form for the Committee on Safety of Medicines (found at the back of the British National Formulary)
- notify this case if not done so already

3 Discussion related to the case

- This case tests the ability of the candidate to make a list of differential diagnoses and to style the history taking appropriately around the symptoms of nausea and vomiting. The history taking should allow the candidate to conclude that the symptoms are related to the antituberculous therapy, particularly as his symptoms eased after cessation of the therapy.
- Other general causes for vomiting include gastrointestinal causes, e.g. peptic ulcer disease (with pyloric outlet obstruction?), gallstones, pancreatitis, small bowel Crohn's disease, oesophageal disorders, (e.g. stricture, achalasia, functional dyspepsia, alcohol or drug-induced and eating disorders) and non-gastrointestinal causes, e.g. bulimia, alcohol or drug-related and psychogenic vomiting.
- As the most serious side-effect of antituberculous therapy is hepatitis, urgent LFTs are required to detect any changes in aspartate (AST) and alanine transaminase (ALT) levels. Modest elevations of these enzymes are not uncommon and, as a general rule, if levels of ALT and AST rise above five times normal or the bilirubin level is elevated, then the medication must be stopped and smaller doses reintroduced individually once the levels have normalized.

- The British Thoracic Society's guidelines on drug challenges, particularly in the case of hepatotoxicity, suggest the following: once LFTs are normal, drugs can be reintroduced sequentially in the order of isoniazid, rifampicin, pyrazinamide, with daily monitoring of the patient's clinical condition and liver function. Isoniazid should be reintroduced initially at 50 mg/day, increasing sequentially to 300 mg/day every 2–3 days, provided no reaction occurs, and then continued. After a further 2–3 days without reaction, rifampicin at a dosage of 75 mg/day can be added increasing to a dosage of 300 mg/day every 2–3 days and then to 450 mg (if weight is <50 kg) or 600 mg (if weight is ≥50 kg) as appropriate after a further 2–3 days without reaction. Finally, pyrazinamide is added at 250 mg/day, increasing to 1.0 g after every 2–3 days and then 1.5 g (for <50 kg body weight) or 2 g (≥50 kg).
- The candidate will be expected to know the side-effects of antituberculous therapy.

Comments on the case

The candidate must be able to decide if the vomiting is drug-induced or not and he or she has to be able to recognize that the patient may have lost all confidence in the therapy, which may endanger future compliance.

Case 46 | Vomiting and forgetfulness

Candidate information

You are the medical SHO on-call. Mr Kenneth French has been referred to you by the surgical SHO. The patient is in the toilet so you decide to speak to his wife for more information.

Please read this letter (it should take no more than 2 min) and then continue with the consultation.

Dear Medical Colleague

Re: Mr Kenneth French, aged 75

Mr French was admitted last night with a 1-day history of vomiting. He lives 200 miles away and is currently visiting his son in this neighbourhood. The casualty officer referred him to the surgeons after suspecting small bowel obstruction, but the consultant surgeon wonders if in fact the patient is suffering from gastroenteritis after eating undercooked chicken the day before at a local pub. The reason for referral is for an opinion on the complicated previous medical history of a pituitary adenoma. His electrolytes are as follows: sodium 133 mmol/L, potassium 5.5 mmol/L, urea 9.2 mmol/L and creatinine 123 mmol/L. Please see and advise.

Yours sincerely

Dr S.H.O. Surgeon

You have 14 min until the relative leaves the room, followed by 1 min for reflection, before the discussion with the examiners. Be prepared to discuss the solutions to the problems posed by the case and how you will respond to your colleague's request.

Patient information

Mr French is a 75-year-old retired librarian. The history is obtained from his wife, Mrs French. Mr French is normally a fit and well, self-caring man who enjoys long walks with the dog. He has a past history of a non-functioning pituitary adenoma for which he first presented 10 years ago to the optician with visual field loss. A CT scan of the head then confirmed the pituitary tumour and this was surgically removed. Since then he has been taking hydrocortisone 20 mg in the morning and 10 mg in the evening, thyroxine 125 µg/day and testosterone patches. Up until his recent illness there has been no suggestion of lethargy, tiredness or fatigue suggestive of adrenal insufficiency, or weight gain, cold intolerance, constipation and voice changes suggestive of hypothyroidism. He has normal body hair distribution including facial hair. Mr and Mrs French live 200 miles away and 4 days ago decided to visit their son who lives in the area. On the day before admission, they went out to lunch at the local pub. Mr French did at the time wonder if the roast chicken was undercooked, but decided it was edible. Next day (day of admission) he began to feel unwell followed by continued bouts of vomiting, approximately every hour with nausea in between. There was some non-specific central abdominal pain, but no blood in the vomitus or any diarrhoea. He could not keep any oral fluids down and the son decided that he should come to the casualty department. Mr French wonders if the chicken was the culprit but no other family member had similar symptoms. Interestingly, Mr French forgot to bring his hydrocortisone tablets when visiting his son but felt he might manage without them as he had been feeling so well recently. He does not have a medic-alert steroid-dependent card with him either; he cannot remember where he keeps it. The treatment so far has been intravenous fluids and Mrs French says that after he had been given intravenous steroids in casualty, he felt much better and his vomiting has improved. However, Mrs French still wonders if the symptoms are related to the possible gastroenteritis as suggested by the consultant surgeon.

Examiner information

1 Data gathering in the interview

A good candidate would be able to elicit:

- an accurate history of the presenting illness: time of vomiting and its frequency, any blood, presence of nausea between vomiting, associated abdominal pain, swelling, diarrhoea or fever. Any possible food poisoning and, if so, how long before the symptoms the food was consumed
- a full history of the pituitary problem: when first presented and with what symptoms, e.g. visual field loss (compression of optic chiasma), any symptoms suggestive of hypothyroidism, e.g. cold intolerance, slowness, weight gain, deepening of voice, skin changes, poor memory, depression, constipation, symptoms suggestive of adrenal insufficiency, e.g. weight loss, malaise, weakness, depression, nausea/vomiting, abdominal pain, syncope from postural hypotension, or symptoms suggestive of hypogonadism, e.g. poor libido, impotence, loss of secondary hair
- the treatment of the pituitary adenoma and whether he keeps a steroid medic-alert card. If not, why, and explain the need for this
- the reasons for the non-compliance. Reinforce the importance of compliance
- what treatment has been given so far in hospital
- any concerns

2 Identification and use of information gathered

The candidate should be able to interpret the history and create a problem list. The objectives for the candidate are to:

- identify the reason for non-compliance
- ascertain the full pituitary history
- decide that the likely cause of the illness is steroid insufficiency and not gastroenteritis (no one else in the family had symptoms suggestive of food poisoning)
- reassure his wife
- reinforce the importance of compliance but accepting the recent lapse was a genuine error as a result of forgetfulness
- suggest issuing a new steroid alert card and counsel for future illnesses; consider having an ampoule of hydrocortisone at home in case oral therapy is impossible. Say that a referral to an endocrinologist will be made and he or she will be able to advise on this matter

3 Discussion related to the case

- This patient presents with steroid insufficiency rather than gastroenteritis as the cause of the vomiting and ill-health. The omission of his treatment, persistent vomiting, the absence of diarrhoea and the improvement of his condition after intravenous steroids are all suggestive of this diagnosis. The raised potassium would otherwise be unusual if the electrolyte disturbance was caused by vomiting alone. It is of note that there was rapid improvement following rehydration and an injection of hydrocortisone. Ongoing management should include intravenous (4-hourly) or intramuscular (6-hourly) hydrocortisone 100 mg or a hydrocortisone infusion together with intravenous rehydration until the vomiting has stopped and the patient is eating. He should then return to his oral hydrocortisone. If there had been a history to suggest an intercurrent illness, then there may be a reason for continuing with a higher dose of an oral steroid for a few days before returning to the patient's standard regimen.

- The candidate will need to be able to discuss the management of acute hypoadrenalism, the role of fludrocortisone, investigations for suspected Addison's disease (synacthen test), and the value of medic-alert cards and bracelet.

Comments on the case

This case highlights the importance of thinking logically for a cause of the illness and not being biased by the surgical colleague's opinion. The history and the urea and electrolytes blood test support the diagnosis of adrenal insufficiency.

Case 47 | **Weakness of an arm**

Candidate information

You are the SHO on call in the general medical emergency clinic. Mr Leonard Williams has been referred to you by his GP.

Please read this letter (it should take no more than 2 min) and then continue with the consultation.

> Dear Doctor
>
> **Re: Mr Leonard Williams, aged 74**
>
> Thank you for your opinion on this gentleman, whom I have just seen as an emergency, with the complaint that he is unable to use his right arm. He has only recently joined my list so I do not have his full records.
>
> He has been taking aspirin for many years, started by a cardiologist when he had palpitations 10 years ago. Eight years ago he had several episodes of weakness in his left arm and was referred to a vascular surgeon who operated on his neck.
>
> He tells me that this current weakness has improved while sitting in the waiting room. On examination, I could detect no weakness or sensory loss in his right arm. His blood pressure is 134/74 mmHg and the pulse is regular. Please see and advise regarding diagnosis and management.
>
> Yours sincerely
>
> Dr G. Practitioner

You have 14 min until the patient leaves the room, followed by 1 min for reflection, before the discussion with the examiners. Be prepared to discuss the solutions to the problems posed by the case and how you might reply to the GP's letter.

Patient information

Mr Leonard Williams is a right-handed 74-year-old retired businessman. He has experienced four recent episodes of a sudden inability to use his right arm; the first was 4 days ago, the next two occurred yesterday and the last one was this morning. The first three lasted between 2 and 3 h and the one this morning seemed to persist much longer so he went to his GP for an emergency appointment. His arm was getting better (after about 4 h) as he waited to see the GP. About 8 years ago a similar episode occurred but he is unsure which arm was affected although his daughter remembers it being the left arm. He was admitted to hospital for scans of the head and neck that were then followed by surgery on the right side of his neck to remove a blockage. Ten years ago he saw a cardiologist because of palpitations and was told that his pulse was intermittently irregular during a 24-h ECG recording. He was started on aspirin and digoxin. He has recently become more aware of his palpitations and on one occasion he could feel his heart beating 'very fast'. He has no other relevant history such as hypertension, ischaemic heart disease or diabetes mellitus. His wife has problems with osteoporosis so she cannot do any heavy work. His caring daughter (a senior nurse) lives away and is fully occupied with her three young children. She does not visit very often. He lives in a moderately sized house that needs a lot of cleaning and maintenance; he thinks that it is all this hard work which has kept him healthy for so long. The neighbours are very helpful but he tends to lead a private life. Mr Williams is worried that there may not be anyone to look after him if he has a stroke or if he needs further surgery.

Examiner information

1 Data gathering in the interview
A good candidate would be expected to elicit:
- a detailed history of the weakness of the right arm, especially the number of recent episodes, which part of the arm first became weak, whether this spread to the rest of the limb, any feeling of numbness, etc.
- the disability as a result of the weakness, e.g. lifting cups, doing up buttons, writing; is he left- or right-handed
- any other associated neurological symptoms, e.g. headache, blurred vision, dysphasia, dysphagia, loss of consciousness, vomiting, seizure, confusion
- a diagnosis of the previous transient ischaemic attack (TIA) with a diagnosis of carotid artery stenosis and carotid endarterectomy
- the frequency of palpitations, their nature and rate, and to elicit the history of the previous cardiology referral and probable diagnosis
- other general risk factors, e.g. family history, hypertension, ischaemic heart disease, diabetes mellitus, hypercholesterolaemia, smoking history
- that it is probably the daughter who more correctly remembers the side of the weakness. Ask about his daughter's input and ability to provide future care
- a history which includes a detailed social history, including the characteristics of the house where he lives (including stairs, access to front door, toilet, kitchen facilities) and his activities of daily living
- the concerns of the patient with regard to future care

2 Identification and use of information gathered
The candidate should be able to interpret the history and create a problem list. The objectives for the candidate are to:
- give a differential diagnosis for the episodes of weakness, which includes TIAs and epilepsy

- consider either paroxysmal atrial fibrillation and/or carotid stenosis/emboli as a cause of the TIAs
- pick up the issue of the side of his previous TIAs and how it relates to his previous surgery
- discuss with the patient the possible diagnosis, confirmatory investigations and possible treatment with warfarin
- appreciate the gentleman's concerns regarding loss of independence and, in particular, his wish not to impose on his daughter

3 Discussion relating to the case
- This case tests the ability of the candidate to take a detailed history of the current and previous symptoms with an assured and accurate record of the chronological order of events. The patient clearly describes TIAs with a past history of atrial fibrillation (AF).
- Further investigations would include a CT scan of the head, carotid artery Doppler and 24-h ECG recording. Treatment will include warfarin and/or he may need further carotid surgery. These procedures will need to be explained to him along with the benefits and risks associated with the warfarin treatment. The patient has had invasive carotid surgery in the past so the candidate would need to appreciate that the patient should be informed of the changes in surgical approach over the last few years. While it is hopeful that further events, especially cerebrovascular, may be avoided by the anticoagulation, the issue of social care along with the various management options may need to be discussed to reassure the patient that his concerns have been noted.
- Because such patients are always at risk of systemic embolization, particularly in the presence of organic heart disease, life-long anticoagulation must be considered. This is particularly important in the elderly, where the attributable risk of AF for stroke approaches 30%. Several studies have now demonstrated conclusively that the incidence of embolization in patients with AF, not

associated with valvular heart disease, is reduced by life-long anticoagulation with warfarin-like agents. Aspirin may also be effective for this purpose in patients who are not at high risk for stroke. Although anticoagulation may be associated with haemorrhagic complications, the risk is largely associated with INRs above the recommended level of 2.0–3.0. Particular relevant risk factors are prior TIAs, systemic embolus or stroke, hypertension, poor left ventricular function, rheumatic mitral valve disease and prosthetic heart valves. All patients with risk factors, and without contraindications for anticoagulation, should be considered for treatment with warfarin. Patients under the age of 65 without risk factors may be considered for aspirin. Patients between 65 and 75 should be considered either for aspirin or warfarin and all patients over 75 should be considered for warfarin.

• The candidate will be expected to discuss the issues of anticoagulation, primary prevention of further events, especially controlling blood pressure, and the role of antiplatelet drugs in cerebrovascular disease.

Comments on the case

While this patient may not be fully abreast of the medical terminology associated with his previous medical history and procedures, he is able to give enough information to allow the candidate to establish his previous diagnoses of intermittent atrial fibrillation, transient ischaemic attacks and carotid artery stenosis. This gentleman has thought ahead as to what might happen if he were to have a cerebrovascular event and is concerned about the possible loss of independence. These issues need to be discussed.

Case 48 | Weight gain

Candidate information

You are the medical SHO in an endocrine clinic. Mrs Patsy Marlow has been referred to you by her GP.

Please read this letter (it should take no more than 2 min) and then continue with the consultation.

Dear Doctor

Re: Mrs Patsy Marlow, aged 44

Thank you for seeing this lady with recent weight gain. She has had type 2 diabetes mellitus for 4 years and, until recently, has had excellent glycaemic control. In the last 6 months her HbA1c has risen from 7.0–9.8% despite maximal oral hypoglycaemic therapy and the diabetes nurses have arranged for conversion to insulin. Her weight has risen during the last year, from 80 up to 91 kg, and she appears to have mainly central obesity. She was found to have a raised blood pressure at her recent annual review and I have started her on ramipril. Her free T_4 and thyroid-stimulating hormone (TSH) are both normal. I have explained to her that we need to be sure that she does not have a gland problem for her weight gain. I wonder if it could be caused by Cushing's syndrome. Please see and advise on management.

Yours sincerely

Dr G. Practitioner

You have 14 min until the patient leaves the room, followed by 1 min for reflection, before the discussion with the examiners. Be prepared to discuss the solutions to the problems posed by the case and how you might reply to the GP's letter.

Patient information

Mrs Patsy Marlow is a 44-year-old housewife who has had type 2 diabetes mellitus for 4 years and is under regular follow-up by the shared primary and secondary care teams. Her main problem is a weight gain of 11 kg, from 80 to 91 kg, over the last year. Most of the obesity is around the abdomen and this is accompanied by striae. She has never had striae except during pregnancy. Her diet and appetite have not changed and she is generally quite careful about what she eats. Other symptoms include general tiredness and fatigue during the day when carrying out household work such as washing and shopping, feeling low in mood, poor sleep, thinning of her skin and easy bruising, particularly when knocking herself on the furniture. She has noticed a change in her appearance, especially with facial acne, hirsutism and her face looks fuller. She has also noticed that her periods are more infrequent with scantier blood loss. Her diabetes has been reasonably well-controlled until the last few months and the GP has noticed a rise in the HbA1c over this time. Her blood sugar testing was usually between 4 and 8 but is now more commonly between 8 and 12. The diabetes nurse has suggested the possibility of insulin, to which she has expressed some concern. Recently, the GP has noticed her blood pressure to be raised and she was subsequently started on ramipril. The GP has explained that there may be a gland overactivity called Cushing's syndrome which could be causing these problems. She was initially quite relieved that there may be a distinct cause for the current problems but further explanations by the GP and warning against the possibility of other comorbidities, such as osteoporosis (if left untreated), has led to considerable anxiety. She is presently on gliclazide 160 mg b.d. and metformin 850 mg b.d. She has never taken steroids, either oral or creams. She does not drink or smoke and is happily married with three children who are in their twenties. Both parents also have diabetes mellitus and her husband works in a petrol station. She is keen to know what investigations will be carried out and whether surgery is needed. Her son is getting married in a few months and she is worried about the changes in her facial appearance.

Examiner information

1 Data gathering in the interview

A good candidate would be able to elicit:

- details of her weight gain, the distribution, any changes in diet to explain this and duration of symptoms
- symptoms suggestive of Cushing's syndrome, e.g. change in appearance (?old photos), skin changes, e.g. thinning and bruising, hair growth/acne, striae, weakness especially climbing stairs or standing up from a sitting position (proximal muscle wasting), depression, amenorrhoea/oligomenorrhoea, poor libido, poor sleep
- other secondary clues, e.g. hypertension, worsening diabetes, bony fractures, osteoporosis
- history of the diabetes mellitus, including medication, glycaemic control, family history
- detailed alcohol history—?pseudo-Cushing's syndrome
- use of steroid medications, including oral, topical and vaginal creams
- her perceptions of the condition, her worries and concerns, particularly about osteoporosis

2 Identification and use of information gathered

The candidate should be able to interpret the history and create a problem list. The objectives for the candidate are to:

- take a clear history of her symptoms and detect other clues suggestive of Cushing's syndrome
- attempt to gain an idea of a possible aetiology, e.g.

alcohol vs. pituitary (Cushing's disease) vs. an ectopic adenocorticotrophic hormone (ACTH) cause
- explain the possible diagnoses
- explain the nature of the investigations, e.g. dexamethasone tests and blood ACTH levels initially, with the possibility of scans (pituitary and adrenal)
- address her concerns regarding facial appearance, osteoporosis, and the long-term prognosis

3 Discussion related to the case

- Screening tests include 24-h urinary free cortisol, cortisol circadian rhythm (only on inpatients), overnight and low-dose dexamethasone suppression tests. If cortisol levels fail to be suppressed by low-dose dexamethasone the diagnosis of pseudo-Cushing's syndrome is unlikely, but further investigations are directed to the cause of Cushing's syndrome. Suppression of cortisol to < 50% on high dose dexamethasone suppression testing would suggest Cushing's disease (pituitary) and non-suppression would suggest either ectopic ACTH or an adrenal adenoma; in the former, ACTH level will be high and in the latter this should be suppressed. Patients with Cushing's disease show an exaggerated ACTH response to corticotrophin-releasing hormone (CRH).
- Patients with ectopic ACTH syndrome may present with a short history of weight loss with pigmented striae and pseudo-Cushing's disease resulting from alcoholism may also present with obesity with all the other features of Cushing's syndrome.
- The candidate will be expected to discuss the possible causes, including excess alcohol intake and iatrogenic

Cushing's disease caused by an excessive use of steroids and be able to discuss the three main types of Cushing's disease—pituitary, adrenal and ectopic—and outline the interventions appropriate for these diagnoses.

- Selective trans-sphenoidal resection is the treatment of choice for Cushing's disease. The remission rate for this procedure is about 80% for microadenomas but <50% for macroadenomas. After successful tumour resection, most patients experience a postoperative period of adrenal insufficiency that may last for up to 12 months. This usually requires low-dose cortisol replacement as patients experience steroid withdrawal symptoms as well as having a suppressed hypothalamic–pituitary–adrenal axis. Biochemical recurrence occurs in approximately 5% of patients in whom surgery was initially successful.

Comments on the case

Cushing's syndrome remains a difficult problem to diagnose and manage. The two difficulties, particularly in a case like this, are: (1) ascertaining whether patients have a pathological cortisol excess or a physiological disturbance of cortisol production; and (2) determining the aetiology of the cortisol excess, which can include iatrogenic administration of glucocorticoids, adrenal adenomas or carcinomas, pituitary adenomas, and ectopic sources of ACTH and CRH.

Case 49 | Weight loss and chronic diarrhoea

Candidate information

You are the SHO in a gastroenterology clinic. Mr Paul Jones has been referred to you by his GP.

Please read this letter (it should take no more than 2 min) and then continue with the consultation.

> Dear Doctor
>
> **Re: Mr Paul Jones, aged 23**
>
> Thank you for seeing Mr Jones who has returned home from India after 4 months of travelling. He complains of loss of weight and chronic diarrhoea. He has no other significant medical history and takes no medication. Please see and advise.
>
> Yours sincerely
>
> Dr G. Practitioner

You have 14 min until the patient leaves the room, followed by 1 min for reflection, before the discussion with the examiners. Be prepared to discuss the solutions to the problems posed by the case and how you might reply to the GP's letter.

Patient information

Mr Paul Jones is a 23-year-old university graduate who has just spent 4 months travelling around India. He complains of pale, bulky stools which he finds difficult to flush away and this has persisted for around 4 months. He may pass this type of stool up to four times a day and this is associated with a progressive loss of weight from around 75 kg down to 68 kg. Closer questioning reveals that he had these symptoms on and off for a few weeks before travelling to India. While in India he was generally well apart from these symptoms but he does remember one acute episode of traveller's diarrhoea 2 months into his travels. Other symptoms include occasional generalized abdominal discomfort, malaise and tiredness, particularly in the last few weeks. He has no mouth ulcers, jaundice, blood in the stools, vomiting, fever, joint pains or iritis. He has not taken any antibiotics recently, there is no family history of tuberculosis or coeliac disease and he is not aware of being in contact with anyone with tuberculosis in India. There has been no previous bowel surgery or radiotherapy and no other history of autoimmune disorders. He is heterosexual and is living with his girlfriend. He has not been exposed to any HIV risks. He does not smoke or drink alcohol.

Examiner information

1 Data gathering in the interview

A good candidate would be able to elicit:

- the timing of the onset of symptoms in relation to his trip to India
- exactly how long the symptoms have persisted for and whether they are deteriorating
- a full diarrhoea history, particularly frequency, consistency of stools, colour, difficulty in flushing away stools, presence of blood, volume (secretory diarrhoea)
- other abdominal symptoms, including pain and weight loss and any other systemic symptoms such as mouth ulcers, iritis, joint pains and fever
- possibility of infective episodes of acute traveller's diarrhoea in India
- antibiotic and laxative usage
- tuberculosis history
- previous gastrointestinal surgery or radiation therapy
- autoimmune disorders, e.g. thyroid disease, insulin-dependent diabetes, fibrosing alveolitis, rashes (e.g. dermatitis herpetiformis)
- dietary intake, especially cereals, wheat, rye and barley (coeliac disease)
- the impact of the symptoms on his life

2 Identification and use of information gathered

The candidate should be able to interpret the history and create a problem list. The objectives for the candidate are to:

- develop a differential diagnosis
- relay these possible diagnoses to the patient
- have a plan of investigations
- address any concerns the patient may have, e.g. regarding the possibility of a neoplasm

3 Discussion related to the case

- This case tests the candidate's ability to obtain a detailed history in order to assimilate a list of possible differential diagnoses. The possibilities here are: (a) malabsorption, e.g. coeliac disease, bacterial overgrowth, tropical sprue, pancreatic disease; (b) infective, e.g. bacterial (*Shigella*, *Yersinia*), protozoan (amoebic dysentery, *Giardia*, *Cryptosporidia*), tuberculosis, parasitic (*Strongyloides*), postinfective irritable bowel; (c) small bowel Crohn's disease causing malabsorption; or (d) colonic neoplasm. Irritable bowel syndrome is unlikely with the loss of weight. From the history, the symptoms started before travelling to India which makes postinfective irritable bowel unlikely—although *Giardia* can occur in the UK. Coeliac disease is the probable cause; it can present at any age.
- Investigations include FBC, U/E, LFT, serum iron, folate, vitamin B_{12}, calcium and autoantibodies for antireticulin and endomysial antibodies (coeliac) and, if positive, small bowel biopsy. If antibodies are negative, consider small bowel barium follow-up to detect Crohn's disease, diverticulae and fistulae/strictures. Stool samples for infective causes and consideration of ^{14}C-glycocholic acid breath test if bacterial overgrowth is suspected.
- All differential diagnoses cannot be fully explained at this stage and hence it will be important to arrange a follow-up appointment in order to discuss the results of investigations.

> **Comments on the case**
>
> This case typifies those clinical consultations where the diagnosis can be one of any number of conditions. It is imperative that the candidate does not bombard the patient with technical jargon and keeps the interview simple and reassuring. Explain that you will do all you can to find a cause with subsequent relevant treatment. As in any clinical situation, you must let the patient know which investigations are being performed and why, and also, if possible, when. Patients find it quite distressing to receive requests through the post for tests they are unfamiliar with.

Case 50 | **Wheeze**

Candidate information

You are the SHO in a respiratory clinic. Mr Jim Barrow has been referred to you by his GP.

Please read this letter (it should take no more than 2 min) and then continue with the consultation.

Dear Doctor

Re: Mr Jim Barrow, aged 31

Thank you for seeing Mr Barrow who has been a baker since leaving school. He had asthma as a child and has been perfectly well until last year when he noticed increasing chest tightness and wheeze, despite a trial of salbutamol and beclomethasone inhalers. Please see and advise.

Yours sincerely

Dr G. Practitioner

You have 14 min until the patient leaves the room, followed by 1 min for reflection, before the discussion with the examiners. Be prepared to discuss the solutions to the problems posed by the case and how you might reply to the GP's letter.

Patient information

Mr Barrow is a 31-year-old baker who works at one of the high street supermarkets. He had asthma as a child but 'grew out of it' at about the age of 9 years. Until a year ago he managed perfectly well with very few symptoms, although a coryzal illness would make him slightly wheezy with a feeling of tightness in the chest. He has not needed any regular inhalers until a year ago when he developed more symptoms, with wheeze and cough particularly during the morning but less so later on in the day. He has minimal sputum and no haemoptysis but has found that he is more tired, with a wheeze, when walking long distances, especially if it is cold. As a baker his shifts start at 3 a.m. and finish at 11 a.m. He was started on a beclomethasone metered dose inhaler (MDI) 200 μg two inhalations b.d. but his symptoms have persisted. His symptoms are definitely worse at work as he finds that he has some relief when he is not at work. When he was away on holiday in Spain 2 months ago, he found he hardly ever needed the inhalers. At work, the most likely allergen to be causing bronchial hypersensitivity is flour. Flour handling, for example when preparing dough, consistently causes him to wheeze and cough, whereas the exposure of flour in the actual baking areas is less troublesome. There are no extraction ventilation systems where he works and he does not wear a mask. He has no other allergic triggers apart from viruses and he does have seasonal allergic rhinitis for which he takes loratadine. He does not have a peak flow meter at home. He has no other past medical history of note and he does not smoke. He lives with his partner who also does not smoke. They have no pets at home and their house is not damp. There has been no exposure to tuberculosis. His major concerns are the continuing symptoms which are occupationally related. He has never thought of leaving his job as a baker.

Examiner information

1 Data gathering in the interview

A good candidate would be able to elicit:
- full history of the recent asthma symptoms, especially wheeze, cough, dyspnoea, haemoptysis. At what time of the day are they worse. Obtain a chronological order of the events. Ascertain any triggers such as viral illnesses, pollen, house dust mite, animal dander, etc.
- if his symptoms are occupationally related and, if so, whether his symptoms improve away from work (e.g. holidays)
- if his symptoms are occupationally related, do they come on immediately or after a time lag during the day
- what the culprit allergen is. Think about other allergens that may cause occupational asthma, e.g. isocyanates (in varnishes, paints, adhesives) and cleaning solvents at work. Ascertain exactly what he does at work, what his job is (desk job most of the time), how much exposure he gets, etc. Have his symptoms become worse over time?
- past history of allergy and atopy, e.g. asthma, allergic rhinitis, eczema. Any exposure to tuberculosis. Any history of oesophageal reflux, sinusitis
- inhaler usage, technique, number of times he has needed the salbutamol as 'rescue inhalations' at work
- other job history since leaving school
- if he has a peak flow meter at home and, if so, what his readings
- if there are any pets at home
- if he is a smoker
- concerns of the patients, e.g. of losing his job because of ill-health

2 Identification and use of information gathered

The candidate should be able to interpret the history and create a problem list. The objectives for the candidate are to:
- identify that the symptoms are occupationally related
- identify a likely allergen — the flour
- compile a list of investigations to prove or disprove occupational asthma

- discuss the consequences of having occupational asthma

3 Discussion related to the case

- Occupational asthma is caused, in whole or part, by agents encountered at work. Once occupational asthma has developed, the worker's asthma is nearly always provoked in addition by other non-specific triggers such as viral infections, cold air and exercise. Individuals with pre-existing asthma are at a higher risk of developing an occupational component and the whole pattern of asthma may be transformed and their livelihoods threatened.
- Looking for trigger factors that precipitate symptoms should be part of the assessment in all patients with asthma. All workers, irrespective of whether they are thought to be exposed or not, should be asked if their symptoms are better on days away from work and on holidays. Workers who have improvement in symptoms away from work may also improve because of avoidance of other allergens such as pets, tree pollen and moulds. Early removal of a sensitized worker from exposure has been shown to improve the prognosis, making early diagnosis particularly important.
- An in-depth occupational history needs to be taken. A chronological account of all jobs, patient exposures to the trigger and the relationship between patient exposure and the onset of symptoms should be documented. The principal points to establish are the materials to which a worker is exposed and the interval between first exposure and the onset of symptoms. If symptoms occur on first exposure, then it is probable that the material is a direct irritant; a period of symptomless exposure would favour occupational sensitization. It is relatively common for bakers to develop symptoms for the first time more than 10 years after first exposure. The problem in this case is chiefly caused by handling flour.
- Measuring lung function with spirometry in the clinic is relatively unhelpful as the individual is away from work. To obtain satisfactory physiological confirmation of occupational asthma, measurements of serial peak flows at work and at home (generally every 2 h),

during weekends and during holidays are necessary to see if the peak flows show an occupational influence.

- If occupational asthma is confirmed, issues regarding changing jobs need to be addressed and referral to an occupational physician is recommended. In an ideal world the material causing sensitization should be substituted but, if not possible, relocation within the workplace is recommended.
- In some patients symptoms may take a long time to reverse and, in a proportion, symptoms with spirometry changes persist.

Comments on the case

This case stresses the importance of taking an occupational history. It should not be underestimated how common occupational disease is, especially occupational lung disease such as asthma. Physicians should realize that one of the most common causes of occupational asthma in the UK is seen in our own workplace—endoscopy nurses exposed to glutaraldehyde.

Section E

This included a discussion about living wills, euthanasia, options for pain control and her anger at the 'delayed/missed' diagnosis
(see Experience 24, p. 314)

Station 4
Communication Skills and Ethics

Section E | **Station 4**

The assessment of communication skills and ethics and a distinct station is a new addition to the MRCP examination. In the early 1990's the Royal Colleges of Physicians started to test candidates' communication skills by including them in the viva part of the examination. The examiners were asked to engage in role-playing with the candidates and to ask them to break bad news or discuss an ethical problem while the examiner played the part of a patient or a relative. An inherent problem with such scenarios was that the examiner often played two or more roles, and changed from being a patient to an examiner and then to the patient's wife — all without notice and all to the chagrin of the candidate. This was compounded by the fact that the examiners, mostly reluctant at playing these roles, could not play them with any degree of conviction. As the entire examination was being reshaped, the Colleges took this opportunity of formalizing the assessment in the form of Station 4. Now you will find a real actor who displays all the appropriate emotions. The examiners watch the interaction for 14 minutes without interfering and then, after a minute for reflection as the person leaves the Station, they discuss the issues raised in the remaining 5 minutes. Although candidates face this Station with considerable anxiety, and the experiment is in its early stages, we have heard few complaints about the conduct and fairness of this encounter.

This Station is about role-playing, both for the actor who plays a patient, relative or a healthcare professional and for you who should have little difficulty in playing a sensitive doctor! You must understant that this Station is not a test of knowledge of the condition under discussion but a test of communication. Although some knowledge of the ethical issues surrounding such scenarios is important, the essence of the interview is that you should conduct it with the appropriate sensitivity and empathy.

The word empathy (from German *einflügen*, penetration) is described in the New Collins English Dictionary as 'the power of understanding and imaginatively entering into another person's feelings'. You have to put yourself in the other person's position and see how you would receive the news that you are about to give him. It is a continuous, four-dimensional process — kinetic (body language: do not appear casual, stiff or uninterested), emotional (appear sympathetic), tactile (e.g. a warm handshake), and verbal (words of comfort). You should not only say that you are sorry, but also show sadness in your countenance and respond sympathetically to any emotional reaction; for example, by holding her hand or offering a box of tissues if she cries.

You will have had some experience of such interviews in your clinical practice and you can now improve upon it by studying and playing out the 50 scenarios given in this Section. We have covered a diverse range of problems that physicians encounter in their clinical practice. Even if you are faced with a problem not given here it will be very similar to one of the scenarios in this book and the principles will be the same. Study each scenario and then play it out with a fellow candidate.

In the exam, in addition to a warm and sympathetic demeanour which you should maintain throughout, there are some basic principles that you should observe when counselling or breaking bad news to a patient. The points listed here apply to all professional interviews but are especially important when discussing a sensitive subject.

- You will be given written instructions during the 5-minute interval before you enter Station 4. Read the scenario carefully, identify the principal problem and work out your approach.
- Greet the person and verify that they are the person that you are supposed to meet. This is the first step in playing this scenario, as you would do in real life.
- Find out how much the person knows about the problem in question. This can be established through a couple of preliminary sentences and provides the base on which you can build your communication. His response can also give you some idea of his level of understanding and conversational ability. For example, you may start by saying, 'Your father was admitted yesterday with pneumonia. May I know what you were told and how much you know about this condition?' His response, whatever it is, will provide you with an easy beginning to detailing subsequent events. For a patient to whom you are going to tell that he has a lymphoma, you may start with a gentle enquiry, 'Since you were told that you had some glands in your chest which were visible on the X-ray, we have done some more investigations. Do you have any idea what we have been looking for?' Even if he says he has no idea you can tell him more about the glands and then build on that.
- Develop a dialogue and encourage the person to ask questions. Do not give information in long chunks as if you want to unburden yourself and be done with it as quickly as possible. Use pauses in strategic places to allow the person to make a guess or to ask a question. For example, you should give a long pause after you say, 'I'm afraid I have some bad news to share with you.' The person may say, 'Is it cancer, doctor?'
- Do not hurry and force the information before the person is ready to receive it. Allow the person to dictate the pace of the interview. A useful method is to give two or three bits of information and then summarize by saying, 'So far I have told you . . . Did you understand all that and do you have any questions?'
- Give bad news with compassion and sensitivity. A useful ploy is to find a 'but' for every piece of bad news. The purpose is not to give incorrect information or to make light of the gravity of a serious disease, but rather to find some words of comfort to accompany the bad news. For example, when telling someone that she has multiple sclerosis, you may add, 'I can't disguise the fact that it is an unpleasant thing to have or that it is incurable, but many people with this live a long and active life.' To someone whom you have just said that he has a lymphoma, you may say, 'Yes, it is a form of cancer but there are many treatment options available.'
- Be honest and accept if either you or one of your colleagues has made a mistake. If you do not know something the person wants to know then say so, 'I'm sorry I do not know this but I will find it out for you.' Explain any legal and ethical issues with honesty and clarity, 'I'm afraid you are barred from driving for one year. This is a legal requirement and I am obliged to advise you that you should inform the DVLA and your insurance company. I will have to write it in your notes that I have advised you.'
- Maintain eye contact throughout the interview.
- Address the tasks set in the message and explain if you have to take any action.
- Make follow-up arrangements so that the person will have an opportunity to ask you more questions after he has had time to consider the problem. If necessary, offer to arrange a second opinion.
- Be polite and courteous throughout.
- Be prepared to discuss the case and its ethical dilemmas with the examiners.

Case 1 | A colleague with hepatitis B infection

Candidate information

You are the medical SHO

Please read this summary (it should take no more than 2 min) and then continue with the consultation.

Re: Dr Alikhan Fahad, aged 26

Your friend, Dr Alikhan Fahad, is a surgical house officer where you work. He's a bright and career-minded young doctor who has recently been appointed to the local teaching hospital surgical SHO rotation. He tells you that an occupational health hepatitis B test has found him to be hepatitis surface antigen (HBsAg) positive. He is from overseas and has never had hepatitis B immunization. His initial jobs were all locums and his vaccination status had never been verified. He is clearly upset and cannot understand how he has acquired the virus. He wants to speak to you for more advice.

Your tasks are to: counsel him about his recent positive finding with an explanation of the results, advise on how this may affect his career and what he needs to do next.

You have 14 min until the colleague leaves the room, followed by 1 min for reflection, before the discussion with the examiners.

Subject/patient/relative information

Dr Alikhan Fahad is a young surgical house officer who has trained overseas. He has shown diligent application and has got on to the local teaching hospital SHO surgical rotation and he intends to take all his postgraduate exams. He had an occupational health hepatitis B test which has shown him to be hepatitis B surface S antigen positive (HBsAg). The results also state that he has no HBe markers but that further tests are necessary. He is clearly upset by this as it may affect his future career. He does not know exactly where he may have acquired the virus, possibly from needlestick injuries while carrying out surgery abroad. His initial vaccination verification had somehow slipped through the net. He is a good friend of the medical SHO (the candidate) and wants further advice. He wants to know the real implications of his blood test and what the effect will be on his career.

Examiner information

1 Communication skills—conduct of interview

- Show empathy and compassion, as he must be concerned for his health and career.
- Ask him if he has any idea where he may have acquired the virus from.
- Ask what type of surgery he has assisted with in the past and whether he has had any needlestick injuries.
- Does he have a partner and, if so, has he or she been immunized?

- Discuss with him the importance of ensuring that his partner is informed and screened.
- Reassure him that confidentiality will be paramount but that the occupational health physician may have to decide on contact-tracing of patients at risk.
- Ask if he knows if he is HBeAg positive, anti-HBe negative or has no HBe markers.
- Explain that if he is HBeAg positive, he would have restrictions imposed on his practice.
- If he is anti-HBe negative or has no HBe markers, he will have hepatitis B virus (HBV) DNA genome levels measured. If this is $>10^3$/ml then restrictions will be imposed. If it is $<10^3$/ml then he will have to have levels tested annually but no restrictions will be imposed.
- Tell him if HBV DNA genome levels are above 10^3/ml, he will be restricted in carrying out procedures where there is a risk that injury to the healthcare worker could result in their blood contaminating a patient's open tissues. This would include where a worker's gloved hands may be in contact with sharp instruments, needle tips or sharp tissues (e.g. bone spicules or teeth) inside a patient's open body cavity, wound or confined anatomical space where hands or fingertips may not be visible at all times. This would obviously include open surgical techniques.
- Tell him that you appreciate how difficult this news is and that it has serious implications for his surgical career. Ask him how this makes him feel.
- Tell him that he would have to tell his consultant and he must cease to perform any surgery until properly assessed by the occupational health physician.
- Explain that he may have to retrain in a low-risk specialty if his practice is restricted.
- He would need to tell medical staff at his future hospital.
- The occupational health physician may advise a referral to a hepatologist for a specialist clinical assessment.

2 Communication skills — exploration and problem negotiation

The candidate should be able to:
- show empathy, as his friend is clearly devastated
- explain the meaning of the results
- reassure him about the maintenance of his confidentiality within the parameters of protecting any patients that he has had surgical contact with
- explain what the occupational health physicians will do next

- advise on the possible impact on his surgical career, suggest that he may want to get emotional support during this process and that Occupational Health may be able to help with this

3 Ethics and the law and other discussion points (recommendations from the Department of Health)

- All hepatitis B infected healthcare workers who are e-antigen negative and who perform exposure-prone procedures or clinical duties in renal units must be tested for viral load (HBV DNA).
- Those who are e-antigen negative and have a viral load exceeding 10^3 genome equivalents per millilitre must not perform exposure-prone procedures in the future. Those workers whose viral load does not exceed 10^3 genome equivalents per millilitre need not have their working practices restricted, but must be retested at 12-monthly intervals. Research has shown that viral loads in some infected individuals may fluctuate over time. If viral load exceeds the specified level or if investigation of a case of hepatitis B in a patient indicates the possibility of a transmission from the healthcare worker, then continuing exposure-prone procedures must cease.
- Hepatitis B infected healthcare workers should not continue to perform exposure-prone procedures while on interferon or antiviral therapy. Those who have undergone a course of such treatment need to show that they have a viral load not exceeding 10^3 genome equivalents per millilitre 1 year after cessation of treatment, before a return to unrestricted working practice can be considered.
- Healthcare workers without the e-antigen, and who are refusing to have their viral load tested, should not be allowed to carry out exposure-prone procedures in the future.
- Arrangements should be made to provide individual healthcare workers with access to a consultant occupational health physician.
- All hepatitis B infected healthcare workers should be given accurate and detailed advice on ways of minimizing the risk of transmission in the healthcare setting and to close contacts.
- It is important that such individuals receive the same right of confidentiality as any patient seeking or receiving medical care. The employer may need to be advised that a change of duties should take place, but hepatitis B status itself will not be normally disclosed without the consent of the individual. However, where patients

are, or have been, at risk it may be necessary in the public interest for the employer to have access to confidential information.

- Employers should make every effort to arrange suitable alternative work and offer retraining opportunities. Postgraduate medical and dental deans also have an important role in retraining or redeploying affected doctors.
- The NHS injury benefits scheme and the Industrial Injuries Disablement benefit scheme provide benefits where hepatitis B has been occupationally acquired.

Department of Health. *Hepatitis B infected health service workers: guidance on implementation of health service circular 2000/020.* 2000.

Comments on the case

This case demonstrates the occupational ethical dilemmas facing a colleague with hepatitis B. One must show sympathy and treat the colleague with the utmost confidentiality. Any careless mutterings in the doctor's mess can be disastrous. In this situation your colleague is entitled to the same respect for privacy and confidentiality that one gives to any patient.

Case 2 | Apologizing for a delay with investigative management

Candidate information

You are the medical SHO in the outpatient clinic

Please read this summary (it should take no more than 2 min) and then continue with the consultation.

> **Re: Mr Terry Palmer, aged 65**
>
> Mr Palmer presented with haemoptysis 5 weeks ago. A chest X-ray showed a right hilar mass and bronchoscopy a week later confirmed the presence of a squamous cell carcinoma in the right upper lobe bronchus. Mr Palmer is a fit man who would be able to tolerate resection. It has been 4 weeks since a staging CT scan of the thorax and upper abdomen was requested. He has not yet had any information about a date. He is naturally angry and wants to show his displeasure to you in clinic.

Your tasks are to: acknowledge the unacceptable delay and propose a plan to rectify this.

You have 14 min until the patient leaves the room, followed by 1 min for reflection, before the discussion with the examiners.

Subject/patient/relative information

Mr Terry Palmer is a fit 65-year-old smoker who has been diagnosed as having right upper lobe bronchial carcinoma. He has been told that he needs a staging CT scan of his chest and abdomen to enable doctors to decide if it would be suitable for resection. He feels fit and ready for surgery but is having to wait for the CT — now having waited for 4 weeks. He is clearly displeased and, as each day goes by, he feels his cancer is spreading. His biggest fear is finding that he is inoperable when he may have been operable 4 weeks ago. He is totally unimpressed with the delay, particularly with the recent media coverage regarding cancer patients waiting for treatment. He feels extremely let down by the system. He is seeing the medical SHO (the candidate) in clinic today to express his disappointment.

Examiner information

1 Communication skills — conduct of interview

- Introduce yourself to Mr Palmer.
- Allow him to voice his anger. Acknowledge the delay and express your concern.

- Tell him you are very disappointed that the scan date has not been arranged, acknowledging that the scan is essential in the work-up of his cancer. Apologize for the delay and make him feel that you are genuinely concerned.
- Check his address (sometimes the wrong address is put on the request card).

- Attempt to speak to a radiologist now while he is in the clinic so that maybe a date can be obtained before he leaves. If you are unable to contact him offer the patient the choice of remaining in clinic until you can do so or take down his telephone number so that you can ring him later *today*.

2 Communication skills—exploration and problem negotiation

The candidate should be able to:
- listen attentively and patiently to the patient's concerns
- agree with the patient that the delay is unacceptable
- formulate a plan of action which is mutually acceptable to rectify the situation

3 Ethics and the law and other discussion points

- Newly diagnosed lung cancer patients who are considered for surgery must have an urgent staging scan to decide if resection is feasible. The staging scan would show metastases (e.g. other lung, liver, renal, adrenal), determine the extent of lymphadenopathy and determine the size of the tumour and its position (e.g. whether adjacent to a large vessel).
- The patient is frightened. He is depending on you for help. Any criticisms are not personal and must not be taken personally.
- You must be seen to care and to take an active role in rectifying the problem, his confidence and trust are already undermined and if you fail he will lose all confidence in you.
- Openly criticizing the radiology department is unprofessional and will be counterproductive. However, Mr Palmer should be free to voice his own opinion.

Comments on the case

Unfortunately this is a very common scenario and all doctors must develop the ability to sit and listen to patients complaining about the health system. We must all be able to show that we care and so acknowledge the complaint with empathy. Listening will go a long way to allow the patient to feel that we are on their side. The doctor dealing with the complaint must provide a plan to tackle the problem/complaint. In this case, there may be a reason for the delay, e.g. request card not filled in, wrong address, patient did not receive scan date, CT scanner broken down, no staff available to perform CT session, scan not reported, etc. Unless the doctor makes an effort to sort it out there and then, nothing will get done. You must let your consultant know, you must speak personally face to face with the radiologist (avoid phone messages), and then ring the patient back immediately to let him know of any resolutions if you are unable to sort it out in the clinic.

A factual note of the situation and your action plan should be written in the notes. Avoid documenting it as a complaint—complaints made by patients should not be held in patients' notes as this could prejudice future care if the patient is flagged as a complainer (however justified).

As there may well be a systems fault an Adverse or Clinical Incident report form must be completed and forwarded to the Trust Risk Manager and this information should be conveyed to the patient.

Adverse Incident reporting is beneficial as it identifies what needs to be done and minimizes the possibility of recurrence.

If the patient wishes to formally complain then obtain the contact information for him to do so.

Case 3 | Asking for a postmortem

Candidate information

You are the medical SHO

Please read this summary (it should take no more than 2 min) and then continue with the consultation.

Re: Mr Stanley Patton, aged 73

Mr Stanley Patton was a 73-year-old man admitted 5 days ago with respiratory failure. He was known to have renal failure, chronic obstructive pulmonary disease (COPD) and ischaemic heart disease and he used to smoke 40 cigarettes a day. A chest X-ray showed a left basal pneumonia which was treated in the usual, appropriate way. Discussions with the patient, the next of kin (his daughter, Mrs Nolan) and the ITU consultant resulted in a decision not to ventilate the patient. Over the next 5 days he remained reasonably stable, but still poorly. Unfortunately, last night he collapsed in the toilet and died, despite attempts at resuscitation. You were quite upset to hear this from your SHO colleague who was on call last night. You decide to review his X-rays and looking at the chest X-ray you feel that there may in fact have been a bronchial carcinoma behind the heart which was technically missed. You speak to your consultant and he suggests asking for the daughter's permission for a hospital postmortem to decide if: (a) Mr Patton died from a pulmonary embolism; and (b) whether Mr Patton had a bronchial carcinoma which was missed by the team. If the daughter refuses permission, your consultant is happy for you to write the death certificate anyway.

Your tasks are to: ask the patient's daughter, Mrs Nolan, for permission to arrange a hospital postmortem.

You have 14 min until the daughter leaves the room, followed by 1 min for reflection, before the discussion with the examiners.

Subject/patient/relative information

Mr Patton has had a long history of renal failure, COPD and ischaemic heart disease. He was admitted 5 days ago with pneumonia. It was decided, with the ITU consultants, that Mr Patton would not be a candidate for assisted ventilation, although he was for resuscitation. Mrs Nolan is his daughter and next of kin. She was aware of her father's poor condition but it came as a real shock to be told that her father collapsed and died last night. She is taking the news bravely and realistically and is very grateful for the care provided. She has been told by the SHO on call last night that the probable cause of death was the pneumonia. She has accepted this and wants no further fuss. She has come to the hospital for the death certificate and she is quite keen to take this to the Registrar of Deaths in town today and to arrange the funeral plans. She is slightly surprised to see the medical SHO (the candidate) who has been looking after her father during this admission. The SHO asks her if she would give permission for a post-mortem. She becomes distressed and says 'No'. However, with gentle persuasion she agrees that you can give her any information she requires. She wants to know when, where and by whom will the postmortem be performed, will the body be disfigured, will she find out the results and whether any organs or tissues will be retained. Despite all the counselling by the SHO, she cannot bear the thought of a postmortem and wants to proceed with the funeral arrangements.

Examiner information

1 Communication skills—conduct of interview

- Tell Mrs Nolan how sorry you are to hear about the sudden death of her father and that all the staff looking after him are saddened by the news. Pause to allow Mrs Nolan to express her emotions.
- Explain that he was very sick when he came in with pneumonia and that despite the medical and nursing teams' best efforts he continued to remain poorly.
- Tell her, however, that you and your consultant were surprised by the suddenness of his death. Explain that it is possible he may have had a pulmonary embolism (explain this with minimal jargon) and that you are also concerned he may have had lung cancer—although you are not sure on either point.
- Pause and give her a chance to absorb this new piece of information. Be prepared for her to challenge why you have only just discovered that he may have had cancer.
- Ask her how important it is for her to find out whether or not her father had cancer.
- Go on to explain that one way of knowing exactly what may have caused the sudden deterioration is a post-mortem—ask her how she feels about this. Ask her what she understands about a postmortem and ask her how much detail she would like you to give her about the postmortem procedure.
- Ask if she knows if the patient himself had any known objection towards a postmortem before this illness.
- Discuss what a postmortem is and what the benefits of one are.
- If she feels uneasy about a full postmortem then explain that if she prefers she could perhaps agree to a limited postmortem of the chest only.
- Tell her when it would be performed, where and by whom.
- Reassure her that the body would not be disfigured.
- Reassure her that funeral arrangements would not necessarily be delayed.

- Explain that if something suspicious is found, e.g. lung cancer, then unless there is a specific objection this organ may be retained to confirm the diagnosis and possibly used for educational or research purposes. If she objects, then reassure her again that in this case another option is for the tissue of interest to be fixed and examined and returned to the body before release. Reassure her again that organs would not be retained.
- Explain that she will be asked to sign a consent form and that she will be informed in writing if any organs or tissues are retained if she agrees.
- Recommendations for changes in the current practice of removal, retention and use of human organs and tissues from postmortem examination has been provided by the Chief Medical Officer.
- Tell her that, if she wishes, she can obtain the results of the postmortem as the results are sent to the consultant looking after her father, and she can arrange an appointment with him to have the findings explained.
- Ask her if she has any other concerns and ask how she feels about a postmortem—she may say 'yes' or 'no'.
- If she says 'no', tell her that you will respect this decision wholeheartedly and will issue a death certificate straight away. Explain what you are going to write on the certificate: 1A respiratory failure; 1B pneumonia; 1C chronic obstructive pulmonary disease; 2 renal failure, ischaemic heart disease.
- Do not forget to let your consultant know of the outcome.

2 Communication skills—exploration and problem negotiation

The candidate should be able to:
- transmit his or her sympathy to the daughter
- explain that it is not absolutely certain what caused the death, giving the possibilities
- counsel the daughter about postmortem procedure, taking care to be led by her as to how specific she wants the information about the procedure to be
- support the daughter whatever her decision

3 Ethics and the law and other discussion points (The Royal College of Pathologists. *Guidelines for the retention of tissues and organs at postmortem examination.* March 2000)

General comments

- Organ and tissue retention at hospital postmortem examinations is currently an issue attracting public attention and is subject to independent inquiries. There are concerns surrounding the standards and practices relating to the retention and disposal of organs and tissue, in particular communication and policies for obtaining 'consent' for the retention of human materials.
- The legislation and guidance for the NHS Trust pathology services is covered by the Human Tissue Act (1961) and the Chief Medical Officer's (CMO) Interim Guidance (May 2000). Chapter 54 of the Human Tissue Act (1961) states the conditions for the removal of body parts and the conduct of postmortem examinations. The person lawfully in possession of the body may authorize the removal from the body of any part or specified part for use in accordance with the request of the deceased made while living OR if there is *no* reason to believe, having made reasonable enquiry, that the deceased expressed an objection or had subsequently withdrawn any request or if the relatives of the deceased object to this.
- The Act does not mention the requirement for the relatives of the deceased to provide their consent to a postmortem examination, only that they do not object, and nor does the Act specify how the wishes of relatives are established or recorded.
- The CMO's Interim Guidance makes a number of recommendations for obtaining consent for hospital postmortems through a signed form which includes:
  (a) clear written information about what the examination entails and why it is required
  (b) agreement to the postmortem and options to limit the examination
  (c) information about why and which organ and tissues may be retained including: (i) an agreement or not to the retention of tissue samples or body fluids for laboratory investigation to establish a cause of death and to study the effects of treatment; and (ii) agreement or not to the retention of organs or body parts and options to specify which organs or body parts relatives would prefer not to be retained
  (d) how this might impact on the funeral arrangements
  (e) clear information about where any retained organs and tissues are stored, why, for how long and arrangements for reunion with the body before the burial or how the relatives want organs, tissues or body parts disposed of following the postmortem examination
  (f) whether retention for longer periods for diagnosis, training, research or legal reason is required or unlimited retention for medical education or research
  (g) details on who is agreeing to the postmortem, their relationship to the deceased, who obtained and witnessed the agreement, their position within the trust and contact details with the date of the agreement.

The Removal, Retention and use of Human Organs and Tissue from Postmortem Examination. Advice from the Chief Medical Officer. Department of Health, 2001.

What is a postmortem examination?

- This is a careful internal examination of the person who has just died and can give valuable information about an illness and its effects on the body. It may tell us more precisely why the person has died but even the most detailed postmortem investigations often leave some questions unanswered.
- Postmortem examinations are carried out by a pathologist, who is a doctor specializing in the laboratory study of disease and of diseased tissue, assisted by a technician who is a person with the specialist training needed to assist pathologists. They are carried out with special facilities provided in the hospital mortuary. Pathologists perform postmortem examinations to standards set by the Royal College of Pathologists in a respectful manner and with regard for the feelings of the bereaved.
- The pathologist will first carry out an external examination of the body. The internal part of the examination begins with an incision made down the front of the body and the internal organs are taken out for a detailed examination. When the brain is examined, an incision is made in the scalp at the base of the head. Small tissue samples are usually kept for further investigation under a microscope. When detailed laboratory investigations require body parts or organs to be kept, the relative will be asked to give their written agreement.

Benefits of a postmortem examination

- A postmortem examination can give valuable information about an illness and its effects on the body and may explain the cause of death. This information can make it easier for the family members to come to terms with the death. Postmortem examinations can provide valuable information which helps doctors to treat other patients with the same kind of illness and can provide vital information for research.

Full or limited postmortem examination

- If the relative agrees to a postmortem examination, the doctor will issue the medical certificate of death before the postmortem so that they can proceed with the arrangements for the funeral.
- A full examination involves detailed examination of all the internal organs including brain, heart, lungs, liver, kidneys, intestines, blood vessels and the small glands which are all removed from the body, examined and returned to the body.
- If relatives feel uncomfortable with a full examination, an alternative is a limited examination where those organs directly related to the illness are examined. This would mean that no information about the other organs, which may have contributed to the death, would be known.

When will the postmortem be carried out and will it delay the funeral?

- As soon as possible within 2–3 working days. The actual examination takes about 3 h. Laboratory investigations, which are carried out after the postmortem, can take several weeks.
- Funeral arrangements need not be delayed. The body will be released to the undertaker on the day of the postmortem, unless the examination is performed late in the afternoon. If relatives wish the organs to be reunited after laboratory analysis, then this may delay the funeral as some laboratory analyses take several weeks.

Will the body be disfigured?

- After the postmortem the technician will prepare the body for relatives to see again if they wish. The internal incision in the centre of the body cannot be seen when the body is dressed. The scalp incision, if the brain has been examined, will be concealed by the hair at the back of the head.

Why may an organ be kept?

- When a postmortem examination is first discussed, the relative may be asked if the pathologist can keep a specific organ, such as the heart, to enable medical staff to carry out further examination. The pathologist, on behalf of the hospital, becomes the custodian of the organ which is kept in a safe place under secure conditions in the hospital. The identity of the organ and the diagnosis are confidential.
- Often the doctors keep the organ indefinitely, which allows the opportunity to learn important information about the underlying condition and its treatment both now and in the future. If in the future relatives change their mind, then the hospital must dispose of the organ in the legal and proper manner or return it to the relative for cremation or burial as they wish.
- The reasons why pathologists may wish to keep an organ, tissue or body parts include:
  (a) to determine the cause of death
  (b) specific current research projects
  (c) archiving for future research projects
  (d) medical museums for the education and training of medical students and doctors
  (e) discussions between other clinicians and pathologists
- Relatives may:
  (a) wish to ask about the implications of agreeing to these uses
  (b) like to ask whether tissue, parts or organs will be sent to medical museums, or used for genetic research
  (c) wish to know whether parts will be sent to another laboratory, to tissue or organ banks or abroad
- If relatives do not wish an organ to be kept indefinitely, they may be asked whether they would allow it to be kept for several weeks so that the pathologist and other doctors can examine it in detail before issuing the postmortem report. The hospital can respectfully dispose of the organ or return it to the relative for cremation or burial.
- It is important that if relatives do not wish an organ to be retained they inform the doctor when permission is obtained for the postmortem examination. It is important to record on a specifically prepared consent form what relatives do agree to.

Comments on the case

Postmortem examinations and tissue/organ retention is an important ethical issue and all candidates must be comfortable at requesting one. The above enables the candidate to develop a script for obtaining consent from a relative.

Ideally, one would wish to devote more than 14 minutes to a relative in these situations. Remember to offer the relatives additional support at this time, a skilled nurse (not necessarily qualified) from the ward or a hospital chaplain or personal spiritual supporter may be very helpful to the relative at this time.

In the wake of the Alder Hey and Bristol heart babies enquiry and reports, many members of the public have become increasingly suspicious about the validity and openness of practices around postmortem and organ tissue retention.

Clinicians should also be aware that a sudden revelation, so soon after death, that a patient may have had an illness which the team 'missed' might invoke more anger and grief. It may be prudent to offer relatives the opportunity to discuss why this may have happened at the time of their choosing and ask your Consultant or Registrar to conduct this meeting.

Another scenario that may arise is requesting a coroner's postmortem (Procurator Fiscal in Scotland) which may be requested to investigate:

- sudden and unexplained death
- deaths where the cause is unknown and the doctor cannot issue a death certificate
- deaths occurring during an operation
- death where the cause of death is known to be, or suspected to be, a result of causes other than natural disease (e.g. accidents, industrial diseases, violence or neglect, drug poisoning, occurring in police custody)

The coroner is an independent officer with statutory responsibility for the legal investigation of the above categories of death. The candidate must explain that the doctor has discussed the case with the coroner, and the coroner will ask a pathologist to carry out a postmortem examination. Details with regard to the postmortem procedure have to be relayed to the relatives concerned. The examination findings will be sent to the coroner who will then issue a death certificate. A representative of the coroner will contact the family to tell them when to proceed with funeral arrangements. If an inquest is required, it will be opened and then adjourned to allow the funeral to take place.

Case 4 | Bleeding varices in a Jehovah's Witness

Candidate information

You are the medical SHO on call

Please read this summary (it should take no more than 2 min) and then continue with the consultation.

Re: Mr Ronald Harrington, aged 61

Mr Harrington is a patient with known chronic liver disease and portal hypertension resulting from haemochromatosis and he has been admitted from clinic because of feeling generally unwell with numerous episodes of melaena over the last 10 days. A clinic blood sample revealed a haemoglobin of 5.0 g/dL. Your consultant has asked you to cross-match him for 5 units and to put him on the endoscopy list. However, the patient tells you that he is a Jehovah's Witness and he has strong views against blood transfusions.

Your tasks are to: explain clearly the nature of the patient's present illness, explain why a blood transfusion is medically in his best interests while taking into account his religious views and discuss any possible alternatives to blood transfusion.

You have 14 min until the patient leaves the room, followed by 1 min for reflection, before the discussion with the examiners.

Subject/patient/relative information

Mr Ronald Harrington is a 61-year-old man who follows the Jehovah's Witness faith. He was diagnosed as having haemochromatosis 10 years ago and now has progressed to cirrhosis with portal hypertension. During the last 10 days he has had numerous episodes of melaena although he did not call the GP or come to casualty as he knew what the outcome would be—a blood transfusion. However, he did keep the outpatient appointment today. The consultant has decided to admit him for an endoscopy for suspected oesophageal variceal bleeding. The result of his haemoglobin test is 5 g/dL and the biggest concern for the consultant is a possible life-threatening haemorrhage in the presence of the anaemia. However, Mr Harrington does not wish to have a blood transfusion because of his faith and he acknowledges that death may result if he does have a massive haemorrhage. He is due to see the SHO (the candidate) with regard to his admission and he or she must explain the seriousness of his condition to him.

Examiner information

1 Communication skills—conduct of interview

- You should interview the patient with a colleague.
- The patient should be offered the opportunity to have a relative or religious adviser present (Jehovah's Witnesses can provide counsellors at short notice if you apply either through a local Jehovah's Witness Hospital Liaison Committee or to the local congregation). If you have difficulty contacting them, then utilize the Hospital Chaplain or ask the switchboard for assistance.
- Explain to Mr Harrington the full nature of his present illness and that the reason he is feeling unwell is because of a low blood count caused by the continuous loss of blood.
- Tell the patient that the best and most efficient way to replete the haemoglobin count is through a blood transfusion.
- Acknowledge his religious position and ask whether or not he will consider a blood transfusion.
- Ask him to let you explain the benefits of the blood transfusion, and the possible hazards if he does not agree to the course of action you recommend, i.e. that he is at risk of dying if he has a large haemorrhage in the absence of a blood transfusion in his present condition. You should attempt to help the patient understand the reasons for your recommendation.
- If he is unable to agree with your recommendation draw his attention to the clause on the consent form giving him the right to list the procedures that he does not consent to.
- You should also make a note of the precise nature of the restriction placed upon you by the patient.
- Tell him that although he is declining to accept a specific aspect of treatment, it does not take away his right to reasonable and proper care.
- The patient may decline treatment when he needs it, either in person or through an advance directive, e.g. the card carried by a Jehovah's Witness.
- Questions occasionally arise about whether the patient's refusal to accept treatment is free of duress from another relative. In these circumstances, consent or refusal could not be said to be voluntary. However, if it is not possible to determine duress his 'choice' remains sacrosanct.
- Document all that has been discussed and talk over the case with your consultant. He or she may want to speak to the defence union for medicolegal advice.

2 Communication skills—exploration and problem negotiation

The candidate should be able to:
- express the reasons for the patient's present illness and explain that a further large gastrointestinal haemorrhage, in the presence of such a low haemoglobin count, may be life-threatening
- explore the patient's religious beliefs with respect
- explain where the patient and carer stand legally if he declines a blood transfusion

3 Ethics and the law and other discussion points

- The courts have ruled that a mentally competent adult has an absolute right to refuse to consent to medical treatment for any reason, rational or irrational, or for no reason at all, even where the decision may lead to his own death. A competent adult has this right even if others, including doctors, believe that the refusal is neither reasonable nor in his best interests.
- Despite the difficulties caused by such restrictions, a doctor's legal and ethical responsibilities towards a patient do not change. Such restrictions do not relieve a doctor of the duty to provide other essential treatment. A refusal to treat the patient would only be acceptable if this posed no additional risk to the patient and a colleague was available to take over the patient's care.
- However, Jehovah's Witnesses' religious understanding does not absolutely prohibit the use of components such as albumin, immunoglobulins and haemophilia preparations; and each Witness may decide individually if he wishes to accept these.
- Witnesses believe that blood removed from the body should be disposed, so they do not accept autotransfusion of predeposited blood. Techniques for intraoperative collection or haemodilution that involve blood storage are objectionable to them. However, many Witnesses permit the use of dialysis and heart–lung equipment (non-blood-prime) as well as intraoperative salvage where the extracorporeal circulation is uninterrupted; the physician should consult with the individual patient as to what his conscience dictates. Under ideal protection of medical confidentiality, decisions on blood transfusion made by a patient who is a Jehovah's Witness would be known only to the patient, their chosen representative, and the medical team. If the patient personally believes that the decision to receive blood com-

ponents, of which the church disapproves, does not violate God's commandment, as some dissident Witnesses do, then he could remain silent about the decision and continue his membership provided that medical confidentiality is fully protected. There is no defence for any member of the clinical team discussing the situation with other members of the congregation. Under the previous policy, any suspicion of receiving blood would prompt a judicial committee which could elicit an involuntary confession from the patient and result in his expulsion from the fellowship.

Comments on the case

A Jehovah's Witness declining a blood transfusion can cause a real ethical dilemma and awareness of the patient's rights in the absence of incapacity must be realized. Support from the consultant and one's defence union is vital. The candidate will be expected to be able to discuss the other possible treatment options, such as recombinant erythropoietin, intravenous iron infusion and nutritional support, e.g. folate and vitamin B_{12}.

Utilizing patient advocates or representatives, Jehovah's Witness Hospital Liaison Committee members, where available, will help to ensure that the patient feels supported and that the clinical team have a factual knowledge base of the patient's position and what alternatives may be available.

Case 5 | Blood transfusion

Candidate information

You are the medical SHO in clinic

Please read this summary (it should take no more than 2 min) and then continue with the consultation.

Re: Mr Edgar Madeley, aged 82

Mr Madeley has been referred because of tiredness and a normocytic normochromic anaemia. His haemoglobin count is 7. 2 g/dL. Investigations have included a normal upper gastrointestinal endoscopy and a barium enema which only revealed mild diverticulosis in the large bowel. The consultant wonders whether the anaemia may be caused by myelodysplasia in the presence of normal haematinics and no obvious gastrointestinal pathology. He suggests offering a blood transfusion of 2 units.

Your tasks are to: explain the results of the tests and offer him a blood transfusion.

You have 14 min until the patient leaves the room, followed by 1 min for reflection, before the discussion with the examiners.

Subject/patient/relative information

Mr Madeley, an 82-year-old gentleman, was found to be anaemic by the GP 3 weeks ago and he was subsequently referred to the clinic for investigations. He is essentially well apart from tiredness but the consultant physician wanted to rule out a gastrointestinal malignancy. A barium enema has shown mild diverticulosis only and an upper gastrointestinal endoscopy was normal. The consultant is keen to give 2 units of blood to the patient. The patient does not have any major objections to the blood transfusion but he wants to be certain that the transfusion is in his best interests and that having a blood transfusion is safe. He wants to speak to the medical SHO (the candidate) to discuss this.

Examiner information

1 Communication skills — conduct of interview

- Introduce yourself to Mr Madeley.
- Ask how he is.
- Explain that now he has had the tests carried out you want to explain the results and discuss with him the treatment plan you want him to consider. (Adopting this approach demonstrates that you are working in partnership with the patient).
- Say that it is unlikely that the diverticulosis itself would have caused the anaemia but it is possible that the bone marrow is not as active as previously and so less blood cells are being produced, contributing to the anaemia.
- Say that the best way to treat this is to give blood through a transfusion. Explain what a normal blood count is and say that, as a result of his anaemia, he has been getting symptoms of tiredness.
- Ask how he feels about having a blood transfusion.
- He says he is not sure and wants to know the risks.

- Reassure him that the blood is being offered in the best interests of his health and that the advantages of having blood is that his improved blood count would help improve the symptoms of tiredness.
- Explain that there is no suitable alternative in terms of tablets to reverse the anaemia.
- Appreciate his concerns but say that in the UK a blood transfusion is safe and that strict regulations are in place to ensure that wrong blood is not given, i.e. checking that the correct blood type is correctly cross-matched, checking patient identification labels with the labels on the blood bag, etc.
- Reassure him that in the UK all blood donated is checked for viruses such as HIV, hepatitis B and C and the risk of contracting an infection is extremely small.
- Other risks with a blood transfusion include allergic reactions to the blood which presents with an itch and weals within minutes of commencing the transfusion. Reassure that if this happens, treatment is available to counter it.
- Again reassure him that a blood transfusion is safe and if he decides to have the blood transfusion then you can arrange a date for this to be carried out with the prospect of going home the same day after a post-transfusion blood test. He will then be seen again in clinic to have the blood count checked. Say that there is a chance that he will become anaemic again and so he may need blood transfusions several times a year.
- Ask if he has any questions and remind him that if he remains unsure he has time to think about it. Offer him a contact point in case he needs more information before deciding whether or not to go ahead.

2 Communication skills — exploration and problem negotiation

The candidate should be able to:
- describe the results of the tests
- explain why the patient may have anaemia
- explain that to treat the anaemia he needs to have a blood transfusion
- demonstrate an ability to negotiate with the patient and work in partnership with him
- discuss the pros and cons of blood transfusion
- give time and space for the patient to decide

3 Ethics and the law and other discussion points

- Adverse effects of blood transfusion include:
  (a) non-haemolytic febrile transfusion reactions, including allergic reaction and anaphylaxis
  (b) acute haemolytic transfusion reaction caused by incompatible transfused red cells
  (c) bacterial contamination of the blood product
  (d) virus infection, although rare, e.g. hepatitis B and C, HIV (1 and 2). *Treponema pallidum* is routinely checked as well
  (e) being given the wrong blood, because of a mix-up in cross-matching, wrong labelling, human error
  (f) late complications of repeated transfusions, e.g. iron overload
  (g) circulatory overload if too much is given
- Recent pressures on the blood transfusion service have arisen because of:
  (a) increased demand for blood compared with the increase of donations
  (b) likely additional demand for blood associated with waiting list initiatives
  (c) the rise in the cost of blood with leucodepletion and nucleic acid testing
  (d) recommendations from the Serious Hazards of Transfusion (SHOT) inquiry on how the safety of patients receiving blood could be improved
  (e) the theoretical risk of new variant Creutzfeldt–Jakob disease
  (f) the implications of clinical governance for the blood transfusion service
- The first SHOT report, published in March 1998, indicated that of the 169 reported serious hazards following blood transfusion, 81 involved a blood component being given to the wrong patient while only eight involved viral and bacterial infections. This endorses the importance of correct handling procedures.

The NHS executive. *Better Blood Transfusion*. 1998.

Comments on the case

This case demonstrates how such a common procedure in hospital is taken for granted. The doctor must be able to allow an informed decision to be made before consent and the patient has every right to decline. Remember that the patient may just need more time and information and that declination on the day of consultation is not necessarily a permanent situation, ensure that your patient knows that they can change their mind at a later date.

Case 6 | Brain stem death

Candidate information

You are the medical SHO

Please read this summary (it should take no more than 2 min) and then continue with the consultation.

Re: Mr Alfred Robinson, aged 57

Mr Robinson was admitted by you 48 h ago with a large intracranial haemorrhage. The next of kin is Miss Robinson, his only daughter. A CT scan has shown midline shift. He was intubated on arrival, started on intravenous propofol and transferred to the ITU. Sedation was completely halted 36 h ago. On admission, the neurosurgeons, intensivists and your consultant felt that the prognosis was extremely poor and that neurosurgical intervention would be inappropriate. Since discontinuing sedation, Mr Robinson has shown no neurological response and now he has been confirmed as brain stem dead by two consultants. Currently, he is in sinus rhythm, is normotensive and the ventilator is artificially providing for his respiration. His daughter has been informed of the poor prognosis and has been told that special 'brain testing' is being performed. She is waiting in the visitors' room for an update. She is unaware of exactly what brain stem death means.

Your tasks are to: explain to Miss Robinson the diagnosis of brain stem death, what this means to the outcome and sensitively approach the idea of organ donation.

You have 14 min until his daughter leaves the room, followed by 1 min for reflection, before the discussion with the examiners.

Subject/patient/relative information

Mr Alfred Robinson is a 57-year-old man who was admitted 48 h ago with a sudden headache. He had been well previously and was working as an electrician. A CT scan of the head showed a large left-sided intracranial haemorrhage with midline shift. On admission, he was unconscious and was promptly intubated, sedated and transferred to ITU. It was felt at the time by the neurosurgeons, intensivists and the medical team that neurosurgery would be inappropriate and that his prognosis was extremely poor. Sedation was stopped 36 h ago and he has made no neurological response to any stimuli. His heart is still functioning but the ventilator is keeping him alive by providing artificial respiration. Without the machine Mr Robinson would not breathe on his own. The next of kin, Miss Robinson, has been fully informed of his condition and is aware of the poor prognosis. She is unaware of the present development, i.e. that brain stem death has been diagnosed by two consultants. She is about to see the medical SHO (the candidate) who will explain what is meant by this. He or she will explain that her father is technically dead but the daughter cannot understand how this can be so when his heart is working and he looks pink, as if 'asleep'. The medical SHO will approach the idea of transplantation but this is all too much for Miss Robinson and she will need more time to think and talk to the family and friends.

Examiner information

1 Communication skills — conduct of interview

- Introduce yourself to Miss Robinson (you would have met her before during the admission).
- Ask her what she thinks her father's condition is.
- Explain gently and with empathy that Mr Robinson has shown no signs of improvement and that there have been no indications of recovering consciousness. Give simple evidence to support the facts.
- Tell her that as a result of the brain haemorrhage, Mr Robinson has suffered irreversible brain damage (there is no easy way to say this — allow a pause for the daughter to take all this in). Explain that the brain cells cannot be replaced once damaged and so these cells will not recover. As a result, her father will never wake up.
- Explain that as a result of the haemorrhage he is now brain stem dead as confirmed by two experienced specialists. Explain what this means and that he is technically dead.
- She will obviously mention that the heart is still working so 'how can he be dead, doctor?'
- Point out gently that her father is relying on the machine to do the breathing for him and that this would instantly cease to function if the machine is stopped and then the heart would stop soon after. Thus, her father's heart and lungs are being artificially maintained and that brain stem death equates with the death of an individual, i.e. her father is clinically dead.
- Explain therefore that the next appropriate step is to stop the ventilation. Explain carefully that this is not to allow her father to die but that continuing ventilation is inappropriate if someone is already dead.
- Explain that the medical team have to make this decision and that it is not the family's responsibility (they may feel they are 'actually causing the death' by allowing the ventilator to be stopped).
- Again allow time for the daughter to come to terms with all this.
- Carefully approach the idea that as her father has died and that there has been no damage to the other organs,

it is common in such situations for the family to be approached about the concept of organ donation.
- Ask if Mr Robinson had any views on this matter and then ask the views of the daughter. Ask if there was any known objection by the patient, the family or of any known religious obstacles.
- If the family are interested, tell them that you will speak to the transplant team who will approach the family about this issue, checking that there is no evidence of medical contraindications, e.g. malignancy, and that there would be routine microbiological screening tests, e.g. for hepatitis B and C.
- Explain that if the family agrees for organ transplantation then the ventilation would be continued until the organs are retrieved.
- Remind the daughter that, as her father is brain stem dead, he will not suffer any distress or pain.
- Ask if there are any queries. The daughter may want time to think and if this is so make sure you all agree to meet again later in the day.

2 Communication skills — exploration and problem negotiation

The candidate should be able to:
- explain, with empathy, the diagnosis of brain stem death and describe what this means
- answer any obvious misunderstandings that the family may have with regard to brain stem death
- approach the subject of organ transplantation

3 Ethics and the law and other discussion points

General comments

- In the clinical setting the diagnosis of brain stem death, the pronouncement of death, and the discussion of organ donation are usually compressed into a matter of hours or a few days. Unlike the persistent vegetative state, which may take weeks or even months to evolve and establish irreversibility, the diagnosis of the irreversible loss of brain stem function can be determined with a high degree of certainty within a short time. Because of this, family members should be approached in steps so that they are able to fully comprehend the process. Where available, utilize the assistance of a skilled nurse, counsellor or chaplain to support the family through the process.

- The first step should be to inform the family of the poor prognosis for recovery of any neurological functions. The second step should be to raise the possibility that the patient may be brain stem dead; at this point families should be told that studies are being performed to determine whether this is the case. The third step should be taken when it seems fairly certain that brain stem death has occurred, and the family should then be told clearly and unequivocally that the usual practice at the hospital is to pronounce a person dead once the neurological criteria have been confirmed. With this approach, a family should be able to understand fully that the pronouncement of death is not their decision and that the conclusion of brain stem death as death is a medical assessment just as cardiorespiratory death is.
- At the same time, practitioners should be sensitive to the feelings of the families who are suddenly confronted with the death of their loved one, who may still look 'alive' and who may have been a healthy and vibrant human being just a few hours ago. Thus, it seems reasonable and humane to give the family some time to understand the process and grasp the concept. But for how long, and under what circumstances should the time be given? There are no clear-cut answers to these questions and there never will be. Under what other circumstances and for how long is it permissible to delay, or hasten, the pronouncement of death and termination of support systems? Should the pronouncement of death be delayed, or not made at all, if the family is in a state of denial and completely unable to accept the concept of brain stem death for religious or other reasons? What should be done in cases where brain stem death has apparently been caused by the actions of the doctors providing treatment, or in cases in which the pronouncement of death will cause charges against an alleged assailant to be changed from attempted murder to murder? Should time be taken to find family members to gain consent for organ donation? Should the need for a bed in the ITU be considered when there is a shortage?
- An essential component of all formal pronouncements by the Royal Colleges and the Departments of Health on this subject is that once a patient is declared brain stem dead that he or she is also legally dead. The Department of Health 1983 code *Cadaveric Organs for Transplantation*, London 1983, HMSO, a code of practice including the diagnosis of brain death, specifically states that the time of death is the time at which brain death is established and not some later time when ventilation is withdrawn or the heartbeat ceases. Clinicians should emphasize this when explaining the situation to relatives, and they should make it clear that ventilation is not being withdrawn to let the patient die but because continued ventilation is inappropriate for a patient who is already dead. The only justification for maintaining ventilation for a short time is to preserve the condition of the organs when it has been agreed that they are to be made available for transplantation.

Code of practice

- The definition of death—it should be remembered that there is no legal definition of death. Hospital doctors are recommended to follow the guidelines produced by the Royal Colleges on Diagnosis of Death and Brain Death, incorporated in the 1983 revised edition of the code of practice on the removal of cadaveric organs for transplantation (Health Departments of Great Britain and Ireland).
- Death entails the irreversible loss of those essential characteristics which are necessary for the existence of a living person. It is recommended that the definition of death should be regarded as the irreversible loss of the capacity for consciousness, combined with irreversible loss of the capacity to breathe. The irreversible cessation of brain stem function (brain stem death) will produce this clinical state and therefore brain stem death equates with the death of the individual.
- Conditions under which the diagnosis of brain stem death should be considered:
  (a) there should be no doubt that the patient's condition is caused by irremediable brain damage of known aetiology
  (b) there should be no evidence that this state is a result of depressant drugs
  (c) primary hypothermia as the cause of unconsciousness must have been excluded
  (d) potentially reversible circulatory, metabolic and endocrine disturbances must have been excluded as the cause of the continuation of unconsciousness
  (e) the patient is being maintained on the ventilator because spontaneous respiration has been inadequate or ceased altogether (relaxants and other drugs need to be excluded as causing respiratory inadequacy or failure)
- The diagnosis of brain stem death means that all brain stem reflexes are absent. The diagnosis must be made by two medical practitioners (one has to be a consult-

ant) who have been registered for over 5 years, who are competent in this field, must not be members of the transplant team and they must test separately. The legal time of death is when the first test indicates brain stem death. Diagnosing brain stem death includes demonstration of the following:

(a) pupils fixed and not responding to light

(b) no corneal reflex

(c) absent vestibulo-ocular reflexes

(d) no cranial nerve motor responses to adequate stimulation

(e) no gag reflex or reflex response to bronchial stimulation (suction catheter placed down the trachea)

(f) no respiratory movements occur when the patient is disconnected from the mechanical ventilator. It is necessary for the arterial carbon dioxide to exceed the threshold for respiratory stimulation, i.e. $Paco_2$ should reach 6.6 kPa (as measured by blood gases). Hypoxia during disconnection should be prevented by delivering oxygen at 6 L/min through a catheter in the trachea.

Organ donation

- The transplant coordinator will be contacted by the medical or nursing staff, ideally before brain stem testing is performed.
- The transplant coordinator will provide local protocols.
- If a patient carries a signed donor card, or has been included in the NHS organ donor register, there is no legal requirement to establish lack of objection on the part of the relatives, although it is good practice to take into account the relatives' views.
- The coordinator should contact the UK Transplant Support Service Authority (UKTSSA) for matching and distribution of organs donated for transplant. As part of its function, the UKTSSA maintains the national transplant database which contains details of all potential organ transplant recipients in the UK and Republic of Ireland. It is responsible for liaison directly with coordinators at transplant centres nationwide to ensure that all potential donor organs are allocated to patients on the waiting list who can benefit the most.

- The NHS Organ Donor registrar can confirm if the potential donor was registered as willing to donate all or some organs.
- Removal of organs is authorized only if there is no reason to believe that the deceased has expressed an objection to his body being so dealt with after death and had not withdrawn this objection, that the surviving spouse, partner or any other surviving relative of the deceased does not object to the body being so dealt with, and that there are no religious obstacles.
- Before removing the organs, the surgeon must personally examine the body of the potential donor and he or she must, on the basis of examination and brain stem tests carried out, be satisfied that the patient is dead. Organs must not be transplanted until microbiological safety to do so has been established.

Department of Health. *A code of practice for the diagnosis of brain stem death: including guidelines for the identification and management of potential organ and tissue donors.* March 1998.

Comments on the case

Discussing brain stem death is never easy, particularly as organ donation may need to be discussed as well. Candidates must be aware of what brain stem death is as it is very likely that they will come across a real case during their medical practice.

In the aftermath of the Alder Hey and Bristol enquiries into the retention of organs by hospital clinical staff, one needs to be conscious that the public may have serious misgivings about the integrity of practices surrounding organ removal for either donation or medical research.

Case 7 | **Breaking bad news**

Candidate information

You are the SHO in a chest clinic and you are about to see Miss Joanne Harrison
Please read this summary (it should take no more than 2 min) and then continue with the consultation.

Re: Miss Joanne Harrison, aged 25

Miss Harrison saw your consultant 4 weeks ago in clinic after presenting to the GP feeling unwell with a fever and loss of appetite. A chest X-ray in the clinic showed bilateral hilar lymphadenopathy. The consultant did not discuss the diagnostic possibilities but arranged for a mediastinal biopsy (mediastinoscopy) which was performed by the thoracic surgeon 10 days ago. Your consultant is away today and Miss Harrison has come back for the biopsy result. Unfortunately, this shows Hodgkin's lymphoma.

Your tasks are to: break the bad news to Miss Harrison and deal with the concerns and questions that she will have.

You have 14 min until the patient leaves the room, followed by 1 min for reflection, before the discussion with the examiners.

Subject/patient/relative information

Miss Harrison is a 25-year-old clerical officer who first presented feeling generally unwell with a fever and weight loss about 6 weeks ago. She thought she had a virus but the GP sent her to the consultant clinic 2 weeks later. A chest X-ray showed bilateral hilar lymphadenopathy. During the initial visit, the consultant did not discuss the possible cause although Miss Harrison could tell by the consultant's language that the chest X-ray was worrying. She was sent to the local thoracic surgery department where she had a mediastinal biopsy. She has come back to obtain the results and she is concerned that this may be cancer.

Examiner information

1 Communication skills — conduct of interview

- Introduce yourself to Miss Harrison. Ensure that this is the correct patient.
- Make sure the clinic room is quiet and comfortable and ask if she has any relatives with her, e.g. partner. If so, ask if she wants him or her to be in the clinic room as well. Normally, a member of the nursing staff would be available but probably not in the exam.

- Start with an open question such as, 'What's been happening to you since you had operation?' She will probably say that she is okay but that her symptoms still persist.
- Ask her whether the consultant explained the possible diagnoses at the first visit or whether she has any ideas of her own. She will probably say no.
- Tell her the biopsy result and then pause. Ask her if she has heard of Hodgkin's lymphoma.
- She may say to you, 'Is that cancer?'
- Say that it is a type of cancer but that it is treatable (be

honest with the patient), then pause to allow this to sink in.

- When the timing feels right, give a brief and concise explanation of what Hodgkin's lymphoma is.
- Explain that there are doctors who specialize in this disease and there are well-established treatments available.
- She may believe that having cancer means dying in agony — it is important to dispel these myths. She may ask if the cancer is inherited. Reassure her on this issue.
- Tell her that you will refer her urgently to the relevant consultant (clinical oncologist) for further staging of the disease and subsequent treatment. Explain to her that the clinical oncologist will arrange a CT scan of the chest and abdomen to stage the disease and to determine the distribution of the nodes.
- She may want to know what treatment options are available. Do not pretend to be an expert when you are not. Do not be afraid to say, 'I do not know the finer details but . . .'. You should give a brief explanation about chemotherapy and radiotherapy, reminding her that it is only after the full assessment and staging have been carried out that one can decide exactly what form of treatment will be the best for her.
- At all times allow her to make her own comments. Listen sympathetically to all of her concerns.
- If a nurse is present, ask him or her for any further comments.
- Ask who is at home to support her. It is wise to inform the GP straight away for primary care support. Check that she is not driving home on her own.
- Offer a contact number if she needs further advice.

2 Communication skills — exploration and problem negotiation

The candidate should be able to:

- ask what she has been told at the previous outpatient appointment
- tell her what the biopsy shows
- explain there are specialists dealing with Hodgkin's lymphoma and that a referral will be made urgently
- explain what the most likely course of events will be, e.g. referral, assessment with CT, decision on therapy and, briefly, the types of therapies available
- address the concerns of the patient

3 Ethics and the law and other discussion points

The candidate should be able to:

- understand that when breaking bad news, it is impor-

tant that he or she confirms who the individual is, otherwise, if the wrong person or partner is given the results without the consent of the patient, he or she will be breaking confidentiality. Remember that a competent patient's partner or relatives should never be told the patient's diagnosis first. In addition, giving the wrong diagnosis will cause that person considerable distress unnecessarily and lead to potential difficulties for the doctor who told them
- know what the individual has been told in the past and how much she knows or suspects so that the depth and detail of the explanation can be judged better
- realize that if personal medical knowledge of the speciality discussed is lacking, he or she must not be afraid to admit this and to refer on to a relevant specialist
- refer the patient to a recognized centre with a full multidisciplinary team approach
- realize that an immediate reaction to bad news of any sort is often numbness and denial. The patient may ask, 'Are you sure? Surely you have got the result wrong.' Once the numbness and denial has diminished a little, the patient may become angry at the news, often with some of the anger pointed towards the bearer of the bad news. The candidate must not take the anger personally. Gradually, over a period of time, there will be sadness, then acceptance and eventually hope.
- The common faults of breaking bad news are:
  (a) avoiding the breaking of bad news in the first place and hoping that someone else will do it
  (b) stalling the breaking of bad news with irrelevant discussion, e.g. 'Nice day today, isn't it?'
  (c) not picking up the patient's cues and body language. If the patient gives no eye contact, maybe this indicates that the patient needs more time
  (d) being dishonest, e.g. 'Don't worry, it's not too serious. You'll be feeling better soon'
  (e) bombarding the patient with too much information
  (f) conveying an aura of impending doom, e.g. 'Oh dear, it really is not good at all and it is worse than I had expected!'
- Useful strategies to aid the breaking of bad news are:
  (a) always be honest and never tell the patient anything that may be false
  (b) do not tell the patient more than he or she wants to know
  (c) give the patient time. Allow for silences. Being told the diagnosis may be too much for the patient and he or she may not be ready to be told any further information, e.g. treatment options. You may find that the acceptance phase takes longer than you expect, so say,

'This must be a great shock for you. You will need time for all this to sink in so I suggest we meet again in a few days so I can answer all your questions.' This next meeting will be a better time to discuss treatment options

(d) never give specific times, e.g. when asked for prognosis

(e) always provide hope; the patient needs you to show support

(f) always be sensitive; never be abrupt and inconsiderate

(g) appreciate the different ways that patients cope with denial

(h) words that are used, e.g. tumour, mass, lesion, malignant or cancer may have a different meaning to the patient, so make sure the language you use is both understandable and interpretable

(i) when dealing with anger, do not allow the anger to be left unexplored. Say to the patient, 'You look upset' or 'Tell me what is bothering you'

- Discuss with the examiners the issues of referral times for cancers, the Calman–Hine report for cancer, the importance of oncology patients entering multicentre clinical research trials, etc.

Comments on the case

This case typifies a common 'breaking bad news' scenario. The candidate has to carry out a consultation properly with empathy, understanding and sharing with the concerns and feelings of the patient. The candidate must not try and be an expert in this field but then again he or she must not admit a total lack of knowledge, thus being totally unhelpful to the patient. Acknowledge to yourself that it is difficult for the clinician and it hurts to break bad news to a patient, but this must not prevent the candidate from conveying the information in an honest manner.

Case 8 | Breaking bad news: a chronic illness

Candidate information

You are the medical SHO in clinic

Please read this summary (it should take no more than 2 min) and then continue with the consultation.

Re: Mrs Paula Reeney, aged 47

Mrs Reeney presented to the clinic 4 weeks ago because of a 4-day history of blurred vision in the left eye which had previously occurred 2 months ago. During that appointment the consultant did suggest the possibility of multiple sclerosis as there was also a history of an episode of facial weakness 8 months ago. Mrs Reeney has blocked out the possibility of multiple sclerosis by 'reassuring herself' that this was very unlikely as she had recovered from her earlier symptoms. An MRI scan performed 2 weeks ago has shown multiple demyelinating plaques in the brain stem and periventricular regions suggestive of multiple sclerosis. Mrs Reeney is now at the clinic awaiting the results.

Your tasks are to: explain the results of the MRI scan and to convey the diagnosis of multiple sclerosis to her.

You have 14 min until the patient leaves the room, followed by 1 min for reflection, before the discussion with the examiners.

Subject/patient/relative information

Mrs Paula Reeney is a 47-year-old secretary who presented to the GP 2 months ago with blurred vision in the left eye. A few months previously she had an episode of facial weakness. She was referred to the consultant physician who wondered if the discs were swollen. The consultant did mention that there was a possibility of multiple sclerosis but Mrs Reeney tried to reassure herself that this could not be possible, as her eye symptoms had resolved. An MRI scan was performed which showed multiple plaques of demyelination suggestive of multiple sclerosis. Mrs Reeney is an active woman and news such as this will be quite devastating for her. She lives with her husband and two children.

Examiner information

1 Communication skills — conduct of interview

- Introduce yourself to her.
- Ask how she has been since her last appointment.
- Ask what she was told at the last appointment. Had the consultant mentioned any possible causes for the blurred vision?
- Explain that the MRI scan findings do suggest multiple sclerosis. Pause to allow this to sink in. Watch for her reactions, e.g. anger, denial.

- When the time is right, ask what she knows about multiple sclerosis.
- She may say she is doomed and the more serious manifestations such as difficulty in walking, incontinence, dementia are inevitable in her case.
- Aim to reassure her that not all patients go on to this type of end-stage disease.
- Point out that there are specialists who look after patients with multiple sclerosis and that they will help her with the best available therapy.
- She will ask questions that will be difficult to answer such as why has she got it, how did she get it, will it go away, her chances of leading a normal life, possibility of a genetic link, etc.
- Be honest and say that it is not possible to answer these questions but what you do know is that many people with multiple sclerosis live very active lives even many years after the diagnosis.
- Be reassuring and explain that patients with relapses and remission, as in her case, may go on for many years without any major disability.
- Tell her about the Multiple Sclerosis Society which will support her through this difficult time. Tell her you will give her the contact number of this society (Multiple Sclerosis Society 0808 800 8000).
- Try to avoid bombarding her with too much information at this stage, unless she asks for it.
- Arrange early follow-up to discuss this further. Say you will also refer her to a specialist and tell her that you will inform her GP. Give her a contact number if she wants to ring you for advice.

2 Communication skills — exploration and problem negotiation

The candidate should be able to:
- explain the findings of the MRI scan
- explain that the likely diagnosis is multiple sclerosis
- provide support and encouragement to enable her to have hope
- allow the patient time and space to enable her to come to terms with the bad news

3 Ethics and the law and other discussion points

- Breaking bad news when it is a diagnosis of a chronic illness such as multiple sclerosis, diabetes mellitus, rheumatoid arthritis or motor neurone disease, usually results in the patient believing the worst is inevitable.
- Despite being asymptomatic, impending doom is a common belief.
- The challenge for the candidate is not to explain all that is known in the literature about the disease but rather to support the patient when giving the bad news, and being aware of the different phases that receivers of bad news go through, i.e. denial, anger, acceptance and hope.
- The impact of having a chronic disease is multiple, i.e. physical, psychological and social. There will be concerns with regard to the family and work as well as health. Coming to terms with the illness and coping with these impacts will take a while and it is the medical team looking after the patient who will help to support the coping mechanisms; particularly on how to deal with setbacks, loss of self-esteem and confidence, dealing with changing goals in life, etc.
- Reassurance and hope is what the patient needs; 15% of patients diagnosed with multiple sclerosis progress to the chronic progressive type of disease and so the vast majority lead quite normal lives.
- Supplying telephone numbers of societies is always helpful. Providing early follow-up will allow further queries to be answered. Always inform the GP.

Comments on the case

Breaking bad news of a chronic illness is a common case. Unless the first breaking of bad news session is done properly, with understanding and empathy, all trust and belief may be squandered. The candidate must take time to allow the patient to take in what has been said; she may remain totally shocked for a while. Avoid besieging her with too much detail on multiple sclerosis (epidemiology, pathogenesis, diagnosis, therapy options, etc.). This is a breaking bad news station and not a multiple sclerosis one.

Case 9 | Concerns over infection control

Candidate information

You are the medical SHO

Please read this summary (it should take no more than 2 min) and then continue with the consultation.

> ### Re: Mrs Gladys Winterburn, aged 91
>
> Mrs Winterburn has been a resident on the ward for 4 months. She was initially admitted after a fall at her home. She has heart failure and has had bilateral chronic leg ulcers for a few years. It has become quite clear that she is unable to look after herself in her own house and so an application for a nursing home place has been made. At present, she can mobilize slowly with the assistance of one person, needs full attention with regard to feeding and toileting and her leg ulcers need regular dressings. Unfortunately, 2 weeks ago a methicillin-resistant *Staphylococcus aureus* (MRSA) screen isolated MRSA in the left leg ulcer, although there is no evidence of any systemic effects or invasive infection of the ulcer. Provisionally, a place may be available at the Lee Bank Nursing Home and one of the senior carers, Miss Brenda Raglan, has come to assess Mrs Winterburn. She has been told about the MRSA and as a result is slightly concerned about the possible impact on the nursing home.

Your tasks are to: speak to the senior home carer, Miss Raglan, explaining Mrs Winterburn's condition, explain the MRSA finding in the leg ulcer and allay any fears she may have with regard to infection control.

You have 14 min until the senior home carer leaves the room, followed by 1 min for reflection, before the discussion with the examiners.

Subject/patient/relative information

Mrs Gladys Winterburn is a 91-year-old lady who was admitted 4 months ago after a fall. She also has heart failure and bilateral chronic leg ulcers for which she needs regular dressings. It has become quite clear that Mrs Winterburn is in need of care for her activities of daily living especially for mobility, feeding, toileting and dressing of the ulcers, and so a request for placement in a nursing home has been put into motion. Miss Brenda Raglan is a senior carer at one particular nursing home. She has come to assess Mrs Winterburn for placement there. The financial arrangements have been sorted out, so all it needs now is for Miss Raglan to see Mrs Winterburn in order to make a general assessment of her suitability. However, to her dismay, Miss Raglan hears about the isolation of MRSA from the leg ulcer. She is particularly concerned about the risk this may have on her staff and on the other patients with regard to possible difficulty in treatment and also the risk of overwhelming infection. She feels that this has jeopardized the placement and wants to speak to the medical SHO (the candidate) for further information about the MRSA.

Examiner information

1 Communication skills — conduct of interview

- Introduce yourself to Miss Raglan from the Lee Bank Nursing Home.
- Tell her about Mrs Winterburn with regard to her needs for daily living: she needs help with mobilizing, feeding, toileting and for the ulcer dressings.
- Explain that MRSA has been isolated from one of the ulcers although this is not causing any problems either locally to the ulcer or systemically to the patient.
- Explain:
  (a) what MRSA is and how long the bacteria has been known to physicians
  (b) what problems MRSA can cause
  (c) why MRSA is so different from some other bacteria with regard to resistance to antibiotics
  (d) how residents with MRSA should be cared for
  (e) what special precautions need to be taken, especially regarding basic hygiene
  (f) whether staff or other patients need screening
  (g) who else to inform
  (h) the procedure if a resident with MRSA needs to be admitted to hospital
  (i) other sources of advice
- Generally reassure.
- Explain that there can be no justification for discriminating against people who have MRSA by refusing them admission to a nursing or residential home, or by treating them differently from other residents.
- Offer to put her in contact with the Infection Control nurse specialist who will be able to offer practical support and advice on any concerns she has about MRSA.

2 Communication skills — exploration and problem negotiation

The candidate should be able to:
- discuss the needs of Mrs Winterburn
- explain the MRSA findings in the leg ulcer
- explain what MRSA is and the implications of having MRSA for the patient

- reassure that MRSA in a nursing home setting should pose little threat to the health of staff and other residents
- demonstrate awareness of the concept of multi-disciplinary team working
- acknowledge that Miss Raglan is likely to require ongoing information and advice

3 Ethics and the law and other discussion points (recommendations from the Department of Health)

What is MRSA?

MRSA stands for methicillin-resistant *Staphylococcus aureus*, a form of *Staphylococcus aureus*. *S. aureus* is the most common type of bacteria that can infect humans; about one-third of the population are colonized with it. 'Colonized' means that the organism lives harmlessly on a person's skin or in the nose and does not cause any infection.

What problems can it cause?

Usually *S. aureus* causes no problems. If it does, the resulting infection is usually trivial and affects the skin, resulting in infected cuts or boils. These are easily treated. *S. aureus* is more of a threat to hospital patients with deep wounds, catheters or drips which allow the bacterium to enter the body. People with severely reduced resistance to infection, e.g. as a result of HIV infection, are also vulnerable. For these groups of patients, the resulting infection can be serious — septicaemia or pneumonia for example.

What is special about MRSA?

MRSA acts in exactly the same way as *S. aureus* and causes the same range of infections. Most people who have it come to no harm at all. What makes MRSA different is its resistance to antibiotics. Some antibiotics are still effective but they may be more difficult to use and cause side-effects. That is why the spread of MRSA in hospitals is a cause for concern and why hospital patients with MRSA may be isolated in side rooms or special wards.

How long has MRSA been around?

MRSA is not a new problem—the strains which can cause outbreaks in hospitals first appeared in the early 1960s. In some countries, where antibiotics are available much more freely than here, the spread of MRSA has now been accepted as more or less inevitable. In the UK, there has been and continues to be a focus on prevention and control.

How should residents with MRSA be cared for?

If good basic hygiene precautions are followed, then residents with MRSA are not a risk to other residents, staff, visitors or members of their family, including babies, children and pregnant women. Good hygiene is important to prevent the spread of all infections, not just MRSA. Like any other resident, those with MRSA should be helped with handwashing if their mental or physical condition makes it difficult for them to wash their own hands. They should be encouraged to live a normal life without restriction and they need not be isolated. They may share a room so long as neither they nor the person with whom they are sharing have any open sores or wounds, drips or catheters. They may join other residents in communal areas such as the sitting and dining rooms, so long as any sores or wounds are covered with an appropriate dressing which is regularly changed. They may receive visitors and go out of the home, e.g. to see their family or friends.

Are any special precautions required?

People with MRSA do not normally require special treatment after discharge from hospital. If a course of treatment does need to be completed, then the hospital should provide all the necessary details. The only special precautions required are that staff:
- with eczema or psoriasis should not perform close-contact nursing care on residents with MRSA
- should complete any procedures on other residents before attending to dressings or carrying out other nursing care for residents with MRSA
- should carry out any clinical procedures and dressings on a resident with MRSA in the resident's own room
- should seek and follow expert infection control advice from the consultant in communicable disease control and/or community infection control nurse for any resident with MRSA who has a postoperative wound or a drip or catheter

In Scotland, seek advice from the consultant in public health medicine (CPHM), and/or community infection control nurse. Affected residents with open wounds should be allocated single rooms if possible.

Good basic hygiene precautions to prevent infections, including MRSA infections
- Good hand hygiene practice by staff and residents is the single most important infection control measure.
- Disposable gloves and aprons should be worn when attending to dressings, performing aseptic techniques or dealing with blood and body fluids.
- Cuts, sores and wounds in staff and residents should be covered with impermeable dressings.
- Blood and body fluid spills should be dealt with immediately according to the locally agreed policy.
- Sharps should be disposed of into proper sharps containers.
- Equipment, such as commodes, should be cleaned thoroughly with detergent and hot water after use.
- Clothes and bedding should be machine-washed, in accordance with the local policy.
- Cutlery, crockery and clinical waste should be dealt with in the normal way.

What about screening?

Residents and staff do not need routine screening for MRSA unless there is a clinical reason; e.g. a wound getting worse or new sores appearing. In that case, the resident's GP should send wound swabs to the local hospital for general microbiological investigations.

Screening of other residents and staff is very rarely necessary and would only be peformed following discussion between the consultant in communicable disease control (CPHM in Scotland) and the microbiologist.

What is the procedure for admitting someone with MRSA?

When a person with MRSA is admitted to a nursing or residential home, the following people should be informed: the manager, matron or designated member of staff with infection control responsibilities and the resident's GP.

What if a resident with MRSA needs to go to hospital?

If an affected resident needs to go to hospital, then the hospital should be informed beforehand that they have, or have had, MRSA: the hospital's infection control doctor or infection control nurse should be contacted if the person is to receive inpatient treatment. They are available through the hospital switchboard and are usually based in the Department of Medical Microbiology. The relevant department should be informed if the person is to receive outpatient treatment.

What if an MRSA infection is diagnosed?

This is uncommon outside hospitals. However, if a resident does become infected with MRSA, their GP should contact the microbiologist at the local hospital for advice on treatment. Meanwhile, any infected wounds or skin lesions should be covered with appropriate dressings.

To find out more, or to get specific advice, you should contact

- your local consultant in communicable disease control (CCDC). This is the person responsible for the control of infectious diseases within the community served by your health authority (in Scotland, contact your local CPHM). You can find the CCDC (or CPHM in Scotland) through the Department of Public Health Medicine at your health authority, or
- your community infection control nurse (CICN). In some areas infection control nurses have been appointed to help provide advice on infection control in the community. They are the best people to consult about writing and implementing infection control policies and about any infection control problems posed by individual residents. The CICN can usually be contacted through the CCDC (or CPHM in Scotland).

Department of Health. *What nursing and residential homes need to know.* November 1996.

Comments on the case

The Department of Health has recommended that there can be no justification for discriminating against people who have MRSA by refusing them admission to a nursing or residential home or by treating them differently from other residents. Long-term residency in hospital with chronic infections encourages emergence of MRSA. It is vital that the candidate understands what is meant by MRSA and its implications. The above information from the Department of Health should be helpful.

Case 10 | Consent for bedside teaching

Candidate information

You are the medical SHO

Please read this summary (it should take no more than 2 min) and then continue with the consultation.

Re: Mrs Edna White, aged 86

For once, time is on your hands and you have agreed to take the third year medical students to see Mrs Edna White, an elderly lady who was admitted 2 weeks ago with a dense right hemiplegia. At present, Mrs White remains unwell with global dysphasia, reduced consciousness and is catheterized. She has no family for support and needs full 24-h nursing care. However, she has excellent neurological signs and the students want these signs demonstrated to them. You have seven students in your group but another group of seven appears on the ward complaining that their teaching has been cancelled. You feel charitable and so ask the second group to join you.

The ward sister (Sister Brennan) is unhappy that you are taking 14 medical students to see Mrs White stating that Mrs White needs some dignity and consideration. She requests that you speak with her in the office.

Your tasks are to: discuss the reasons for her dissatisfactions and come to a compromise.

You have 14 min until Sister leaves the room, followed by 1 min for reflection, before the discussion with the examiners.

Subject/patient/relative information

Mrs Edna White is an 86-year-old lady who was admitted 2 weeks ago with a dense right hemiplegia, global dysphasia and reduced consciousness. She remains unwell with no signs of improvement, needing full 24-h nursing care and she is catheterized. The consultant's impression is that her prognosis is poor. Mrs White has no family. The medical SHO (the candidate) has agreed to take 14 students to see Mrs White to demonstrate her physical signs. The ward sister (Sister Brennan) is unhappy that the SHO is taking so many students to see her because: (a) she feels so many students would disrupt the running of the ward; (b) Mrs White would be unable to consent for physical examination; (c) Mrs White would be indecently exposed to the students as she has no undergarments on; (d) Mrs White would be unable to state whether she has any discomfort during the examination; and (e) most importantly, she feels that the teaching is not in the best interests of the patient. Sister Brennan feels quite strongly about this and wants to discuss this privately with the SHO. Sister Brennan does appreciate that students must learn and one possible solution is to have the students present in smaller groups during the SHO's or the consultant's ward round, which would allow them to watch the SHO or consultant carrying out an examination of Mrs White to assess her present medical state.

Examiner information

1 Communication skills — conduct of interview

- Sit and listen to what Sister Brennan has to say; do not be confrontational, the ward sister is senior and experienced and is not 'anti medical students'.
- She tells you that she is unhappy that so many students are around the bedside for the teaching; she feels that this may overtire Mrs White and disturb the other patients unduly.
- Sister also tells you that Mrs White would be unable to consent for physical examination, would be indecently exposed to the students as she has no undergarments on, would be unable to state whether she has any discomfort during the examination and she also feels that the teaching is not in the patient's best interests.
- Sister also tells you that she does understand that students need to learn, but in this case one possible solution would be to observe the consultant or yourself examining the patient during a ward round when assessing her medical state/progress.
- You agree and decide that this is the best solution.
- Apologize to her for any misunderstanding.

2 Communication skills — exploration and problem negotiation

The candidate should be able to:
- sit down and listen to Sister Brennan's concerns
- appreciate these concerns
- agree on a solution or compromise

3 Ethics and the law and other discussion points

- It is a general legal and ethical principle that valid consent must be obtained before starting treatment or physical investigation, or providing personal care for a patient. This principle reflects the right of the patient to determine what happens to their own bodies, and is fundamental to good clinical practice.
- For a person to have capacity, he or she must be able to comprehend and retain information and material relevant to the decision, especially as to the consequences of having or not having the intervention in question.
- To give valid consent the patient needs to understand in broad terms the nature and purpose of the procedure. Any misrepresentations of these elements will invalidate consent. Where relevant, information about anaesthesia should be given as well as information about the procedure itself.
- Clear information is particularly important when students or trainees carry out procedures to further their own education. Where the procedure will further the patient's care (e.g. taking blood sample for testing) then, assuming the student is appropriately trained in the procedure, the fact that it is carried out by a student does not alter the nature and purpose of the procedure. It is therefore not a legal requirement to tell the patient that the clinician is a student, although it would always be good practice to do so. In contrast, where a student proposes to conduct a physical examination which is not part of the patient's care, then it is essential to explain that the purpose of the examination is to further the student's training and to seek consent for that to take place.
- During an operation it may become evident that the patient could benefit from an additional procedure that was not within the scope of the original consent. If it would be unreasonable to delay the procedure until the patient regains consciousness (e.g. because there is a threat to the patient's life), it may be justified to perform the procedure on the grounds that it is in the patient's best interests. However, the procedure should not be performed merely because it is convenient. For example, a hysterectomy should never be performed during an operation without explicit consent, unless it is necessary to do so to save life.
- Video recordings of treatment may be used both as a medical record, treatment aid and tool for teaching, audit or research. The purpose and possible future use of video recordings must be clearly explained to the person before their consent is sought for the recording to be made. If the video recording is to be used for teaching, audit or research, patients must be aware that they can decline without their care being compromised

and that when required or appropriate their identity in the video can be hidden. As a matter of good practice the same principles should apply to clinical photography.

- The clinician providing treatment or investigation is responsible for ensuring that the patient has given valid consent before treatment begins, although the consultant responsible for the patient's care will remain ultimately responsible for the quality of medical care provided. The task of seeking consent may be delegated to another health professional, as long as that professional is suitably trained and qualified. In particular, they must have sufficient knowledge of the proposed investigation or treatment and understand the risks involved in order to be able to provide any information to the patient that is required. Inappropriate delegation (e.g. where the clinician seeking consent has inadequate knowledge of the procedure) may mean that the consent obtained is not valid. Clinicians are responsible for knowing the limits of their own competence and should seek the advice of appropriate colleagues when necessary.

- If the patient has capacity but is illiterate, the patient should, if able to, make their mark on the form to indicate consent. It is good practice for the mark to be witnessed by a person other than the clinician seeking consent and for the fact that the patient has chosen to make their mark in this way to be recorded in the case notes. Similarly, if the patient has capacity and wishes to give consent but is physically unable to mark the form, this fact should be recorded in the notes. If consent has been validly given, the lack of a completed form is no bar to treatment. In practice, patients need to be able to communicate their decision although consent may be expressed verbally or non-verbally. A non-verbal consent would be where a patient, after receiving appropriate information, holds out an arm for their blood pressure to be taken. In the case of Mrs White verbal and non-verbal consent is impossible. It is important to be aware that not all patients are aware of teaching practices and cannot be assumed to have agreed implicitly to them.

- If consent has been obtained a significant time before undertaking the intervention, it is good practice to confirm that the person who has given consent (assuming he or she retains capacity) stills wishes the intervention to proceed, even if no new information needs to be provided or further questions answered.

- A patient with capacity is entitled to withdraw consent at any time, including during a procedure. Where a patient does object during treatment, it is good practice for the practitioner, if at all possible, to stop the procedure, establish the patient's concerns and explain the consequences of not completing the procedure. At times an apparent objection may reflect a cry of pain rather than withdrawal of consent and appropriate reassurance at that point may enable the practitioner to continue with the patient's consent.

Department of Health. *Reference Guide to Consent for Examinations or Treatment.* March 2001.

Comments on the case

This case highlights the need to ensure that patients' rights to privacy and dignity are maintained, as well as the ethics of consent for examinations and treatment. Medical practitioners must be aware of the consent procedure. The Department of Health website provides useful guidelines.

If patients decline an examination or the presence of students, the clinician should respect their choice with good grace!

Case 11 | Consent from a patient who does not have the capacity to give consent

Candidate information

You are the medical SHO

Please read this summary (it should take no more than 2 min) and then continue with the consultation.

> ### Re: Mr George Andrews, aged 77
>
> Mr George Andrews is a patient with dementia who was admitted from a nursing home with a right basal pneumonia. He was started on intravenous antibiotics but it was quite clear that he had problems with his swallowing, and so it was felt that Mr Andrews probably had an aspiration pneumonia. His routine blood tests show an albumin of 28 g/L, suggestive of poor nutrition. He mobilizes with one helper and needs help with feeding, dressing and washing. He has no other comorbidities. A speech therapy assessment has now shown poor swallowing coordination with aspiration of fluids (dementia-related pharyngeal phase dysphagia). It is now felt that his swallowing is unsafe and that feeding by other means should be introduced. A nasogastric tube has been tried with the permission of the next of kin who is the eldest daughter, Mrs Jean Fawkes. However, despite strapping with tape, the nasogastric tube was pulled out each time by Mr Andrews. Mr Andrews has a tendency to pull drips out as well. During the ward round, the consultant decided to get the gastroenterologists to insert a percutaneous endoscopic gastrostomy (PEG) tube for feeding. You have spoken to the gastroenterology registrar who has kindly put the patient on the afternoon list. Because of the patient's dementia, you have called Mrs Fawkes to the ward to obtain her consent for the PEG tube insertion.

Your tasks are to: discuss why a PEG tube is being considered and to obtain consent from the patient's daughter.

You have 14 min until the daughter leaves the room, followed by 1 min for reflection, before the discussion with the examiners.

Subject/patient/relative information

Mr George Andrews is a 77-year-old man who lives in a nursing home. He has dementia which manifests as poor memory and poor orientation in time and space. He was admitted with a pneumonia which is most likely caused by problems with swallowing. Mr Andrews mobilizes with one helper and needs help with feeding, dressing and washing. There is no doubt that he is malnourished. His daughter, Mrs Jean Fawkes, has been told that the poor swallowing (resulting from the dementia) will put her father at further risk of developing aspiration pneumonia, as well as continued malnutrition. One option is to try a nasogastric tube for feeding. This has been tried but was unsuccessful. Another option is a percutaneous endoscopic gastrostomy (PEG) tube which is inserted using an endoscope by the gastroenterology specialists. It is performed under sedation, and her father would then be fed through a tube in the abdominal wall, which directly feeds the stomach. This means that Mr Andrews would not need to take feeds orally. The daughter is concerned that as her father has dementia it is not clear if he would ever consent to such a procedure. She is worried that this procedure is too invasive and feels reluctant to support the medical plan. She is to see the medical SHO (the candidate) to discuss these issues further. After a full explanation of the risks of oral feeding, she expresses an understanding of the legal position and the rationale for the clinician's decision.

Examiner information

1 Communication skills—conduct of interview

- Introduce yourself to the patient's daughter, Mrs Fawkes.
- Establish that she is her father's nominated next of kin.
- Ask her what she knows so far to get an idea of how to start your explanations.
- Explain why her father came into hospital and remind her that a problem with the swallowing has been found. Explain that this leads to aspiration pneumonia and malnutrition.
- Explain what aspiration pneumonia means. You may draw a diagram to illustrate how incoordination of swallowing can cause spilling of food into the trachea.
- Tell her that the ward staff have tried nasogastric tube feeds but that her father keeps pulling the tube out. Explain that he has a similar tendency to pull out the drips so only when he is asleep does he get any fluids. The saline bag is taken down in the morning before waking and the venflon wrapped securely with a bandage. Explain this situation is of no benefit to Mr Andrews.
- Ask her if she understands all of this.
- Tell her that one other option is for PEG feeding. Explain (with the help of a diagram) what this is in terms of the purpose, who carries out the procedure, and where, how long it takes, the invasiveness of the procedure, feeding carried out through a tube in the abdominal wall rather than orally, etc. Let her know the possible complications, e.g. displacement of the PEG tube and cellulitis around the wound. Explain that the medical team feels that this would, however, be the best solution to his swallowing problems. Ask her how she feels about this.

- She may agree or she may refuse—if she disagrees ask for her reasons and appreciate her concerns. You may need to clarify the legal situation with her if it is appropriate at this stage. She may want to discuss the matter with other members of the family and the consultant in charge.
- If she requests a second opinion you must tell her that this can be arranged.

2 Communication skills—exploration and problem negotiation

The candidate should be able to:
- give an update of the present situation
- explain the problem with the patient's swallowing and the long-term consequences of poor swallowing
- explain the procedure (PEG) and its pros and cons
- if she concurs with the clinical decision explain that the consultant will be signing the 'Best Interest' document and that she will be provided with a copy of it

3 Ethics and the law and other discussion points

Most relatives will agree to the PEG feeding if it is medically indicated. However, ethical issues arise if: (a) consent is not available from a patient without the capacity to give a consent; and (b) the concepts of acting 'in the best interests' for this incapacitated person. The guidelines from the BMA are as follow.

Adults' consent

The assessment of an adult patient's capacity to make a decision about his own medical treatment is a matter for clinical judgement guided by professional practice and subject to legal requirements. It is the personal responsibility of any doctor proposing to treat a patient to judge whether the patient has the capacity to give a valid consent. Even where capacity to give consent may be limited, the doctor has a duty to give the patient an account, in simple terms, of the benefits and risks of the proposed treatment and to explain the principal alternatives to it and the possible consequences.

In deciding what options may be reasonably considered as being in the best interests of a patient who lacks capacity to decide, you should take into account:
- options for treatment or investigation which are clinically indicated
- any evidence of the patient's previously expressed preferences, including an advance statement
- your own and the healthcare team's knowledge of the patient's background, such as cultural, religious or employment considerations
- views about the patient's preferences given by a third party who may have more knowledge of the patient, e.g. the patient's partner, family, carer, tutor-dative (Scotland), or a person with parental responsibility
- which option least restricts the patient's future choices, where more than one option (including non-treatment) seems reasonable in the patient's best interest

The concept of necessity

Not only is a doctor able to give treatment to an incapacitated patient when it is clearly in that person's best interests, but it is also a common law duty to do so. Nevertheless, this still only applies to treatment carried out to ensure improvement or to prevent deterioration in health. If a person is now incapacitated but is known to have objections to all or some treatment, then doctors are not justified in proceeding, even in an emergency. If the incapacity is temporary because of an anaesthetic, sedation, intoxication or temporary unconsciousness, doctors should not proceed beyond what is essential to preserve the person's life or prevent deterioration in health. Where incapacity may be reversible then every effort should be made to do so. Where there is dispute or doubt amongst either professionals or the next of kin/carers, then a *senior* psychiatric opinion is strongly advised in accordance with the BMA best practice guidelines and usually with the Trust's policy.

Best interests

The doctrine of necessity, which underpins the treatment of people lacking capacity, is essentially made up of two components. First, there must be some necessity to act and, secondly, such action must be in the best interests of the person concerned. Under the current law, the second limb of the necessity concept means that a doctor who acts in accordance with an accepted medical opinion will be acting in the best interests of the patient and will not be negligent in providing such treatment.

General principles

The following general principles should be taken into account when considering the medical treatment of a patient lacking capacity. The patient has a right to:
- be free from discrimination and should not be treated differently solely because of the condition that gives rise to the incapacity
- privacy—the patient should be free from any medical procedures unless there are good therapeutic reasons for them
- confidentiality of personal health information— disclosure only to the nominated next of kin
- liberty—patients should be free from interventions that inhibit liberty or the capacity to enjoy life unless such intervention is necessary to prevent a greater harm to the patient or to others. However, end stage situations or cases such as 'Miss B' who no longer wished to be supported by artificial ventilation need to be examined on their individual merit and expert opinion should always be sought. Appropriate justification must be shown for the use of restraints and it is inappropriate for restrictive measures to be used as an alternative to adequate staffing levels.
- dignity—the patient's social and cultural values should also be respected. They should have their views taken into account even when they are considered legally incapable of determining what happens.

As a matter of good practice it is advisable to obtain a second opinion from another doctor, such as a psychogeriatric physician, in cases where a complex decision is contemplated. This can both assure the doctor proposing to treat the patient that the patient does lack capacity to consent and that the treatment is in the patient's best interests. It is recommended that for any serious procedure doctors should follow a series of basic steps:
- consider whether there are alternative ways of treating the patient, particularly measures which might be less invasive
- discuss the treatment with the healthcare team
- discuss the treatment with the patient in so far as this is possible
- consider any anticipatory statement of the patient's views
- consult other appropriate professionals involved with the patient's care in the hospital or community
- consult relatives and/or carers

- obtain a second opinion from a doctor skilled in the proposed treatment
- ensure that a record is made of the discussions

Views of relatives

Informing and asking the next of kin and other family members to consider the proposed interventions deemed appropriate by the consultant in charge is in accord with the best practice guidelines. It has long been accepted medical practice to consult people close to the patient, to help the medical team assess what the patient would have wanted. The views of relatives are important in so far as they reflect what the patient would have chosen if in a position to decide. It is, however, illegal in England, Wales and Northern Ireland, to ask another adult to consent for any other adult regardless of the patient's incapacity or otherwise. The consultant with responsibility for the patient's best interests may override relatives wishes if they (the consultant) can prove they are acting in the patient's best interest and are not wittingly overriding a patient's previously stated position on this regard. (British Medical Association. (2000) *Withholding and Withdrawing of Medical Treatment–Best Practice Guidelines*.)

PEG feeding in severe dementia

The practice of PEG feeding in patients with severe dementia (those who have become bedridden and dependent in all activities of daily living) has been recently reconsidered. Various experts feel that the practice of PEG insertion should be discouraged on clinical grounds and on the basis that there is no clear evidence of a benefit, e.g. in survival, reduced risk of infection or pressure sores, improved function or improved palliation. Many experts now believe that in such patients a comprehensive, motivated, conscientious programme of hand-feeding is the proper treatment. However, in this case, the patient is not at an end-stage state of dementia and the aspiration pneumonia should be taken into consideration. The BMA (2000) document suggests that it is acceptable to initiate an intervention such as PEG feeling with the caveat that the situation can be regularly reviewed and that if it is not beneficial to the patient it is then appropriate to withdraw the intervention. The principle ethos in this situation is to ensure that *effective, consistent and accurate* lines of communication are maintained during this process between clinicians, multi-disciplinary team (where appropriate) and family.

Comments on the case

This case illustrates the complexities of decision making when a patient is unable to give consent. This type of scenario is extremely frequent and it may be easy for doctors to forget the ethical issues surrounding it.

The reality of the understandable concerns and potential pressures from family members illustrate the need to ensure that you are fully conversant with the contemporary legal and professional position of this complex area of medical care. If you are in any doubt you should discuss these issues with the following people:
Your consultant or Clinical Director
The Trust legal department
The Medical Defence Union, BMA or GMC.

Case 12 | Consent to participate in a clinical trial

Candidate information

You are the SHO in a cardiology clinic

Please read this summary (it should take no more than 2 min) and then continue with the consultation.

Re: Mr Ronald Stevens, aged 65

You see Mr Stevens in your clinic. He has heart failure and you decide that he would be suitable to enter a double-blind randomized controlled trial looking at the effect of treatment 'X' against placebo. This is being carried out by your department as part of a multicentre trial. Treatment 'X' is a new anti-heart-failure drug and is given in a dose of 10 mg o.d. for 1 year. Previous phase I and II trials have only revealed rare side-effects such as a rash, ankle swelling and headaches. The endpoint is left ventricular ejection fraction as measured on the echo. Your consultant is the main supervisor for the project in your department. At present, the patient is taking frusemide (furosemide) and an angiotensin-converting enzyme (ACE) inhibitor and he should remain on these throughout the trial.

Your tasks are to: consider if Mr Stevens would like to enter the trial and counsel him for this.

You have 14 min until the patient leaves the room, followed by 1 min for reflection, before the discussion with the examiners.

Subject/patient/relative information

Mr Stevens is a 65-year-old man who has moderate left ventricular dysfunction as a consequence of ischaemic heart disease and an anterior myocardial infarction 4 years ago. At present he is reasonably well-controlled on frusemide 40 mg o.d. and an ACE inhibitor. He manages to carry out his usual activities of daily living quite well although he becomes more tired by the end of the day. He has never entered a clinical trial before but is willing to try it in the hope that it might improve his condition. His main queries are the side-effects of the new tablet, why there must be a placebo arm to the trial, what happens if he changes his mind halfway through the trial, and whether he can remain on the present medication. He is about to see the SHO (the candidate) who is to consider recruiting him into the trial on behalf of the consultant.

Examiner information

1 Communication skills—conduct of interview

- Introduce yourself and ask the patient what he understands about his condition.
- Tell him you would like to invite him to take part in a 'research' study, explaining the aims and purpose of the study and why he is a suitable candidate.
- Explain that he would be given either the tablet being tested or a dummy (placebo) once a day for 12 months. Which tablet he will receive is decided at random (like tossing a coin). Explain the need for having a placebo in the trial: to test whether there is a benefit from the new treatment i.e. taking a placebo would allow a controlled comparison which would eliminate bias in the handling and assessment of patients. Explain neither he nor you will know what medication he has received (double-blinded). However, the information would be immediately available if required for medical reasons.
- Explain what would be measured and tell him that the advantage of taking part in the study is that his condition would be monitored by the same doctors more closely than usual. It is also possible that his condition may improve—although there is no guarantee—and it may be helpful in developing a new therapy for others with similar conditions.
- Explain the possible side-effects and reassure him that he will be regularly reviewed for this. Explain that the drug has been tested before and the side-effects are rare. He would remain on all his present medication as well.
- Explain that participation is totally voluntary and he does not have to decide now. If he decides not to take part then his management by the team would not be altered in any way. If he does decide to take part, he can still withdraw at any time and this would not affect the future conduct of his treatment.
- His identity in the study would be treated as strictly confidential. Records identifying him would not be made publicly available. If the results of the trial are published, his identity would remain confidential. If reference to him is made, this would only be done by using code numbers. However, in order to meet legal obligations, records identifying him may be inspected by representatives of the sponsor and could be reviewed by the registration authorities or hospital ethics committee. His GP would be informed about his participation in this study.
- Explain that monitoring would include echocardiograms and blood samples.
- Explain there are other patients in other centres taking part in the study.
- Should any illness arise from the trial then he would be treated in the usual appropriate way.
- Tell him that you will give him your telephone number for any queries or worries and that you will provide an information sheet. If he decides to take part he would sign a consent form which is attached to the information sheet.
- Invite him to ask any questions he has now and also after he has studied the information sheet.

2 Communication skills—exploration and problem negotiation

The candidate should be able to discuss clearly and openly:
- what the study is about
- what the patient has to do
- what are the benefits of the study
- what are the discomforts of the investigations and risks (side-effects of therapy)
- the options if he does not want to take part; would the patient be treated in the usual way if he refuses to enter?
- what happens to the information obtained and the issue of confidentiality
- who else is taking part
- what if something goes wrong; would he be treated in the appropriate way?
- who to contact for further information (usually the chief investigator or member of the local ethics committee)

3 Ethics and the law and other discussion points (general guidelines adapted from the General Medical Council)

- Research involving clinical trials of drugs or treatments and research into the causes, or possible treatment for a particular condition is important in increasing doctors' ability to provide effective care for present and future patients. The benefits of the research may, however, be uncertain and may not be experienced by the person participating in the research. In addition, the risk involved for research individuals may be difficult to identify or to assess in advance. If you carry out or participate in research involving patients or volunteers, it is particularly important that you ensure, as far as you are able, that the research is not contrary to the individual's interests and that individuals understand that it is research and that the results are not predictable.

- You must take particular care to be sure that anyone you ask to consider taking part in research is given the fullest possible information, presented in terms and a form that they can understand. This must include any information about possible benefits and risks, evidence that a research ethics committee has given approval and advise that they can withdraw at any time. You should ensure that individuals have the opportunity to read and consider the research information leaflet. You must allow them sufficient time to reflect on the implications of participating in the study. You must not put pressure on anyone to take part in research. You must obtain the person's consent in writing. Before starting any research you must always obtain approval from a properly constituted research ethics committee.

- You should seek further advice where your research involves children or adults who are not able to make decisions for themselves. You should be aware that in these cases the legal position is complex or unclear, and there is currently no general consensus on how to balance the possible risks and benefits to such vulnerable individuals against the public interest in conducting research.

General Medical Council. *Seeking Patient's Consent: the Ethical Considerations*, Section 35–37. Consenting to research. November 1998.

Comments on the case

Never put pressure on a patient when enrolling into a clinical trial and be informative without using jargon. Candidates must realize that consenting to research is not just the patient 'signing on the dotted line'. Any recruiting to research carried out in a wayward manner can and will lead to serious consequences. You are relying on the patient's goodwill and so they deserve honesty and openness from you.

Case 13 | Dealing with poor compliance

Candidate information

You are the medical SHO in clinic

Please read this summary (it should take no more than 2 min) and then continue with the consultation.

Re: Mr Stephen Morley, aged 19

Mr Morley was diagnosed as having pulmonary tuberculosis 2 months ago (smear positive). He is being reviewed in clinic by yourself. He is not unwell but his cough and sputum persist and he has not gained any weight. His chest X-ray is no better either. He works in a nightclub collecting glasses, drinks about 8 pints of strong lager a day and smokes 40 cigarettes a day (including cannabis). He does not have HIV infection. He lives in a home for the homeless. He migrated from Galway when he was 12, and essentially comes from a sad family background. His father is in prison and his mother committed suicide 4 years ago. You have spoken to the TB health visitor and she is not convinced that Mr Morley is taking the antituberculous tablets every day. In fact, the TB health visitor has confirmed with the GP that Mr Morley has only picked up one prescription (2 weeks' supply) on the first day of treatment 2 months ago. At present he should be on Rifinah 300 two tablets a day, pyrazinamide 2 g/day, ethambutol 800 mg/day and pyridoxine 10 mg o.d. You are concerned that he is still symptomatic, that he is poorly complying with the medication and that he is still infectious. Mr Morley has let it be known that he would not want to be admitted to hospital.

Your tasks are to: approach Mr Morley on the issue of non-compliance and discuss ways of improving his compliance.

You have 14 min until the patient leaves the room, followed by 1 min for reflection, before the discussion with the examiners.

Subject/patient/relative information

Mr Morley is a 19-year-old Irishman who was diagnosed 2 months ago with pulmonary tuberculosis which presented with cough, sputum and loss of weight. The chest X-ray showed shadowing and the tuberculosis was confirmed by a sputum sample which was microscopically positive (smear positive). Cultures revealed fully sensitive *Mycobacteria tuberculosis*. He settled in the UK when he was 12 and comes from an unsettled background; his mother committed suicide 4 years ago and his father is in prison. At present he lives in a hostel for the homeless and works part-time as a glass collector in a nightclub. He drinks too much and smokes heavily as well. He has been started on Rifinah 300, pyrazinamide, ethambutol and pyridoxine, in total nine tablets a day. His compliance has been poor, in fact non-existent over the last 2 months. He finds the pyrazinamide difficult to swallow (chalky, white tabs) and felt sick with the others (especially the Rifinah — the orange tabs). His hours are nocturnal and, because he drinks heavily, he forgets to take his tablets. He has seen the TB health visitor only once because each time she visits the hostel he is not in. He is usually at someone else's house drinking heavily. He has failed to attend clinic four times but has turned up today. His symptoms of cough and sputum persist and he has not gained any weight. He is in denial of his illness and will not admit to poor compliance. He is due to see the medical SHO (the candidate) in clinic. After being given a full explanation he agrees to participate in a programme of direct observed therapy (DOT).

Examiner information

1 Communication skills — conduct of interview

- Introduce yourself to Mr Morley.
- Ask how he is with regard to his symptoms.
- Ask him how he is finding taking the tablets and has he had any problems — first give him every opportunity to tell you himself that he is having difficulties complying.
- If he says he has not been taking them, then ask why. Ask about the possible reasons, e.g. side-effects (real or perceived), forgetfulness, inability to get hold of the tablets, poor information about how to take the tablets, the purpose of taking the medicine is not clear, perceived lack of efficacy, unpleasant taste/difficult to swallow (pyrazinamide is notorious for this), complicated regimen, etc.
- If he says 'everything is fine', then say that there does not seem to be any improvement in his health and that the most common reason for this is usually because the tablets are not being taken correctly. If necessary then tell him that you are aware that he has not picked up his prescriptions for the past two months. He may then admit to non-compliance. (Be careful about attributing suspicions about his non-compliance to a specific person, with some patients this may wreck their relationship with the 'informer'.)
- Discuss with the patient how important it is to treat TB properly and acknowledge that it can be difficult for patients who have been on antibiotics for a long time. Explain that in such situations a new plan must be generated to help him take his medication correctly.
- Explain that you will be speaking to your consultant and to the TB health visitor and that one of the options is to arrange directly observed therapy (DOT) where ingestion of every dose is witnessed. Tell him this will be done three times a week with the doses of the tablets altered to accommodate this change in frequency.
- Advise him that he should not work in the nightclub because of the risk of infecting others. Acknowledge that this is obviously difficult news for him as it is his livelihood. Suggest that he may want to discuss with his TB health visitor what alterative employment options may be available to him.

2 Communication skills — exploration and problem negotiation

The candidate should be able to:
- make an assessment of the patient's current health
- approach the issue of compliance in a non-confrontational manner
- discuss and negotiate ways to improve compliance
- acknowledge the personal impact on the patient and offer a route for them to obtain continuing support

3 Ethics and the law and other discussion points

- The doctor in the clinic *must* involve the GP immediately. Do not wait for the letter to be typed by the secretary. Ring the GP from clinic and inform him or her of the problems. The GP may be able to carry out the DOT using a practice health visitor if the practice has had any such experience before.
- Non-compliance to medication is very common and the factors causing this are stated above. Every consultation should have some assessment of compliance.
- Ways to help compliance include better education, explanation of side-effects, alternative regimens and simplified drug regimens. In antituberculous therapy, rifampicin, isoniazid and pyrazinamide can be taken as a combination product, Rifater, which is much easier to swallow.
- DOT in tuberculosis therapy is where ingestion of every drug is witnessed. Cohort studies with historical controls receiving self-administered therapy have shown improved cure rates from DOT. In the UK, where tuberculosis is usually managed by experienced

physicians with the help of specialized nurses, DOT is recommended in non-compliers, particularly the homeless, alcoholics, drug abusers, drifters, the seriously mentally ill, patients with multiple drug-resistance, a history of non-compliance either in the past or during the present treatment and should be considered in refugees, especially from countries where multidrug resistance is particularly high (e.g. Eastern Europe).

- DOT can be daily but an intermittent regimen is more convenient. A common regimen is rifampicin, isoniazid, pyrazinamide and ethambutol (or streptomycin) three times weekly for 2 months then rifampicin and isoniazid three times weekly for 4 months.

Comments on the case

Poor compliance is a huge problem in clinical practice and this case highlights one particular scenario where non-compliance can be really difficult. Do not be confrontational towards a patient who does not admit to non-compliance. Many patients will bluff their way through the consultation. Use your investigative skills to work out the degree of compliance, e.g. clinical and radiological improvement. Colour of urine can sometimes help to check if the patient has taken rifampicin the same day. Do not necessarily go for the easy alternative and admit the patient to hospital; circumstances will not change when he is discharged.

Case 14 | Deliberate self-harm

Candidate information

You are the medical SHO in the emergency admissions unit

Please read this summary (it should take no more than 2 min) and then continue with the consultation.

> ### Re: Mr William Bremner, aged 49
>
> Mr Bremner was admitted today by the house officer following a paraceta-mol overdose. He took 10 500-mg tablets 24 h ago with the intention of committing suicide. His paracetamol levels are under the treatment level and he does not have any symptoms suggestive of hepatotoxicity. He is sitting alone in the day room watching television. The ward nurse is worried that this episode was a genuine suicide attempt. She wants you to assess him.

Your tasks are to: explore the reasons behind the suicide attempt and assess Mr Bremner's suicide risk.

You have 14 min until the patient leaves the room, followed by 1 min for reflection, before the discussion with the examiners.

Subject/patient/relative information

Mr Bremner is a 49-year-old information technology consultant. He has recently lost his job as a result of poor business and his wife left him 2 months ago after 27 years of marriage. They had been incompatible for a number of years but one day his wife just decided to leave. As a result he is convinced that his life is now hopeless and worthless and that the future is very bleak. He had never really thought about killing himself until now. Over the last month he has been having suicidal thoughts most days, but yesterday was his first real attempt. He took 10 tablets of 500 mg paracetamol in one go with two glasses of vodka. He wrote a damning note to his wife before the attempt. He went to bed but woke up this morning with a slight headache and nausea. He told his neighbour who brought him straight to casualty. He does not have any paranoia or persecutory delusions. He has always been a heavy drinker (especially spirits, usually three bottles a week) but more recently his consumption has increased. He does not suffer from any physical illnesses and he has had no other bereavements. Currently, he is clearly depressed with low mood and poor sleep, appetite and concentration. He feels life is not worth living but is not sure if he really wants to kill himself. What he does realize is that he wants some help. He is about to see the medical SHO (the candidate).

Examiner information

1 Communication skills—conduct of interview

- Introduce yourself to Mr Bremner.
- Explain how sorry you are that he is in hospital and that you realise things must be very hard for him to attempt to kill himself.
- Reassure him that you are there to help him.
- Ask him how he is feeling physically at the moment. Ask if he has any symptoms of nausea, abdominal pain or headaches (from the paracetamol poisoning).
- Then ask him to go through with you what tablets, how many, all at once, with alcohol, planned self-harm, was he alone, timed so that no one could intervene, suicide note, recent change in his will. Did he inform anyone after the act, intend to kill himself?
- Ask him if he still wants to die.
- Tell him you realise it must be painful and difficult but is he able to explain the reasons for attempted self-harm and the problems faced by Mr Bremner: job loss, marital problems, financial difficulties, legal problems, alcohol and drugs problem, present psychiatric disorders, bereavement or impending loss and social isolation.
- Assess Mr Bremner's mental state: suicidal thoughts, feeling of hopelessness, worthlessness and despair, lowering of mood with symptoms of poor sleep, poor appetite and poor concentration, persecutory delusions, paranoia and any auditory hallucinations.
- Is there a present or past psychiatric history including previous suicide attempts?
- Assess family and social support.
- Explain again that you are there to help. Ask if he understands why he needs help (insight?). Say that you will look after him medically as he gets over the paracetamol poisoning and will arrange further liver function tests. Then he will be seen by the psychiatrist who may consider transferring him to the psychiatric unit to start antidepressant therapy and to protect him from any further self-harm. Ask how he feels about seeing a psychiatrist.
- Ask if he has any other questions.

2 Communication skills—exploration and problem negotiation

The candidate should be able to:

- understand and sympathize with Mr Bremner's present psychological state

- obtain a detailed history of the suicide event without being judgemental
- assess the other factors important in assessing an attempted suicide
- assess the risk of further suicide attempt
- reassure him that help is available

3 Ethics and the law

Factors suggesting a suicidal intent

- act carried out in isolation
- act timed so intervention unlikely
- precautions taken to avoid discovery
- preparation made in anticipation of death (e.g. making a will)
- active preparation made for the attempt (e.g. saving up tablets)
- extensive premedication
- leaving a suicide note
- failing to inform potential helpers after the act
- admission of suicidal intent

Assessing a patient following an attempted suicide should include

- the events that preceded the act
- reasons for the act, including suicide intent
- the problems faced by the patient
- any psychiatric disorders and psychiatric history, including previous suicide attempts
- family and personal history
- the risk of suicide
- the coping resources and support
- whether the patient is ready to accept help

Factors associated with a risk of a further attempt include

- male
- under 19 or over 45 years old
- unemployment
- separated, widowed, divorced or living alone
- chronic physical ill-health
- previous attempt with hospital admission
- problems with alcohol and drugs
- psychiatric disorder, especially depression, schizophrenia, alcoholism

An important minority of patients attempting suicide are uncooperative with medical treatment and they attempt to self-discharge. These patients are in a particularly high-risk group for self-harm and although patient autonomy is paramount, doctors must be aware of their duty of care. If the patient is suffering from a mental disorder, there may be grounds for treating them under the Mental Health Act. An urgent psychiatric opinion is necessary. Where there is no evidence that the patient is mentally disordered, the patient's capacity to make decisions needs to be assessed. The doctor must determine if the patient is able:

- to comprehend and retain information on the proposed treatment including its indications, main benefits and the consequences of non-treatment
- to believe the information
- to use the information and weigh it up as part of the process of arriving at a decision

---

Comments on the case

While the situation of an attempted suicide is complex, it is important to make an initial psychosocial assessment, including the patient's mental state, as soon as possible. All doctors in medicine must be able to do this.

Patients who repeatedly present with parasuicide may have fallen through the support network. Where they are not diagnosed as having a mental disorder, then advice and support should be sought from psychology or counselling services if the patient is willing to explore these options.

Case 15 | Deep vein thrombosis in pregnancy

Candidate information

You are the SHO in the medical admissions unit

Please read this summary (it should take no more than 2 min) and then continue with the consultation.

> **Re: Mrs Stacey Charlton, aged 28**
>
> Mrs Stacey Charlton is a 28-year-old lady who is 32 weeks pregnant with her first child. She presents with a 1-week history of left calf swelling—so much so that she finds walking difficult. She has been sent in by the GP and an ultrasound scan performed this morning has confirmed a left calf deep vein thrombosis (DVT). The femoral veins are patent. She is on folate 0.5 mg/day. She is in the waiting room waiting for the results; she was told that if the scan was normal, she could go home.

Your tasks are to: explain the results of the ultrasound scan and decide on a plan of management.

You have 14 min until the patient leaves the room, followed by 1 min for reflection, before the discussion with the examiners.

Subject/patient/relative information

Mrs Stacey Charlton is a 28-year-old housewife who is 32 weeks pregnant with her first child. She has been well until 1 week ago when she started complaining of swelling in the left calf; there was no previous history of a fall or any trauma. The left calf is quite painful now and she has difficulty in walking. The GP suggested that this may be a DVT and so arranged for her admission for an ultrasound scan. She is worried that any therapy might harm the fetus and so she is hoping that the scan is normal. She has had no previous history of thromboses and she does not have any chest pain or breathlessness. She is in the waiting room expecting to see the medical SHO (the candidate) with the ultrasound result. She is expecting to be able to go home.

Examiner information

1 Communication skills—conduct of interview

- Introduce yourself to Mrs Charlton.
- Show sympathy for her symptoms.
- Explain the result of the ultrasound scan, that it con-

firms a DVT in the left calf but that there is no extension of the clot above the knee. Acknowledge that the news will obviously concern her, particularly because she is pregnant, and that you want to explain the treatment plan and discuss any anxieties she may have.

- Ask what she understands by a deep vein thrombosis and whether she has any previous history of a DVT.

- Determine if there has been any history of clotting abnormalities (family history as well) or recurrent miscarriages in the past (antiphospholipid syndrome?).
- Ask if there are any symptoms which may suggest a pulmonary embolism, such as pleuritic chest pain, dyspnoea or haemoptysis.
- Reassure her that the DVT is treatable but explain that it needs to be treated with anticoagulation.
- Describe the types of anticoagulation available: warfarin (tablet) and low molecular weight heparin (LMWH).
- Explain that warfarin is contraindicated in pregnancy, despite the ease of administration, because of the risk of placental and fetal bleeding.
- The safest option is daily subcutaneous injections with LMWH. Explain that she will be on therapy for 12 weeks. When she is at term (about 8 weeks into therapy), she will stop the LMWH for 24 h (to reduce the risk of bleeding during labour) and the obstetrician will induce labour. Once delivered safely, she can be recommended on LMWH and started on warfarin with about 5 days of overlap, after which the LMWH can be discontinued. She should continue on the warfarin for another 4 weeks postpartum. Warfarin and LMWH are safe during the postpartum period.
- Explain that you will ask for the opinion of her obstetrician and the haematologist for further advice and that she will be closely followed-up by these two teams.
- Reassure her that, with LMWH, the fetus will be safe and she will find that her swelling will reduce with treatment.
- Suggest pain relief such as paracetamol and advise her to wear support stockings.
- Ask if she has any further worries or questions.
- Reassure her again.

2 Communication skills—exploration and problem negotiation

The candidate should be able to:
- explain the ultrasound results
- explain what a DVT is and acknowledge that she is going to be especially concerned because of the pregnancy
- investigate the possibility of a pulmonary embolism
- provide a management plan with a description of the available anticoagulants and an explanation as to why LMWH is indicated during pregnancy rather than warfarin

3 Ethics and the law and other discussion points

- A hypercoagulable state is characteristic of pregnancy and so a DVT is a common complication. The risk is particularly great during the third trimester and for a few weeks postpartum. A pulmonary embolism is not an uncommon reason for maternal death in the UK. Activated protein C resistance caused by the factor V Leiden mutation increases the risk for DVT and pulmonary embolism during pregnancy. Approximately 25% of women with a DVT during pregnancy carry the factor V Leiden allele. The presence of the factor V Leiden mutation also increases the risk for severe pre-eclampsia. If the fetus carries a factor V Leiden mutation, the risk of extensive placental infarction is high.
- Anticoagulant therapy with heparin is indicated in pregnant women with a DVT. Warfarin crosses the placenta with a risk of placental or fetal haemorrhage. Warfarin therapy is contraindicated in the first trimester because of its association with fetal epiphyseal haemorrhage. In the second and third trimesters, warfarin may cause fetal optic atrophy and mental retardation. However, warfarin is safe during breastfeeding.
- In the initial treatment of a DVT, LMWH, which does not cross the placenta, may be administered subcutaneously according to body weight. LMWH is not contraindicated in breastfeeding women. Recent concerns about LMWH use and epidural haematomas suggest that caution must be used in the anaesthetic management of patients who had been receiving LMWH near the onset of labour.
- Difficult decisions arise when patients are on long-term warfarin therapy because of prosthetic valves or recurrent pulmonary embolism. Any change over to LMWH must be carried out with care and under the multidisciplinary care of the obstetrician and the haematologist.
- During the third trimester, increased blood volume with obstruction of venous return by the gravid uterus makes non-invasive assessment of the deep veins difficult. In cases where a pulmonary embolism is suspected, pulmonary angiography is possible with precautions.
- Ventilation–perfusion scanning of the lungs can be carried out in pregnancy. The procedure must be explained carefully to the patient. Generally, the technetium-labelled microaggregated albumin (for perfusion) is of a low radioactive dose (especially when compared to a bone scan) and the krypton gas used

(for ventilation) has a very short half-life (seconds). However, these risks must be weighed up against the importance of having adequate information to diagnose a pulmonary embolism.

Comments on the case

This case shows how complicated a thromboembolism in pregnancy can be. Having a secure plan of management is vital to reassure the mother, who is particularly concerned about any possible harm to the fetus. Therefore it is important for the candidate to win over the patient's trust early in the consultation with maximum reassurance.

Case 16 | Eligibility for coronary artery bypass surgery

Candidate information

You are the cardiology SHO

Please read this summary (it should take no more than 2 min) and then continue with the consultation.

> ### Re: Lawrence Boon, aged 74
>
> Mr Boon had a subendocardial myocardial infarction 6 months ago and a subsequent coronary angiogram was performed because of persistent angina. The angiogram revealed three-vessel disease, particularly in the distal ends of the arteries. The cardiac surgeons decided that there was no distinct artery amenable to grafting or stenting and so a decision for optimum medical therapy was made at a recent cardiology/cardiac surgery combined meeting. Mr Boon is relatively fit apart from the angina. He smokes 20 cigarettes a day and does not intend to give up. The smoking habit was also an issue raised at the meeting. Regrettably, Mr Boon had to be away on the day of the combined meeting: he has come to see you in clinic to discuss the decisions made. He is keen to undergo bypass surgery to relieve his symptoms. His recent medication includes aspirin 75 mg o.d., simvastatin 20 mg, atenolol 50 mg and Imdur (isosorbide mononitrate) 60 mg o.d.

Your tasks are to: explain the decisions made regarding the bypass surgery and address the disappointment that he will have.

You have 14 min until the patient leaves the room, followed by 1 min for reflection, before the discussion with the examiners.

Subject/patient/relative information

Mr Boon is a 74-year-old retired salesman who had a subendocardial myocardial infarction 6 months ago. Since then, he has continued to have angina which may come on after walking 100 m on the flat. He does not have any rest pain. An angiogram confirmed three-vessel disease, particularly in the distal areas, but no vessel was amenable for grafting or stenting. At a recent joint cardiology/cardiac surgery meeting it was felt that optimum medical therapy would be the most appropriate management for him. Mr Boon is relatively fit apart from the angina and has been told that a decision will be made regarding the possibility of an operation. He is keen for the operation as he feels a graft will cure all his cardiac ailments. He has been a heavy smoker for many years and does not intend to give up. He feels very strongly about the prejudice medical staff have against smokers and if he is told he is unsuitable for a bypass graft, he has no doubt that the main reason would be his smoking.

Examiner information

1 Communication skills — conduct of interview

- Introduce yourself to Mr Boon.
- Ask what has been discussed with him so far.
- Explain the main reason for the consultation.
- Convey to him that it has been decided by the surgical team that bypass grafting is not technically possible.
- Explain the reasons; none of the vessels were amenable for bypass grafting or stenting.
- Listen to Mr Boon and appreciate how he feels about it. He may challenge you by asking if his smoking influenced the decision.
- Explain that the decision is made by numerous experts in the meeting, based on technical grounds. Any decision made by the team is in the best interests of the patient.
- Address Mr Boon's challenge that although smoking does affect post-bypass prognosis, this did not influence the decision on the bypass grafting. It was simply a question of technical feasibility.
- Tell him the plan of management for his angina, explaining that optimizing the medical treatment is the main treatment objective.
- Ask how his angina is at present and go through the list of medications he is on with a view to increasing the dosage.
- Address the issue of cessation of smoking.
- Address any persisting grievances and offer him the opportunity to discuss the decision with a consultant involved in the decision making process.

2 Communication skills — exploration and problem negotiation

The candidate should be able to:

- ascertain what has been explained to the patient before

- discuss the decision made by the cardiac teams with an explanation of why
- address any concerns and grievances made by the patient
- convey a plan of management for the patient with the aim of optimizing his medical therapy

3 Ethics and the law and other discussion points

- The patient is concerned that he has been denied surgery because of lifestyle issues and that he has been discriminated against because of his smoking habit.
- While it should be explained that discrimination on such issues is unacceptable, it is still important to make the patient aware of the deleterious effect of continued smoking when he already has significant coronary heart disease.
- Even if the surgeons were amenable, bypass grafting cannot be denied because of lifestyle, age, gender, income and religion ('The NHS — our commitment to you': the new NHS charter).

Comments on the case

It is not uncommon for physicians to be faced with a situation where a patient is being denied treatment for whatever the reason, e.g. unsuitability (e.g. cancer resection), poor outcome of surgery (e.g. unfit for surgery), lack of funds (e.g. certain chemotherapy regimens) or lack of expertise (specific specialized surgical procedures, e.g. multiorgan transplantation). The skill of addressing the disappointment and anger will be thoroughly tested here.

Case 17 | Fitness to drive

Candidate information

You are the SHO in a general medical clinic

Please read this summary (it should take no more than 2 min) and then continue with the consultation.

> ### Re: Mr Robert Wills, aged 39
>
> Mr Wills is in clinic today after being discharged from hospital 4 weeks ago. He was admitted with a solitary fit. There were no precipitating factors and an EEG and CT scan of the head were normal. Legally, he is barred from driving for 1 year with a medical review before restarting driving. He was given this information at the time of discharge.

Your tasks are to: determine if Mr Wills has had any more fits and discuss the issue of driving.

You have 14 min until the patient leaves the room, followed by 1 min for reflection, before the discussion with the examiners.

Subject/patient/relative information

Mr Robert Wills is a single, 39-year-old man who was admitted from casualty 4 weeks ago with a solitary fit. A CT scan and EEG were both normal. There was no particular precipitant for the fit and he does not drink alcohol. He has had no more fits since discharge and he feels well. He does not take any medication. He works for British Telecom (BT) as a maintenance technician which involves a lot of driving to visit residents who have reported a fault. He was told that he must not drive for 1 year when he left hospital but as he was feeling so well and, with the risk of losing his job, he has decided to go back to full-time work. He has not considered placement elsewhere within British Telecom. He is about to see the medical SHO (the candidate) in the clinic who will approach him regarding the subject of driving. At the end of the consultation Mr Wills will agree to talk to the BT personnel department to discuss placement elsewhere within BT.

Examiner information

1 Communication skills—conduct of interview

- Ask how he has been since discharge. Ask if he understands why he was admitted and reassure him that the EEG and CT scan of the head were both normal. Remind him, however, that there is no doubt that he did have a fit. Find out if he has had any more fits.
- Discuss what his occupation is and whether this involves driving.
- Ask him if he is back at work and still driving (Mr Wills says yes).
- Ask him if he was informed before discharge that after a solitary fit patients are legally banned from driving for 1 year until there has been a medical review to determine if driving can recommence; as recommended by the Drivers Medical Unit, DVLA, Swansea.

- Mr Wills tells you that he cannot stop driving as this is essential for his work.
- You reply by saying that very often it is those patients who drive for a living who are at greatest risk both to themselves and to the public at large as they spend more time on the road.
- Tell him he must notify the DVLA and that he should not drive until he fulfils their guidelines.
- Point out that whether he notifies the DVLA or not, his insurance policy is now invalid (this may persuade him).
- Mr Wills thinks for a short while and tells you that he still intends to drive.
- Tell him that you appreciate being barred from driving is very difficult for him especially as his livelihood depends upon it.
- Tell him that if he does not inform the DVLA then you are acting within reason to inform them yourself. Furthermore, you will record this advice in the notes.
- Ask him if he would like to see the consultant and ask if there is any opportunity for placement elsewhere within BT during the ban. Mr Wills says that he will speak to the BT management.
- Suggest that it is important for him to negotiate with his employer to see whether or not he can be given alternative work for the duration of the bar. Offer to contact his occupational health doctor.
- If he remains adamant that he will continue to drive and doubts the veracity of the information you have given, offer him an opportunity to see the consultant.
- Make sure you arrange to see Mr Wills again soon to reinforce the advice.

2 Communication skills — exploration and problem negotiation

The candidate should be able to:
- determine if the patient has had further fits
- obtain details of whether Mr Wills is back at work and driving
- explain to Mr Wills that legally he is banned from driving for 1 year
- inform Mr Wills of the risks and persuade him to inform the DVLA
- know the doctor's rights if Mr Wills refuses to consider stopping driving

3 Ethics and the law and other discussion points

- The legal basis of fitness to drive lies in the Road Traffic Act 1988 and subsequent regulations including, in par-

ticular, the Motor Vehicles (Driving Licences) Regulations 1996. A **prescribed disability** is one that is a legal bar to the holding of a licence unless certain conditions are met (e.g. epilepsy). A **relevant disability** is any medical condition that is likely to render the person a source of danger while driving (e.g. a visual field defect). A **prospective disability** is any medical condition which, because of its progressive or intermittent nature, may cause the driver to have a prescribed or relevant disability in the course of time (e.g. insulin-treated diabetes mellitus). A driver with a prospective disability may only hold a driving licence subject to a medical review every 1, 2 or 3 years, depending upon the circumstances.
- It is the duty of the licence holder or applicant to notify the DVLA of any medical condition which may affect safe driving. There are some circumstances in which the licence holder cannot, or will not, do this. Under these circumstances the GMC has issued clear guidelines.
- The DVLA is legally responsible for deciding if a person is medically unfit to drive. They need to know when holders of a driving licence have a condition which may, now or in the future, affect their safety as a driver. Therefore, where patients have such conditions, you should:
(a) make sure that the patient understands that the condition may impair their ability to drive. If a patient is incapable of understanding this advice, e.g. because of dementia, you should inform the DVLA immediately
(b) explain to patients that they have a legal duty to inform the DVLA about the condition
(c) if the patient refuses to accept the diagnosis or the effect that this condition has, or may have, on their ability to drive, you can suggest that the patient seeks a second opinion, and make appropriate arrangements for the patient to do so. You should advise the patient not to drive until the second opinion has been obtained (in this case there is no doubt about the diagnosis, i.e. a solitary fit)
(d) if patients continue to drive when they are not fit to do so, you should make every reasonable effort to persuade them to stop. This may include telling their next of kin
(e) if you are unable to persuade a patient to stop driving or you are given, or find, evidence that the patient is continuing to drive contrary to advice then you should disclose the relevant medical information immediately, in confidence, to the medical adviser at the DVLA
(f) before giving information to the DVLA you should

inform the patient of your decision to do so. Once the DVLA has been informed, you should also write to the patient to confirm that a disclosure has been made. Inform the GP as well (copy letter) and document all discussions accurately in the notes

- Another common scenario that physicians come across is the issue of driving for diabetic patients with poor eyesight. The law states that a licence holder or applicant is suffering from a prescribed disability if unable to meet the eyesight requirements, i.e. to read in good light (with the aid of glasses or contact lenses if worn) a registration plate fixed to a motor vehicle at a distance of 20.5 m and containing letters and figures 79.4 mm high. If unable to meet this standard, the driver cannot drive and the licence must be refused or revoked. In practice, with regard to poor visual acuity, e.g. those with cataracts, this usually corresponds to between 6/9 and 6/12 on the Snellen chart. The minimum field of vision for safe driving is defined as 'a field of at least 120° on the horizontal measured by the Goldmann perimeter using III4e settings'.

Drivers Medical Unit, DVLA. *For medical practitioners: at a glance guide to the current medical standards of fitness to drive.* March 2001.

> ### Comments on the case
>
> This is another case where most patients react sensibly and advise the DVLA themselves and seek a possible change of placement at work. However, there will be occasions where you will be put in a tricky situation such as this, so it is vital that you should know the rules and regulations. The DVLA are very helpful in providing further information and it is important that you are factual and avoid giving inaccurate information, it is not fair to feign ignorance or false hope and pass the responsibility for imparting this bad news to either your consultant or the DVLA. Patients may use alcohol as a cause for the fit but the DVLA does not use alcohol or drugs as an excuse.

Case 18 | Genetic counselling

Candidate information

You are the SHO in a neurology clinic

Please read this summary (it should take no more than 2 min) and then continue with the consultation.

> **Re: Miss Jackie Cromwell, aged 23**
>
> Miss Cromwell has come to see you in clinic today with her father who has recently been diagnosed with Huntington's disease. There is no apparent family history. The daughter wants to speak to you privately about the possibility of a genetic blood test to determine whether she is at risk of developing this disease in later life and possibly passing this condition to her future children.

Your tasks are to: obtain her reasons for a genetic test and counsel her for this.

You have 14 min until the daughter leaves the room, followed by 1 min for reflection, before the discussion with the examiners.

Subject/patient/relative information

Miss Jackie Cromwell is a 23-year-old lady attending the neurology clinic with her father who has recently been diagnosed as having Huntington's disease. She has been reading various leaflets which have highlighted the autosomal dominant nature of the condition, with children of an affected parent having a 50% chance of inheritance. She is aware of the symptoms and the progressive nature of the disease leading to dementia. Although she is fit and well, she has been considering long and hard as to whether or not she should have a test to determine her chance of developing the disease. She does not have much idea about the procedure of the test and so has asked the SHO (the candidate) for more information. She has one younger brother and she is unmarried with no children. She is concerned about the risk of possibly passing this condition on to any future children.

Examiner information

1 Communication skills — conduct of interview

- Ask if she has a partner. If so, try to encourage her to bring them to participate in the counselling.
- Try to obtain a family tree: number of sisters, brothers, aunts, uncles, cousins.

- Ask if there is anything about Huntington's disease that she is unsure of. If not, explain briefly the nature, treatment and prognosis of the disease and ask if there is anyone else in the family with Huntington's disease who might already be affected.
- Explain the purpose of the screening and that a genetic make-up is ascertained to see if she has the genetic

mutation seen in this illness (mutation of distal short arm of chromosome 4).

- Explore her rationale for wanting the test in case she is being forced to have it.
- Explain the nature of the test and the possibility of false positive and negative results.
- Discuss any significant medical, social or financial implications of screening.
- Reassure her that there will be time to decide if she is unsure about proceeding and that at the next appointment you will provide her with addresses of support services.
- Say that you could refer her to a regional genetic centre if she decides to go ahead with the testing.
- Keep the conversation simple and comprehensible. Encourage questions.

2 Communication skills—exploration and problem negotiation

The candidate should be able to:

- determine why she wants the test
- determine her understanding of the disease
- explain the nature of the test, i.e. blood test looking at the genetic make-up

3 Ethics and the law and other discussion points

General comments

- All individuals who may wish to take this test should be given up-to-date, relevant information so that they can make an informed, voluntary decision.
- The subject must choose freely to be tested and must not be coerced by family, friends, partners or potential partners, physicians, insurance companies, employers or others.
- The test is available only to subjects who have reached the age of maturity (according to the laws of the respective country).
- Subjects should not be discriminated against in any way as a result of genetic testing for Huntington's disease.
- Extreme care should be exercised when testing would provide information about another person who has not requested the test. This issue arises when an offspring with 25% risk requests testing with full knowledge that his or her parent does not want to know his or her own status.
- Testing for Huntington's disease should not be part of a routine blood investigation without the specific permission of the subject and such specific permission

should, in principle, also be required for symptomatic subjects.

- Ownership of the test result remains with the subject who requested the test. Legal ownership of the stored DNA remains with the person from whom the blood was taken.
- The consent form should address this issue. Local legal guidance policies may be helpful.
- All laboratories are expected to meet rigorous standards of accuracy. They must work with genetic counsellors and other professionals providing the test service.
- Lay organizations can provide an inestimable service in enquiring about the standards of the laboratory and can assist subjects who want to be, or have been, tested with their enquiries and concerns.
- Counsellors should be specifically trained in counselling methods and form part of a multidisciplinary team.
- Such multidisciplinary teams should comprise, e.g. a geneticist, a neurologist, a social worker, a psychiatrist and someone trained in medical ethics.
- The subject should be encouraged to select a companion to accompany her throughout all stages of the testing process: the pretest stage, the taking of the test, the delivery of the results and the post-test stage.
- This companion may be the spouse/partner, a friend, a social worker or any individual who has the confidence of this person. It may not be appropriate for the companion to be another at-risk person.
- The counselling unit should plan, with the subject, a follow-up protocol that provides support during the pre- and post-test stages, regardless of whether this person chooses a companion.
- Neither the counselling centre nor the test laboratory should establish direct contact with a relative whose DNA may be needed for the purpose of the test without the permission of the subject.
- Information should be presented both orally and in written form and be provided by the team responsible for the testing service.

General information

- Information on Huntington's disease must be given to the subject, including the wide range of its clinical manifestations, its social and psychological implications, its genetic aspects, options for procreation, availability of treatment and so forth.
- It must be pointed out that, at this time, neither prevention nor cure is possible.
- Genetic testing may show that the putative parent is not the biological parent; this should be brought to the

attention of the subject and discussed. With the availability of techniques such as *in vitro* fertilization, etc., even cases of non-maternity may occasionally be discovered.
- Psychosocial support and counselling must be available before the test procedure commences.

Information about the test
- Explain how the test is carried out.
- Explain the possible need for DNA from one other affected family member and the possible problems arising from this.
- Asking an affected subject who may be unaware, or unwilling to acknowledge, his or her symptoms to contribute a blood sample may be considered an invasion of privacy.
- The limitations of the test (error rate, the possibilities of an uninformative test and so forth).
- The counsellor must explain that, although the gene defect has been found, at the present time no useful information can be given about age at onset or about the kind of symptoms, their severity or the rate of progression.

Consequences
- All consequences have to be discussed — those related to the presence or absence of the gene defect as well as those related to not taking the test. Consideration should be given to the subject, the spouse/partner and children, the affected parent and the spouse.
- Socioeconomic consequences of the test result including potential employment, insurance, social security, data security and other problems.

Alternatives the applicant can consider
- not to take the test for the time being
- to deposit DNA for research
- to deposit DNA for possible future use by family and self

Important preliminary investigations
- It is important to verify that the diagnosis of Huntington's disease in a family member of the subject is correct.
- Neurological examination and psychological appraisal are considered important to establish a baseline evaluation of each subject. Any other specialized tests are always non-compulsory; refusal may not affect participation in the test.
- Refusal to undergo these and other additional examinations will not justify the withholding of the test from subjects.

The test and delivery of results
- Excluding exceptional circumstances, there should be a minimum interval of 1 month between presentation of the pretest information and the decision whether or not to take the test. The counsellor should ascertain whether the pretest information has been properly understood and should take the initiative to be assured of this. However, contact will only be maintained at the subject's request.
- The result of the predictive test should be delivered as soon as possible after completion of the test, on a date agreed upon in advance between the centre, the counsellor and the subject.
- The manner in which the result will be delivered should be discussed by the counselling team and the subject.
- The subject has the right to decide, prior to the date fixed for the delivery of the result, if he or she does not want to be told.
- The result of the test should be revealed in person by the counsellor to the subject and his or her companion. No result should ever be revealed by telephone or by post. The counsellor must have sufficient time to discuss any questions with the subject.

Post-test counselling
- The frequency and the form of post-test counselling should be discussed by the team and the subject prior to the performance of the test, but the subject has the right to modify the planned programme. Although the intensity and frequency will vary from person to person, post-test counselling must be available at all times.
- The counsellor should have contact with the subject within the first week after delivery of the result, regardless of the nature of the result.
- If there is no further contact within 1 month of the delivery of the test result, then the counsellor should initiate the follow-up.

International Huntington Association. *Guidelines for the molecular genetics predictive test in HD*. 1994.

Comments on the case

Genetic counselling is a massive subject but candidates must have a grasp of the basic principles involved rather than leaving it all to the local genetics department.

Case 19 | HIV testing

Candidate information

You are the SHO in an infectious diseases clinic and your consultant in HIV infection has asked you to see Mr John Whittle with regard to having an HIV test

Please read this summary (it should take no more than 2 min) and then continue with the consultation.

> ### Re: Mr John Whittle, aged 28
>
> Mr Whittle is known to have been an intravenous user of heroin in the past but he has abstained for the past two years. He has been sent to the clinic with a 3-week history of dyspnoea and oral thrush. He has had a chest X-ray which is very suggestive of *Pneumocystis carinii* pneumonia. The consultant has spoken to the GP over the phone and both suspect that he may have HIV infection with an AIDS-defining illness. In order to confirm this, your consultant has asked you to discuss an HIV test with Mr Whittle in clinic.

Your tasks are to: explain the most likely cause for his breathlessness, approach the possibility of HIV infection and counsel him for an HIV test.

You have 14 min until the patient leaves the room, followed by 1 min for reflection, before the discussion with the examiners.

Subject/patient/relative information

Mr Whittle is a 28-year-old unemployed man who used intravenous heroin for a total of 8 years up until 2 years ago. He used to inject over 100 mg/day of diamorphine and admits to having shared needles. He was well until 3 weeks ago, since when he has been complaining of dyspnoea, particularly going uphill, with a dry cough. He has also complained of a sore mouth, which the GP confirmed as being caused by thrush. He has come to the clinic after having had a chest X-ray arranged by the GP. He has never thought about HIV infection because the friends he used to inject heroin with have always told him that they were HIV negative. As he has been abstinent from intravenous abuse for 2 years, he feels that the likelihood of acquiring HIV is now negligible. He has no other HIV risk factors; he is heterosexual and has never come into contact with prostitutes. He has never had an HIV test. He believes his breathlessness is caused by bronchitis as he smokes 15 cigarettes a day. He is living with his partner and their two children.

Examiner information

1 Communication skills—conduct of interview

- The consultation should be unhurried and confidential.
- Briefly ask him about the breathlessness.
- Explain the findings of the chest X-ray (a pneumonia). Tell him you are concerned that his presentation may be related to HIV infection and the reason why you think this.
- Ask him how he feels about this.

- Ask him if he has ever considered the possibility of HIV infection.
- Ask him about his previous heroin addiction; whether he injected heroin and whether he shared needles. If he did, were any of his associates known to be HIV positive? Has he been abstinent from injecting heroin and, if so, for how long?
- Confirm whether he has other risk factors for HIV infection.
- Ask him if he has ever had a test for HIV.
- Ask him if he would consider one.
- Reassure him that the test is confidential to the staff looking after him and that the result would not be released to anyone without his consent.
- Explain that the test is not a test for AIDS but a test for the HIV virus. Emphasize the difference.
- Explain that a sample of blood is taken and that the result should be available by the next day at the latest.
- He may ask if he has AIDS. Explain that if the HIV test is positive and the pneumonia is confirmed as being pneumocystosis, then he has AIDS as *Pneumocystis* pneumonia constitutes an AIDS-defining illness.
- He may ask you about life insurance. Explain if the test is negative then generally an individual should not be discriminated against. If the test is positive then all insurance policies taken out prior to this will be honoured, although he may find difficulty taking out future policies.
- Ascertain if he has a regular partner and emphasize the importance of safe sex.
- Explain to him that if the test result is positive it is essential that he tell his partner. Also explain to him why it is important for him to consider telling his GP.
- Tell him that he doesn't have to decide about the test immediately and should not feel pressurized. Reinforce the benefits of knowing whether he is HIV+ or not.
- Acknowledge that hearing this information must be hard for him.
- If he does decide to have the test, ask him who he would like to give him the result and who he wants with him at the time.
- He may want time to decide; if so, tell him you still need to do further tests for his pneumonia and that you recommend a bronchoscopy.
- Tell him that there is a full counselling service available and he is free to see a member of staff anytime during the day.
- Tell him there is an array of leaflets that would answer any questions he may think of later.
- Provide a contact number.
- Ask if he has any concerns that have not been addressed.

2 Communication skills—exploration and problem negotiation

The candidate should be able to:
- carry out a tricky consultation showing understanding and empathy without rushing
- explain the findings of the chest X-ray
- take a detailed HIV risk factor history
- counsel for an HIV test with reasonable insight about what the test involves
- detail a plan of action, i.e. HIV testing, when and by whom, and bronchoscopy to confirm *Pneumocystis carinii* pneumonia

3 Ethics and the law and other discussion points

General advice for counselling
- Ask what impact he thinks the test result will have on him.
- Address the question of whom he ought to tell the result to.
- Describe the test and how it is performed.
- Explain what AIDS is and the ways in which HIV infection is spread.
- Discuss ways to prevent the spread of HIV.
- Explain the confidentiality of the test results.
- Discuss the meaning of possible test results.
- Discuss the importance of telling his sex and/or drug-using partner(s) if the result indicates HIV infection.

Important elements of HIV counselling
- Confidentiality—strict protection of client confidentiality must be maintained for all persons offered and receiving HIV counselling services.
- Risk assessment—allows the individual to identify, understand and acknowledge his personal risk for acquiring HIV.
- Prevention counselling—allows a critical opportunity to assist the patient in identifying his risk of acquiring or transmitting HIV. It provides an opportunity to negotiate and reinforce a plan to reduce and eliminate behavioural risk.
- The test results—pretest counselling should prepare the individual for receiving, understanding and managing the result. Providing the test result to an individual involves an interpretation that is based on the result, and the individual specific risk for HIV infection. Skilful counselling will allow assessment of behavioural risks and it is not uncommon for individuals to focus on the actual results rather than the broader behavioural and preventative messages.

- Testing should always be accompanied by pre- and post-test counselling. The counsellor should be knowledgeable about this process.

Because the results of tests for HIV infection have profound consequences and raise many questions, individuals should give written informed consent for the testing procedure, and should understand the choices implied by the test results. Counselling should include information about the test, HIV infection and AIDS, as well as risk behaviour associated with the transmission of HIV. Discussion about the consequences of a positive or negative result for the individual being tested (e.g. pregnancy, employment and insurance, family, lovers and friends), as well as the need for appropriate follow-up in the event of a positive test result should also be addressed. Explanation of equivocal results that require additional tests may be necessary. Even for a person whose result is negative, counselling is recommended to allay a false sense of security and to promote future risk-reducing behaviour. If the clinical suspicion of infection is high, based on risk behaviours and/or symptoms, then follow-up testing should be recommended. Professionals who request HIV antibody tests should be familiar with these counselling issues.

Benefits of testing

- If you know you are HIV positive, you can take advantage of monitoring with early treatment and intervention.
- By taking the test, you can find out whether or not you can infect others.
- Regardless of the result, testing often increases your commitment to improving healthy habits as counselling also provides general information about sexually transmitted diseases.
- If you test negative, you may feel less anxious after testing.
- Women and their partners considering pregnancy can take advantage of treatments that potentially prevent transmission of HIV to the baby.

Negative aspects of testing

- If you test positive, you may show an increase in anxiety and depression.
- When testing is not strictly anonymous, you risk job and insurance discrimination. You can prevent this by ensuring that you are tested at an anonymous testing site.

Interpretation of test results

A **positive** result means that:

- you are HIV positive (carrying the virus that causes AIDS)
- you can infect others and therefore must take precautions to prevent doing so

A **positive** result does *not* mean that:

- you have AIDS
- you will necessarily get AIDS
- you are immune to AIDS, even though you have antibodies
- no HIV antibodies were found in your blood at this time

A **negative** result does *not* mean that:

- you are not infected with HIV (you may still be in the 'window period')
- you are immune to AIDS
- you have a 'resistance' to infection
- you will never get AIDS. You may wish to consider avoiding unsafe activities in order to protect yourself

An **indeterminate** result (which is rare) means that:

- the entire HIV test must be repeated with a new blood sample, usually several weeks after the first blood test
- indeterminate results usually occur if the test is performed just as the person begins to seroconvert

The above guidelines are from: US Department of Health and Human Services, Public Health Service Centres for Disease Control and Prevention (CDC). *HIV counselling, testing and referral standards and guidelines.* May 1994.

Comments on the case

HIV medicine is a minefield of ethical issues. All issues cannot be covered totally in this section and the candidate is advised to refer to specialized texts. Ethical issues which cause particular discussion points include: informed consent for HIV testing, confidentiality, postpositive testing counselling, informing sexual partners, informing the GP, life insurance and general health education, especially with practising safe sex.

Don't forget to make use of specialist clinicians and nurses working in the field of sexual health as well as reputable organizations such as the Terrence Higgins Trust who are able to provide ongoing information, support and advice to people with HIV or AIDS and their families.

Case 20 | Hormone replacement therapy

Candidate information

You are the medical SHO in a medical follow-up clinic

Please read this summary (it should take no more than 2 min) and then continue with the consultation.

> **Re: Mrs Jacky Lorimer, aged 55**
>
> Mrs Lorimer was admitted 6 weeks ago for a community acquired pneumonia. She was treated with amoxicillin and made a full recovery. The chest X-ray today shows complete resolution of the pneumonia. Her main concern now is about her intermittent hot flushes. She suspects that she is menopausal and wants advice on whether she should try hormone replacement therapy (HRT). She is a little concerned about the risk of thromboembolism in light of the scares she has read about in the press.

Your tasks are to: determine whether Mrs Lorimer would benefit from hormone replacement therapy (HRT) and discuss the pros and cons of HRT.

You have 14 min until the patient leaves the room, followed by 1 min for reflection, before the discussion with the examiners.

Subject/patient/relative information

Mrs Lorimer is a 55-year-old housewife who was admitted 6 weeks ago with a community acquired pneumonia. She has made an excellent recovery and has no more respiratory symptoms. While in clinic, she thought she would get some advice from the medical SHO (the candidate) about the use of HRT. She has been getting intermittent hot flushes over the last 5 months. She has noticed some vaginal dryness but no urinary symptoms. There is also reduced libido. She is otherwise well and has no past history of thromboembolism, cardiovascular disease or breast cancer. There is no significant history of these illnesses in the family either. However, she did have a hysterectomy 14 years ago for uterine fibroids. She feels as if she is coming towards her menopause but she cannot be totally certain because of the lack of menstrual periods. She is quite keen to try HRT but is unsure about the risks of thromboembolism. She has been reading a few women's magazines recently and the articles on HRT seemed to have scared her. She does not smoke or drink and she lives with her husband.

Examiner information

1 Communication skills — conduct of interview

- Introduce yourself to Mrs Lorimer. Ask how she is. Tell her that her chest X-ray is normal and that the pneumonia has fully resolved.
- She tells you that she may be menopausal but is not sure if she should have HRT.
- Ask her why she thinks she is menopausal. She tells you that she has had a hysterectomy and so she does not have any periods but she tells you about the hot flushes.
- Ask her what other symptoms she has been having, e.g. urogenital atrophy (vaginal dryness, dyspareunia, dysuria, urinary frequency and urgency), mood changes, loss of libido.
- Ask what she knows about HRT.
- Explain what the menopause is: declining ovarian function with falling levels of oestrogens. Tell her that you can confirm this by testing her blood oestrogen levels. So, explain that the reason for giving HRT is to increase the oestrogen levels and so prevent or treat clinical features associated with the menopause.
- Describe the components of HRT: natural oestrogens with or without progesterones.
- Explain that for women with a uterus, progesterone is added to ensure that the endometrium ('lining of the womb') does not become overactive (endometrial hyperplasia and thereby possible carcinoma).
- Describe how HRT can be given: systemically or topically. Systemically includes tablets by mouth, on the skin (transdermal) or a subcutaneous oestrogen implant. Topically is via vaginal creams, rings, tablets or pessaries.
- She asks about the advantages of HRT. Say there will be an improvement of the menopausal symptoms. Tell her that the risk of coronary heart disease and strokes may be reduced in those women on treatment and that HRT helps to prevent the development of osteoporosis.
- She asks about the disadvantages of HRT. She is particularly worried about thromboembolism. Explain that there is a suggestion that the risk of developing venous thromboembolism is 2–4 times higher in women on HRT (whichever route of administration) but reassure her that, even on HRT, the risk of developing a deep vein thrombosis is very small. Inform her that women on long-term HRT (over 10 years) have a slightly increased risk of developing breast cancer although this needs to be confirmed by further long-term studies.
- Ask if she has a past history of thromboembolism, breast cancer or coronary heart disease. Family history as well. Ask if she smokes.
- Reassure her again that in those without risk factors, the benefits outweigh the disadvantages.
- Explain that as she does not have a uterus, she can have the oestrogen-only preparation.
- Inform her of the side-effects of HRT: oestrogen-related unwanted effects such as breast swelling and tenderness, nausea, increased appetite with weight gain, and vaginal discharge, but these tend to resolve within 3 months.
- Say that the optimum length of time a woman should be on HRT is not known and usually the individual makes an informed choice.
- Ask if she has any other queries. Say that you will try to get some leaflets from the gynaecology and bone clinics and that you will send these to her in the post. Tell her you will let the GP know of today's discussion.

2 Communication skills — exploration and problem negotiation

The candidate should be able to:

- reassure the patient that the pneumonia has fully resolved
- obtain the history of symptoms the patient has that are suggestive of the menopause
- determine any contraindications to HRT
- discuss the pros and cons of HRT
- be aware that progesterone is not needed in those without a uterus

3 Ethics and the law and other discussion points

- Specific issues related to misperceptions and fears regarding HRT need to be clarified and specific, patient-focused educational pamphlets help to address common concerns about HRT. Doctors should communicate effectively with the patient. Doctors must focus on the emotional and physical aspects of HRT choices and tailor any therapies to the individual patient. It is important to discuss frankly the very serious concerns a woman may have regarding the association with breast cancer and endometrial cancer. Discussing and preparing women for possible side-effects helps patients to cope better if and when side-effects occur. Finally, offering a wide variety of HRT therapies provides women with a broader choice if an initial regimen is unsuccessful.
- The Heart and Estrogen/Progestin Replacement Study

(HERS) showed no reduced risk of coronary heart disease in those using HRT. There is biological plausibility and supporting evidence from epidemiological studies despite the lack of data from confirmatory clinical trials. Because of this, recommendations for HRT should be made on an individual basis with emphasis on informed decision making.

- A woman who has undergone a hysterectomy can take oestrogens without a progesterone. An oestrogen implant is one option, although the individual may wish to take tablets or patches. A woman who still has a uterus must take a progesterone with an oestrogen. This also applies to a woman who has undergone an endometrial ablation procedure because some endometrial tissue may not have been destroyed. The progesterone can be given cyclically or continuously. During a 28-day cyclical treatment, progesterones are given for 10–14 days so producing monthly withdrawal bleeding. During 3-monthly cyclical treatment, progesterones are given for 14 days with the aim of producing a quarterly withdrawal bleed. The cyclical progesterone therapy minimizes the development of oestrogen-induced endometrial hyperplasia.

Comments on the case

This case highlights the importance of informing the patient of the pros and cons of a therapy. The patient must be able to make an informed decision. It is not uncommon for patients to exhibit fears originating from the media.

Case 21 | Industrial benefits

Candidate information

You are the medical SHO in clinic

Please read this summary (it should take no more than 2 min) and then continue with the consultation.

> ### Re: Mr Alan Clarke, aged 74
>
> Mr Clarke has been seeing you in clinic because of breathlessness. A chest X-ray has suggested pulmonary fibrosis with pleural thickening and plaques over both lungs. Lung function testing has confirmed reduced lung volumes and impaired diffusion. A CT scan of the thorax has confirmed interstitial lung disease with pleural thickening and plaques. All this is suggestive of asbestos lung disease. However, Mr Clarke is unaware that he can claim industrial disablement benefit.

Your tasks are to: explain the findings of the lung function tests and the CT scan, explain the diagnosis of asbestos lung disease and help him to claim industrial disablement benefit.

You have 14 min until the patient leaves the room, followed by 1 min for reflection, before the discussion with the examiners.

Subject/patient/relative information

Mr Alan Clarke is a 74-year-old retired plumber. He has worked for a number of firms including work at the local hospital. He has been a plumber all his life and has been exposed to asbestos from pipe lagging/insulating material during most of his working life. He has been coming to the clinic after a 6-month history of increasing breathlessness. Investigations (chest X-ray, lung function tests and a CT scan of the thorax) have confirmed the diagnosis of asbestosis with pleural thickening as a result of the previous asbestos exposure. He is about to see the medical SHO (the candidate) for the results. He is unaware that compensation is available in the form of industrial disablement benefit from the Department of Social Security.

Examiner information

1 Communication skills—conduct of interview

- Introduce yourself to Mr Clarke.
- Ask how he is.
- Start off by explaining the results of the tests. Explain that the tests suggest scarring of the lung tissue (as

bestosis) with thickening of the lining around the lung (pleural thickening) with calcified plaques (hardened patches). Say that all this is a result of asbestos exposure.
- Ask what his occupation was and whether he has been exposed to asbestos. Take details of the length and degree of the exposure.
- Explain that unfortunately treatment is limited

and that the asbestosis does tend to progress slowly.
- Reassure him that there is no evidence of lung cancer or cancer of the lining of the lungs which can occur in asbestos lung disease (mesothelioma).
- Ask if he is aware that as he has an occupational lung disease and that he is able to claim for industrial disablement benefit.
- Say that he must go to his local social security office where he should ask for a B1(100Pn) form which covers occupational/industrial lung diseases.
- Explain that he will be visited by a Department of Social Security medical officer who will judge the degree of 'disability'. Based on this, the benefit per week can be determined.
- He is allowed to have this back-dated (by 3 months).
- If he disagrees with the disability verdict (i.e. feels he should receive more benefit) the patient can appeal, although only within 1 month of the date of the letter confirming the decision.
- Ask if he has any other questions.

2 Communication skills—exploration and problem negotiation

The candidate should be able to:
- explain the findings of the results
- explain the diagnosis of asbestos lung disease
- inform the patient that he is allowed to claim benefit
- inform the patient how to go about claiming this benefit

3 Ethics and the law and other discussion points

- Many industrial countries have arrangements for compensation for affected workers by the State. In the UK, the conditions for which compensation might be awarded are mesothelioma, asbestosis, bilateral diffuse pleural thickening (to a thickness of 5 mm or more at any point within the area affected as measured by a plain chest X-ray) and primary carcinoma of the lung where there is accompanying evidence of asbestosis and/or diffuse pleural thickening. The amount of industrial injuries disablement benefit one can get depends on how badly the individual is disabled. It can be paid 15 weeks from the first day the individual was disabled by the disease, unless it is for a mesothelioma when it can be paid from the first day of disability from this disease. Other industrial diseases for which claims can be made include silicosis, byssinosis, coal worker's pneumoconiosis.
- The patient must go to the local social security office for a form B1(100Pn) which should be filled in as soon as possible because the date when the completed form is received by the social security office is the date of the claim. Benefit cannot be paid for a period of more than 3 months before the date of the claim (except for mesothelioma).
- A medical officer will meet the patient and estimate the degree of disability which will then determine the amount of weekly benefit that can be claimed. For asbestosis, or mesothelioma, benefit can be awarded if the disability is deemed as 1% or above.
- Other allowances available include the constant attendance allowance for a patient who is 95% or more disabled where the effects of the disease means care and attention is needed for most of the time, and reduced earnings allowance which is awarded to those who first suffered from the disease 10 years ago, or cannot go back to their normal job, or cannot do another job of the same standard with similar pay. These industrial benefits do not affect other national insurance benefits such as incapacity benefit or the retirement state pension.
- Patients can appeal to a tribunal within 1 month of the date of the benefit decision.
- Patients who wish to sue an employer may do so with the help of legal representation. However, as many patients will have worked for several different employers, establishing responsibility for the disease by a specific employer is difficult. In many cases the previous employers no longer exist and most patients are unable to afford the legal expenses.

> ### Comments on the case
>
> This case highlights the importance of being aware of industrial diseases and the availability of compensation. All too often patients miss out on benefits because doctors are unaware that they exist.

Case 22 | Informed consent for an emergency operation

Candidate information

You are the medical SHO on-call. You are about to see Mrs Collins who is the daughter of Mr Watkins.

Please read this summary (it should take no more than 2 min) and then continue with the consultation.

> **Re: Mr Bill Watkins, aged 75**
>
> Mr Watkins is a previously fit 75-year-old man who is brought to casualty unconscious after being involved in a hit and run accident. He has been intubated and sedated in casualty by the anaesthetists. A CT scan of the head shows a large extradural haematoma with midline shift. He also has a fractured left tibia. After discussing the case with your neurosurgical colleagues, it has been decided that it is in the patient's best interest to take the patient to theatre directly from casualty to evacuate the haematoma. As he remains intubated and sedated, you decide to speak to his daughter, Mrs Collins, who is waiting in the relatives' room, for consent. However, Mrs Collins is unsure whether her father would ever want to undergo a risky operation, particularly when there is a risk of neurological deficit.

Your tasks are to: explain Mr Watkin's condition to his daughter, explain that an operation is needed to evacuate the haematoma and explain the neurosurgeon's rationale. If possible gain the daughter's agreement.

You have 14 min until his daughter leaves the room, followed by 1 min for reflection, before the discussion with the examiners.

Subject/patient/relative information

Mrs Collins is the daughter of Mr Watkins, a previously fit 75-year-old, who has just been admitted with a serious head injury after a hit and run accident. He also has a broken left tibia. Mrs Collins is the next of kin and lives two streets away from him. When told by the doctors that her father has to have an operation to remove a blood clot from his head, she becomes unsure if her father would ever want to undergo such a serious operation, particularly with the risk of possible neurological sequelae. He has always been a strongly independent man who has stressed that he would never want to live if he ever had a serious neurological deficit, e.g. after a stroke. However, he never wrote a living will or an advanced directive to support this. Mrs Collins is unsure whether surgery should be carried out. She is about to see the medical SHO (the candidate) to discuss her father's condition.

Examiner information

1 Communication skills—conduct of interview

- Introduce yourself to Mrs Collins, checking that she is the daughter of the patient. In a real situation, having a member of the nursing staff present during the consultation would be prudent.
- Establish that your information about previous fitness is correct.
- Explain how sorry you are that her father is in such a critical situation, explaining that he has been in a car accident as a pedestrian and describe exactly what has been found on the CT scan without using any medical jargon.
- Pause to allow this information to sink in.
- Explain that her father is intubated (explain what this means) and under sedation to keep him free from distress in the emergency room in casualty.
- Explain how critical the situation is and that you have spoken to your neurosurgical colleagues who all believe that without an operation to remove the haematoma, Mr Watkins will die.
- The daughter asks you about the operation and the risks involved, especially about any possible neurological sequelae.
- Explain the basics of the operation, including the opening of the skull and removing the clot. Explain that the procedure is relatively straightforward but one cannot wholly guarantee a 100% recovery. Explain that there may be neurological sequelae and deficit as a result of neuronal ('brain cell') damage secondary to the haemorrhage or from any other intracranial haemorrhage that cannot be rectified by the operation.
- The daughter tells you that her father would never want to consent to such an operation if there was a risk of neurological deficit, even if *not* having an operation could result in death. She asks you to respect this decision.
- Ask Mrs Collins if Mr Watkins has ever written a living will or an advanced directive with a solicitor which can be used as a legal document if the need ever arises. She says no.
- Clarify with her that the responsibility for proceeding with the surgery rests with the consultant in charge.
- Explain that legally, when consent is not available, one has to offer such treatment as is necessary to save life (as in this situation), particularly when the team feels that this decision is in the best interests of the patient.
- Mrs Collins is not happy with the decision and you tell her that you will call your consultant to discuss the situation further.
- Suggest that it may be useful for her to have support from other family members to discuss the situation with the team.

2 Communication skills—exploration and problem negotiation

The candidate should be able to:
- break the bad news to the daughter clearly but with compassion and understanding
- explain that her father is in a critical condition and give the reasons why
- explain the need for emergency surgery to remove the haematoma
- understand the daughter's feelings with regard to her father's wishes of never wanting to undergo surgery with a risk of neurological sequelae
- ask if there has been a living will or an advanced directive made by Mr Watkins or clear and repeated wishes
- explain, however, that although one cannot totally eliminate the risk of neurological sequelae, neurosurgery is the only way in which to save his life
- involve the consultant in this case

3 Ethics and the law and other discussion points

- In an emergency the consultant may provide medical treatment to anyone who needs it, provided the treatment is limited to what is immediately necessary to save life or to avoid significant deterioration in the patient's health (General Medical Council. *Seeking patient's consent: the ethical considerations.* Section 18: Emergencies. November 1998).
- Consent to operate is assumed by the medical carer unless the patient would have withheld consent. Such evidence may be in the form of a living will or an advanced directive.
- It is imperative that doctors should seek such substantial evidence before curtailing treatment, and it may be prudent to include patient's GP, minister or priest.
- When speaking to the daughter, have a senior nurse to accompany you and involve your consultant early.
- It is important to ask for other members of the family to be involved, as different individuals express different views on a situation.

Comments on the case

This is a tricky case. The daughter's concerns that her father would not wish to live with a neurological deficit and her 'responsibility' to him place her in a difficult position. One has to remember always that it is the patient's life at risk and legally, in order to save life, one has to do what is necessary, unless there is legal evidence to the contrary. This case tests the candidate's ability to be diplomatic—appreciating the daughter's views but trying to convey the primary concerns for the patient balanced against the clinician's belief that surgery is potentially in the patient's best interest.

Case 23 | Informed refusal of therapy

Candidate information

You are the medical SHO

Please read this summary (it should take no more than 2 min) and then continue with the consultation.

> ### Re: Mr Ronald Higgenbottom, aged 79
>
> Mr Higgenbottom has been admitted to hospital with palpitations and has been found to have atrial fibrillation. An echocardiogram has also revealed moderate left ventricular dysfunction. Your consultant felt that it would be wise to anticoagulate Mr Higgenbottom but, after explaining in depth the pros and cons of anticoagulation, he has made an informed decision not to undertake this and to remain on aspirin. His main reasons are that he does not wish to have his coagulation tested every few weeks for the rest of his life and that he is frightened of having a stroke (cerebral haemorrhage) as he has a tendency to have falls. His daughter, Mrs Anderson, wants to speak to you about this issue. She firmly believes that her father should be anticoagulated as a stroke prevention measure. Having approached Mr Higgenbottom and gained his permission for you to speak to his daughter, you are now meeting with her to discuss his condition.

Your tasks are to: speak to Mrs Anderson about her father's refusal to have anticoagulation and discuss the legal issues surrounding this.

You have 14 min until the daughter leaves the room, followed by 1 min for reflection, before the discussion with the examiners.

Subject/patient/relative information

Mr Ronald Higgenbottom is a 79-year-old gentleman who was admitted a few days ago with atrial fibrillation. An echocardiogram has shown moderate left ventricular dysfunction and it was felt that anticoagulation with warfarin should be offered in order to reduce the risk of a stroke. Mr Higgenbottom was fully informed of the pros and cons of anticoagulation by the medical SHO (the candidate) but eventually the patient decided not to accept anticoagulation and to stay on aspirin. The daughter, Mrs Anderson, is upset that her father is not being anticoagulated for stroke prevention. She wants to talk to the medical SHO (the candidate) about this issue. She states that she is the next of kin and therefore has the right to overrule her father's decision.

Examiner information

1 Communication skills—conduct of interview

- Introduce yourself to Mrs Anderson.
- Ask her what she knows about her father's condition.
- Ask her what her views are on this matter.
- Explain that you appreciate her feelings but the issue of anticoagulation was fully discussed with her father in terms of the advantages (reducing the risk of a future stroke) and, at the same time, he was informed of the possible risks of anticoagulation. As a result of the information given he has made an informed decision not to be anticoagulated.
- Explain that you did explore all the reasons why he may not want to be anticoagulated and that you did try to counter any possible misconception. Tell her why her father did not wish to be anticoagulated.
- His daughter may challenge this by saying that she is the next of kin and that her father is old and cannot make decisions for himself.
- Explain that there is no evidence that her father cannot make an informed decision because of incapacity and that her father is legally allowed to refuse treatment. As a result of this, physicians are unable to enforce treatment to such patients even if the next of kin tries to overrule their decision.
- Try to reassure her that her father is receiving effective treatment and that he remains on aspirin which has been shown to be almost as good in reducing the risk of strokes, although admittedly warfarin would have been the treatment of choice.

2 Communication skills—exploration and problem negotiation

The candidate should be able to:

- ascertain the feelings and wishes of the patient's daughter
- convey that her father has made an informed decision and that you did explore in depth any possible misconceptions about the therapy
- explain that patients who show no incapacity to make an informed decision have the right to decline treatment
- explain that despite declining warfarin, her father will remain on aspirin which will provide some protection against strokes

3 Ethics and the law and other discussion points

- In most cases, health professionals cannot legally examine or treat any adult without their valid consent (the management of minors is not addressed here). The principal exception is treatment provided under the Mental Health Act 1983. This authorizes assessment of individuals, their admission to hospital or reception into guardianship and, if necessary, treatment for mental illness. Apart from such compulsory treatment, it is unlawful and unethical to treat a person who is capable of understanding and willing to know without first explaining the nature of the procedure, its purpose and implications and obtaining that person's agreement. Some people consent to treatment while choosing not to be told the full details of their diagnosis or treatment. Their uninformed consent is nevertheless valid as long as they had the option of receiving more information.
- Competent adults have a clear right to decline medical diagnostic procedures or treatment for reasons which are 'rational, irrational or for no reason'. The person's capacity to refuse in a valid manner must be assessed in relation to the specific treatment proposal. It is irrelevant whether refusal is contrary to the views of most other people if it is broadly consistent with the individual's own values.
- If an individual appears to be choosing an option which is not only contradictory to that which most people would choose, but also appears to contradict that individual's previously expressed attitudes, then health professionals would be justified in questioning in greater detail that individual's capacity to make a valid refusal in order to eliminate the possibility of a depressive illness or a delusional state.

British Medical Association. *Assessment of Mental Capacity*, Chapter 10. Capacity to consent to and refuse medical treatment. December 1995. Further advice in Scotland is highlighted in the BMA report: *Medical treatment for adults with incapacity: guidance on clinical and medico-legal issues in Scotland.* Second edition. BMA. October 2002.

Comments on the case

This is a common case where the next of kin may blame the physician for not initiating certain therapy for their relative. It is important for the physician to be aware of their legal rights as well as the rights of the patient in order to allow patients to choose whether they want treatment or not.

It is likely that the offspring of such patients are likely to remain unhappy that their wishes cannot override those of the patient and it can be useful to engage the patient and offspring in dialogue together with the clinician as sometimes the support of a third party may enable them to discuss issues they have been finding it difficult to address to one another.

Case 24 | Internet therapy

Candidate information

You are the medical SHO in clinic

Please read this summary (it should take no more than 2 min) and then continue with the consultation.

> ### Re: Mr Harry Webberley, aged 62
>
> Mr Webberley is a patient who regularly attends clinic for his severe asthma. He has been on high-dose corticosteroids, long-acting beta-agonist inhalers and antileucotriene medication for many years. He is well known to have multiple allergies to common allergens such as house dust mite, cat dander and pollen. He is regularly on steroids and as a result of long-term usage, he has become Cushingoid. He is desperate to try anything. He is seeing you in clinic today and he tells you that he saw an advertisement on the Internet regarding a new portable breathing device, which claims to cure asthma and which he has ordered from California for $65. He seems convinced that this device will cure all his asthma problems.

Your tasks are to: discuss the pros and cons of Internet information technology, discuss the likelihood or not of a possible cure from this new device and remind him of the essential treatment principles of asthma.

You have 14 min until the patient leaves the room, followed by 1 min for reflection, before the discussion with the examiners.

Subject/patient/relative information

Mr Harry Webberley is a 62-year-old man who has had asthma for many years and is on maximum inhaler and antileucotriene therapy. He has been taking oral steroids on and off for many years and has now become Cushingoid. He is desperate for a cure and recently saw an advertisement on the Internet for a breathing device which is claimed cures asthma. He has ordered one for $65 from California and is eagerly awaiting its arrival. Currently, his asthma remains troublesome with interrupted sleep and wheeze in the mornings. His peak flow rate is never above 150 L/min. He has no pets at home. He is about to see the medical SHO (the candidate) and wants an honest opinion about this device.

Examiner information

1 Communication skills—conduct of interview

- Introduce yourself to Mr Webberley.
- Ask how his asthma is at present.
- He tells you about the device he has ordered over the Internet and asks your opinion.
- Tell him that the purpose of the Internet should be to provide general medical information and to allow

communication with societies such as the asthma societies.

- Explain that it is prudent to research how valid the information is, indicators such as peer-review/assessment by the reputable academic groups may be an indicator of its validity. Also tell him that there is no control over the legitimacy of material put on websites.
- Tell him that he should be prepared that the device he has bought may not be successful but there is no harm in trying. Also tell him that you have not seen any randomized controlled trials using this device in asthma.
- Remind him of the importance of continued allergen avoidance and anti-inflammatory therapy in the management of asthma.
- Emphasize that the basic principles of asthma control remain the same.

2 Communication skills—exploration and problem negotiation

The candidate should be able to:

- listen to the patient's view on the new device he found on the Internet
- tell him the pros and cons of the Internet
- tell him your views on the possible success of the device
- remind him of the important principles of asthma management

3 Ethics and the law and other discussion points

- The Internet can be a useful source of medical information but many sites are not peer-reviewed. It is not unusual for patients to see their physician and ask about an article on the Internet which claims to be genuine. Unless the website is from a reputable source, physicians must remain sceptical and they must convey this to their patients.
- Further ethical issues have arisen from the Internet, particularly physicians being asked for medical advice over the Internet (by e-mail), the trading of pharmaceutical drugs over the Internet, and medical advertising on the Internet. Below are the views held by the Medical Defence Union regarding use of the Internet.

Referral between physicians

When a physician sends an ECG, pathology slide or X-ray to a specialist, does the specialist have duty of care? If he or she does, the specialist must share liability if some-

thing goes wrong but, generally, the physician taking the advice from the specialist would assume most of the liability.

Who makes a record of the consultation?

As in any doctor–doctor interaction, it makes sense for each doctor to make his or her own record. The record might take the form of a video recording of the telemedical consultation kept on disc or tape.

Who is responsible for confidentiality and security of the system?

Doctors have a duty to ensure that information they obtain from patients is kept secure and is not available to those not entitled to see it. As with equipment, if doctors have doubts about the medium then they should not be using it. A patient's personal identity details should not be divulged on the Internet. Any e-mail exchange with or about the patient should only take place with the patient's full agreement and understanding that e-mails are potentially not a secure form of communication.

An e-mail exchange

E-mail exchange between a doctor and one of his or her patients is essentially an exchange of letters electronically. If the doctor begins the exchange, he or she should make sure that the patient is happy to continue using the medium.

Medical websites

The purpose of a website can be to provide general medical information, to advertise a practice or to offer medical advice. The intention of the site should be clear to the reader. If the site is simply for information or education it should clearly say so. If the site is advertising a practice it should conform to the law and the guidance issued by the Advertising Standards Authority and the General Medical Council (*Good Medical Practice.* May 2001).

If the site offers advice

The site might need an appropriate disclaimer—it might say, for example, that it is *not* the intention to establish a doctor–patient relationship. If this is so, it raises the question as to why the advice is being given in the first place. The usual answer is that the site is a commercial enterprise. Nevertheless, if a doctor gives personal medical advice he or she establishes a duty of care and thus potential liability. The site should be as secure and confidential as possible.

Selling/prescribing drugs on the Internet

Doctors who prescribe drugs on the Internet may have to justify to their registration body why they are prescribing to someone they do not know, have not seen, have not examined and cannot effectively follow-up. Such doctors need to ask themselves if they are serving the unknown patient's interests by prescribing and they must be prepared to justify their actions.

Comments on the case

This case demonstrates the potential ethical dilemmas faced by physicians from the Internet and, as more and more patients gain access to the Web, more and more will be asking for and questioning new therapies on topics that physicians may not have kept up to date with.

The physician has a responsibility to be open-minded enough not to instantly dismiss the potential benefit of therapies presented to them by patients who have sought out internet information, but to make rational decisions as to whether or not they may need to support the patient by further investigation of the validity of the information presented.

Case 25 | Lifestyle adjustments after an anterior myocardial infarction

Candidate information

You are the medical SHO on the postcoronary care ward

Please read this summary (it should take no more than 2 min) and then continue with the consultation.

Re: Mr Johnny Giles, aged 73

Mr Giles was admitted 5 days ago with chest pain. An ECG and cardiac enzyme tests revealed an anterior myocardial infarction (AMI). He was successfully treated with streptokinase and he is now 5 days past the episode. He has never been in hospital before and all this has come as a bit of a shock to him. He has been started on aspirin, atenolol, ramipril and simvastatin. He is sat in the day room waiting for a taxi to take him home. He sees you and summons you over to speak to him. He has a few unanswered questions.

Your tasks are to: answer his queries regarding his MI and give him advice on adjusting his lifestyle relevant to having had an MI.

You have 14 min until the patient leaves the room, followed by 1 min for reflection, before the discussion with the examiners.

Subject/patient/relative information

Mr Johnny Giles is a 73-year-old retired painter and decorator who was admitted 5 days ago with an anterior myocardial infarction (AMI). He has never been in hospital before and never previously took any medication. The suddenness of his illness has taken him by surprise. He is about to go home but he does not really understand what has been happening. He has got to know the medical SHO (the candidate) quite well over these last few days and sees him walking through the ward. Mr Giles calls him over to ask him a few questions. His first query is whether he really has had a heart attack. No one has actually sat down with him and explained what a heart attack is. His next query is that he cannot understand why he is on so many tablets when he feels so well. Finally, he wants to know what happens next. Will he see the specialist again and should he change his lifestyle and, if so, in what way. He used to smoke 20 cigarettes a day 5 years ago and he does admit to having an unhealthy diet, especially with fried food, and he never does any exercise. He is not overweight.

Examiner information

1 Communication skills—conduct of interview

- Say hello to Mr Giles. Ask how he is.
- He asks you if he has had a heart attack.
- Explain in simple language what a heart attack is, i.e. that doctors and nurses call it a 'myocardial infarction' or 'MI', that it is caused by a blockage of a blood vessel that supplies blood to the heart and that this results in damage to part of the heart muscle which causes chest pain. Reassure him that he has had the correct and best treatment available (streptokinase), which would have helped to clear some of the blockage. Reassure him that many people do well after a heart attack and that the reason for the tablets is to offer some prevention from a second attack.
- He asks you why he is on so many tablets.
- Explain why he is on aspirin, atenolol, ramipril and simvastatin, with individual drug descriptions. Explain the importance of simvastatin in secondary prevention of ischaemic heart disease. Reiterate the need to take these tablets.
- He asks what happens next.
- Say that you will arrange a special walking ECG test in the next few weeks and that he will receive a letter in the post telling him where and when to go for this test. Explain what the exercise ECG test entails. Say that this test will detect if there are any possible serious blockages to the arteries. If so, further treatment can be given to help this.
- He asks whether he should change his lifestyle.
- Ask him what his diet comprises, whether he smokes and whether he does any exercise.
- Say that you are pleased that he no longer smokes and that he is not overweight. However, he ought to cut down on his fat intake. Emphasize that he is on simvastatin for a high blood cholesterol level and having a high fat diet will contribute to keeping it high. Say that you will ask a dietitian to give him advice at an outpatient appointment.
- Point out that regular exercise has benefits for preventing further heart attacks and encourage him to go for walks, recommending that he gradually increases his activity with an eventual aim of a 30-min brisk walk at least five times a week.
- Say that you will speak with the cardiac rehabilitation nurse who will arrange a rehabilitation programme for him.
- Determine if there is an element of anxiety or depression. Tell him that the cardiac rehabilitation pro-gramme will allow him to meet other people like himself, enabling him to share his experiences with them. Reassure him that a rehabilitation team will be there to look after him and to answer any other queries. Reassure him that the rehabilitation programme will consist initially of simple basic exercises which will be slowly increased as he gains more confidence in his exercise ability. Tell him that if he has any problems with anxiety and stress, then the programme will give him relaxation therapy.
- Offer him pamphlets from the rehabilitation team and the British Heart Foundation. Say that he should not drive for a month (longer if he has any difficulty in co-ordinating or braking, etc.) and he can have sex only after increasing his activity level, say to going briskly up two flights of stairs.
- Ask if he has any other queries. If not, reassure him again and say you will see him in clinic after the walking ECG test.

2 Communication skills—exploration and problem negotiation

The candidate should be able to:
- explain what a myocardial infarction is
- explain why he is on the drug regimen
- reassure him that with these medications and lifestyle improvements, his outlook is promising
- assure him that referrals will be made for an exercise ECG, dietetic advice and for cardiac rehabilitation
- establish if there is an element of anxiety or depression

3 Ethics and the law and other discussion points

- Secondary prevention includes managing medical co-morbidities associated with ischaemic heart disease, e.g. hypercholesterolaemia, hypertension and diabetes mellitus.
- Improving outcome in patients with an MI includes not only the acute management but also the aftercare following this major life event. Cardiac rehabilitation gives attention to physical remedies, education and psychological support. Cardiac rehabilitation reinforces advice to adopt a healthier lifestyle and so achieve secondary prevention.
- Patients should not drive for a month, longer if they feel that their activity and reflexes are not back to their usual level. They should inform the DVLA and their insurance company.
- Patients should be able to cope with the stresses of sex after 2–4 weeks of the exercise programme.

- Rehabilitation includes strong encouragement to smoking cessation, physiotherapy-led exercise programmes with an initial warm-up followed by 'individual exercise prescription' consisting of the cycle and/or floor circuits. Close observation of the heart rate is performed, with particular reference to reaching target heart rates and maintaining these heart rates during exercise. Such exercise regimens are best undertaken three times a week.
- Stress management, particularly in a group setting, can be undertaken after the exercise class. High levels of depression and anxiety are common in patients after having an MI.
- Education is also an important component, with practical advice on lifestyle changes, help with going back to work and discussion of delicate topics such as sex.
- Studying information leaflets given by the cardiac rehabilitation team should be encouraged.

Comments on the case

This case highlights the importance of post-MI rehabilitation. This case is not a test of knowledge of an MI but a test of counselling for a patient's fears and worries after such a life event.

Case 26 | Managing a complaint after an adverse incident

Candidate information
You are the medical SHO

Please read this summary (it should take no more than 2 min) and then continue with the consultation.

Re: Mrs Irene Singleton, aged 79

Mrs Singleton was admitted from a nursing home earlier today with a history of reduced activity and a cough. A chest X-ray revealed a left lower lobe pneumonia. One of the carers relayed a message to the casualty triage nurse that Mrs Singleton is allergic to penicillin. Unfortunately, because of various breakdowns in the communication pathway, this message was not passed on to you. The GP letter had no mention of the allergy and inadvertently intravenous amoxicillin 500 mg (first dose) was prescribed and given by yourself. As a result Mrs Singleton developed a rash and vomiting which was then treated with intravenous chlorpheniramine (chlorphenamine), hydrocortisone and metoclopramide. Mrs Singleton remains rather delicate but the vomiting has settled. Mrs Singleton's daughter, Mrs Edwards, is upset about this incident and wants to make a complaint. You decide to speak to her first.

Your tasks are to: speak to Mrs Edwards acknowledging the mistake, listen to her grievances and explain what you will do about the incident.

You have 14 min until the daughter leaves the room, followed by 1 min for reflection, before the discussion with the examiners.

Subject/patient/relative information
Mrs Irene Singleton is a 79-year-old lady who lives in a nursing home. She has dementia but over the last 3 days she has had a cough and reduced general activity. The GP came to visit and suspected pneumonia. This was confirmed on the chest X-ray in the casualty department. She was accompanied by a carer and was immediately seen by one of the triage nurses. The carer passed over the nursing details, including the known allergy to penicillin. If given penicillin, Mrs Singleton develops a rash and becomes nauseated with vomiting. The casualty department is, as ever, extremely stretched and the triage notes stating the allergy were not received by the medical SHO on call (the candidate). As the patient was unable to give a proper history, all the SHO had was a GP's letter which did not state the allergy. The SHO, in managing the pneumonia, gave the first dose of intravenous amoxicillin 500 mg (prescribed by him or her) but within 20 min Mrs Singleton came out in a rash and started vomiting. The SHO promptly realized what had happened and reacted appropriately by giving intravenous hydrocortisone, chlorpheniramine and metoclopramide, arranging observations every 15 min for any deterioration. The SHO crossed off the intravenous amoxicillin from the chart and

wrote in big capital letters in the notes and on the cover 'ALLERGIC TO PENICILLIN'. The patient's daughter, Mrs Edwards, who arrived after the treatment was started, is angry that although the carer had relayed the message with regard to the allergy, no one took notice and that this has led to further suffering for her mother. She wants an explanation and is prepared to make an official complaint. She is about to see the SHO (the candidate) to make her feelings known.

Examiner information

1 Communication skills—conduct of interview

- Provide the daughter with space and do not make her feel threatened. Ideally, in the real situation, you would have a member of nursing staff with you.
- Introduce yourself and make sure you know who you are speaking to.
- Allow her to say what she wants without interrupting her. Do not take any criticism personally. Find out the exact nature of her complaint.
- Acknowledge her feelings with empathy. Look her in the eye as you are listening.
- Offer an apology, saying how sorry you are that this incident has occurred. The daughter will want to know how and why the penicillin was given. Explain that there was a breakdown in communication which should not have happened, that you sincerely did not know that Mrs Singleton was allergic to penicillin and that, most importantly, the antibiotic was given in good faith in the best interests of her mother: it was the best treatment and was given when you did not know she was allergic.
- Explain that you spotted the mistake as soon as symptoms appeared and that the situation was managed correctly by administering the appropriate drugs.
- Tell her what you are going to do about it. Tell her that you will bring the issue up with the consultant, that you will report this mishap as a 'critical incident' to the risk management team, who will let one of the hospital managerial staff know, and that endeavours will be made for this not to happen again, e.g. by better staff awareness and reporting of drug allergies.
- Document everything in the notes and draw up an incident report.
- Again apologize for the grievance.
- Hopefully, she will be a little happier and she may accept your apologies or may take this further by making a written complaint. If she does want to do this, then give her the name and address of the appropriate person she should write to.

2 Communication skills—exploration and problem negotiation

The candidate should be able to:
- acknowledge that a mistake has been made
- apologize for the incident
- explain how the incident has been managed and what is going to be done about it

3 Ethics and the law and other discussion points

General comments

- In 1985 the Health and Safety Executive defined untoward incidents (or adverse incidents) as events that give rise to, or have the potential to produce, unexpected or unwanted effects involving the safety of patients. The definition therefore includes near misses.
- It should be made clear that an untoward incident is a serious event in which a patient, or patients, were harmed or could have been harmed; the event was unexpected and that the event would be likely to give rise to serious public concern or criticism of the service involved.
- Adverse incidents can have devastating consequences for individual patients and their families, can cause distress to the usually very committed healthcare staff involved, and can undermine public confidence in the services that the NHS provides.

What the GMC recommends

The GMC recommends that patients (and relatives) who complain about the care or treatment have a right to expect a prompt, open, constructive and honest response. This will include an explanation of what has happened and, where appropriate, an apology. You must not allow the complaint to prejudice the care or treatment you provide or arrange for that patient, *and* you must cooperate fully with any formal inquiry into the treatment of a patient as well as with any complaints procedure which applies to your work. You must give, to those who are entitled to ask for it, any relevant information in connection with an investigation into your own, or another healthcare professional's conduct, performance or health. General Medical Council. *Good Medical Practice*, Sections 29–32. Complaints and formal inquiries. May 2001.

How to avoid and manage complaints

- Every effort must be made to avoid dispute and altercations with patients and their relatives. Many complaints and claims of negligence are prompted by a lack of good communication between doctors and their patients. Most of these could be avoided if practitioners took the time and trouble to establish good rapport with patients, to explain details of their care to them and to listen to them and their relatives.
- In circumstances where complications and errors arise it is proper that patients (or, in this case, the next of kin) should be given prompt, objective, factual information with appropriate clinical reassurance. Adequate explanation from a senior clinician assists in reducing the fear and uncertainty that may give rise to complaints and claims. *Withholding objective factual information or expressions of sympathy or to retreat behind 'walls of silence' is regarded as counterproductive.*
- If an apology is warranted it should be sincerely given. However, it would be inappropriate for you to speculate or, worse, to assign blame unless and until all the relevant facts have been carefully established by a proper and thorough inquiry. An ill-considered remark made to a patient or relative could lead him or her to misleading conclusions and prejudice the interests of other members of the clinical team, both medical and non-medical, who themselves have a right to be consulted and given an opportunity to comment and seek advice.
- Avoid criticizing colleagues in front of patients but do not dismiss or excuse what the patient or relative is saying. All too often a casual remark, perhaps intended in jest, is misunderstood and leads to a claim or complaint against a colleague.

Typical content of an adverse incident report form (as recommended by a defence body)

The form should be confined to a single side of A4 and kept within the department with a top copy being sent to the manager. It should include the following:

- date and time of the report
- date and time of the event
- location of the event
- identification of the person affected
- condition of the person affected
- identity of person(s) witnessing the event
- identity of the person preparing the report
- identity of the person to whom the incident is reported and action taken
- the factual details of the adverse incident
- details of any equipment/drug/vaccine involved, including the manufacturer, model and lot number where applicable

Non-punitive reporting system

To encourage staff to report untoward incidents they need assurances that the system will not be used for disciplinary purposes. On the contrary, it should be made clear that the system is about prevention, education and improving quality of care. The material reported is necessary, not for apportioning blame but to inform staff at meetings for educational purposes, to improve systems and avoid future problems. Involving practice staff in this way will lead to a more open and blame-free culture.

Legal aspects of the report form

In the context of litigation, an untoward incident report is a discoverable document. This means that, if a clinical negligence claim were to arise from the incident, the report would have to be disclosed as evidence. Concerns about this possible use of reports should not dissuade people from instituting an active and effective reporting system. However, it is always wise to ensure that the details of an incident are confined to purely factual events and do not stray into opinion giving.

Claiming clinical negligence

To succeed in a claim of clinical negligence against a doctor, the patient or the next of kin (if the patient is unable to, and who would then become the claimant) has to prove, on the balance of probabilities, that:

- the doctor owed a duty of care
- there was a breach of that duty
- harm followed as a result (that causation is established)

Examples where claims of clinical negligence against a doctor have been made (as stated by a medical defence body)

- Communications
  (a) a conciliatory approach may defuse a potential complaint
  (b) give a prompt sympathetic account of care and treatment
  (c) apologize where appropriate
- Medication/injections

Complaints arise for various reasons:
  (a) unfamiliarity with prescribed medication
  (b) being unaware of all existing medication taken by a patient
  (c) ignorance of drug interactions, side-effects and known contraindications
  (d) no systems in place for regular monitoring of patients on long-term medication
  (e) not reviewing repeat prescriptions, the type of medication or the treatment time
  (f) telephone prescribing
  (g) not checking prescriptions written by others on your behalf and requiring your signature, including those generated by computer
- Medical records

Accurate, complete and contemporaneous medical records can help to refute complaints and claims. They ensure continuity of care and treatment. It is wise to make an entry in the medical record after every consultation and telephone conversation.

- Failure to diagnose and follow-up

Many patients have ambiguous or non-conclusive symptoms and thus one must:
  (a) re-evaluate if there is no improvement following initial treatment
  (b) record the plan of medical treatment along with a time scale in the clinical notes
  (c) do not discount a diagnosis merely because of a patient's age

---

Comments on the case

Unfortunately, the above case is all too common and, unless handled in the proper way, will lead to preventable distress for all parties involved.

Most patients/relatives will appreciate prompt information giving, a sincere apology and the assurance that the error or omission will be properly recorded and reported.

Case 27 | Medical opinion for fitness for anaesthesia

Candidate information

You are the medical SHO in a general medical clinic

Please read this summary (it should take no more than 2 min) and then continue with the consultation.

> ### Re: Mr Tom Watson, aged 82
>
> Mr Watson is an elderly man who is under the care of the urologists for benign prostatic hyperplasia. He is known to have heart failure and COPD. The urology consultant wants to know if this patient is fit for a general anaesthetic and has asked for a medical opinion, hence the patient's referral to the medical outpatients. His current medication includes: aspirin, ramipril, Combivent nebulizer 2.5 mL q.d.s., beclomethasone 200 μg b.d. inhaler.

Your tasks are to: give a medical opinion to the urologist.

You have 14 min until the patient leaves the room, followed by 1 min for reflection, before the discussion with the examiners.

Subject/patient/relative information

Mr Watson is an elderly 82-year-old man who lives in warden-controlled accommodation. He has been under the care of the urologists for benign prostatic hyperplasia and his symptoms of prostatism are now so severe that a transurethral resection of the prostate is recommended. The urologist is worried about his medical condition, particularly with regard to tolerating a general anaesthetic. He is known to have COPD and heart failure. He has not managed to get out of his flat for the last year and the warden does all the shopping and most of the cleaning. He gets breathless walking upstairs and has a chronic cough and phlegm. He has no chest pain but does have ankle swelling as a result of his heart failure. For these conditions he takes a nebulizer, a diuretic and an ACE inhibitor (he cannot remember the names). He used to smoke 30 cigarettes a day but stopped 6 months ago. He had a previous femoral neck fracture 5 years ago after a fall and then he remembers undergoing a spinal procedure (an injection in the back and both his legs went numb and floppy as a result). He is not allergic to any medication and he is unaware of any allergy to anaesthetic gases as he has never had a general anaesthetic before. He understands the need for the operation but he is worried about having the anaesthetic.

Examiner information

1 Communication skills — conduct of interview

- Explain why you are seeing the patient; he may think you are the urologist or an anaesthetist.
- Explore his symptoms caused by the heart failure and COPD. Ask about other medical problems, e.g. diabetes, cerebrovascular disease.
- Ask about previous operations: general, local or spinal anaesthesia.
- Are there any allergies to medication or anaesthetics.
- An anaesthetist would, as a rule, ascertain the state of the teeth and any possible indications of difficult intubation, e.g. short immobile neck, malpositioning of teeth, high-arched palate, receding mandible, poor mouth opening.
- Address any concerns.
- Explain that you are a physician and your job is to give a medical opinion but not to decide on your own whether he is fit for an anaesthetic.

2 Communication skills — exploration and problem negotiation

The candidate should be able to:
- carry out a medical assessment
- ascertain a drug history and any previous allergies
- arrange a list of investigations which would be useful for the urologist and the anaesthetist, e.g. FBC, U/E, glucose, resting ECG, oxygen saturations on air, spirometry, chest X-ray

- discuss the case with the consultant as a courtesy and write back to the urologist about the medical opinion

3 Ethics and the law and other discussion points

- It is common for physicians to be asked for an anaesthetic opinion from surgeons. Remember you are a physician and not an expert in anaesthesia.
- It is important that you give a medical opinion and relay the results to the urologists. If investigations are performed but the results are not available that day, e.g. spirometry, biochemistry, haematology, etc., you must let the urologist know that the results are to follow.
- Patients will ask 'Am I fit for an anaesthetic, doctor?' You must be honest and say that you are not the right person to judge that, but you can give your medical opinion to the patient concerning the level of his COPD and heart failure.

Comments on the case

Remember where you stand in cases like these; giving advice beyond your expertise. You can assess the cardiovascular and respiratory system and arrange relevant investigations, all of which will help the anaesthetist to make the final decision.

Case 28 | Needlestick injury from an HIV patient

Candidate information

You are the medical SHO on call with your recently qualified house officer

Please read this summary (it should take no more than 2 min) and then continue with the consultation.

> **Re: Dr Alison Mariner, aged 24**
>
> Dr Mariner is your new house officer and you are both on-call today. A patient with known HIV has been admitted with dyspnoea? cause. Dr Mariner has clerked the patient and has arranged all the appropriate investigations, including blood tests which she took herself (using gloves). However, she comes back to you extremely upset as she has just had a needlestick injury while taking the blood.

Your tasks are to: calm the situation, to advise her about the management of a needle-stick injury and discuss the need for antiretroviral therapy.

You have 14 min until the house officer leaves the room, followed by 1 min for reflection, before the discussion with the examiners.

Subject/patient/relative information

Dr Mariner is a recently qualified house officer working on-call with the medical SHO (the candidate). She was asked to see an HIV positive patient, well-known to the infectious diseases department and who is already on numerous therapies including zidovudine, didanosine, indinavir and Septrin. The patient has been admitted for queried dyspnoea and its cause, possibly *Pneumocystis carinii* pneumonia. The house officer wore two pairs of gloves but, after taking the blood and with the syringe full, she had a needlestick injury with the green needle entering about 0.5 cm into the pulp of her right index finger. She panicked and disposed of the whole syringe and needle into the sharps bin. She has carried out the correct initial procedure of washing the contaminated area with water and soap, avoiding scrubbing and allowing the injury site to bleed freely. She is obviously panicking because this is an injury involving an HIV positive patient. She has only a vague idea about the possible risk of spread of HIV in such cases. She lives with her boyfriend and she is 4 months pregnant. She has been fully immunized against hepatitis B.

Examiner information

1 Communication skills—conduct of interview

- Ask the house officer exactly what has happened. She also tells you she is 4 months pregnant.
- First, calm her as continued panic will impair her thought processes.
- Tell her that her concerns for the baby will be dealt with and that you will speak to her obstetric consultant about this incident.
- Show empathy and reassure her that the risk of contracting HIV in this type of circumstance is low (around 0.3%). Also explain that there is a risk of contracting hepatitis B and C.
- Ask if she has been immunized against hepatitis B.
- Tell her she must immediately wash the contaminated area thoroughly with soap and water. Avoid scrubbing and allow the wound to bleed freely. She tells you that she has done this.
- Establish the type and size of needle in question, the depth of penetration, the amount of bleeding produced and the exact time of the needlestick injury.
- Establish who the patient is and confirm their HIV, hepatitis B and C status.
- If unsure what treatment to give to the house officer, say to her that you will ring occupational health immediately for advice on any established hospital guidelines.
- If this fails or the incident has taken place out of normal working hours, the senior nurse in the casualty department should know what the guidelines are and where the anti-HIV triple therapy starter pack is kept. This should be given within the first hour.
- Explain that treatment will be for 4 weeks and that she must watch out for side-effects such as sickness and a rash. The candidate must know of any medication that the house officer is on to assess potential drug reactions.
- Warn her of the potential risk of any drug interactions.
- She should be followed-up regularly by the occupational health team.
- She should also watch out for symptoms suggestive of seroconversion (rash, fever, malaise, myalgia, lymphadenopathy).
- Tell the house officer that zidovudine and lamivudine are not contraindicated in pregnancy. Experience with other therapies, e.g. indinavir is limited. Explain that the advantages outweigh the risks and also that therapy is known to reduce the risk of vertical transmission.
- Explain to the house officer that she should be encouraged to undertake an HIV test, explaining that without it, it would be difficult to claim compensation (industrial injuries disablement benefit) if she was found to be HIV positive at a later date.
- Counsel her for the HIV test, explaining what the test involves and give a reassurance of confidentiality (see Case 19 for further details).
- Explain that blood taken will also be tested for hepatitis B and C.
- Also tell her that you will explain to the patient what has happened and that you will counsel the patient for a hepatitis B and C test with consent.
- Explain that HIV retesting will be repeated 6 months after stopping prophylaxis.
- Until then she should decide how to tell her partner what has happened with consideration of practising safe sex using barrier methods (condoms).
- Ask the house officer if there is anything that she is not sure about.
- Suggest that she should go off duty and that you will try and arrange some cover.

2 Communication skills—exploration and problem negotiation

The candidate should be able to:

- assess, support and counsel the individual who has been put at risk with empathy and understanding
- know when to recommend postexposure prophylaxis (PEP). Four factors increasing the risk of occupationally acquired HIV infection are:
  - (a) deep injury
  - (b) visible blood on the device causing the injury
  - (c) injury with a needle that has been placed in the patient's vein or artery
  - (d) terminal HIV-related illness in the source patient
- know which PEP drugs are used: zidovudine 250 mg b.d., lamivudine 150 mg and indinavir 800 mg t.d.s. (or nelfinavir 1250 mg b.d.). Combination drugs have proven superior efficacy than zidovudine alone and also, because of increasing zidovudine resistance, combination therapy for prophylaxis is recommended
- relay the importance of close follow-up by a senior occupational health physician with further counselling and postexposure HIV testing

3 Ethics and the law and other discussion points (guidelines from the Department of Health)

- Confidentiality is paramount.

- If the HIV status of the patient is unknown but suspected, then HIV test counselling should not be undertaken by the individual exposed (in this case the house officer).
- Patients with unknown HIV status cannot have HIV testing without their consent and so an assessment of the likelihood of infection may have to be made.
- Pregnancy does not preclude the use of HIV PEP therapy. Zidovudine and lamivudine are not contraindicated in the second and third trimester; such evidence for other drugs is limited.
- Healthcare workers exposed should be given the chance to discuss the balance of risks with appropriate psychological support, including information about the potential toxic side-effects and the risk of passing HIV to the baby if pregnant, and so allowing the individual to make an informed decision about whether or not to undergo PEP therapy.
- It would be wise to inform the house officer's consultant.
- Pending follow-up and absence of seroconversion, healthcare workers are not obliged to be the subject of work modifications, e.g. avoidance of exposure-prone procedures.
- All individuals exposed must be given advice on safe sex and avoiding blood donation.
- The occupational health physician is encouraged to report the case (in absolute confidence) to the Public Health Laboratory Service (PHLS) Communicable Disease Surveillance Centre (or Scottish Centre for Infection and Environmental Health in Scotland).

> **Comments on the case**
>
> This is quite a complicated case, but one that can happen to anyone working in acute medicine. There are many ethical complexities that the candidate must be appreciative of and, unless adequately prepared, can lead to a badly conducted station. More guidance can be obtained from the Department of Health website.

Case 29 | Obesity—'It must be my glands, doctor'

Candidate information

You are the medical SHO in an endocrine clinic

Please read this summary (it should take no more than 2 min) and then continue with the consultation.

> **Re: Miss Kathryn Beagle, aged 30**
>
> Miss Beagle was referred to the clinic 2 months ago because of obesity and the GP queried the possibility of an endocrine cause. The body mass index (BMI) measured at her first appointment was 32 kg/m^2 and she has subsequently gained another 2 kg. She has seen the dietitian who agrees that while her diet is not excessive it is not a weight-reducing diet. She works as a secretary and sits at a desk all day with little exercise. Initial investigations have shown normal thyroid function tests, and a normal fasting plasma glucose, luteinizing hormone (LH), follicle-stimulating hormone (FSH) and testosterone levels. Following her last appointment she underwent a dexamethasone suppression test, which was also normal. Your consultant has reviewed her results and assures you that she does not have a recognized endocrine cause for her obesity. She has come to the clinic for the results and is keen for help.

Your tasks are to: explain the findings, reassure her that there are no obvious endocrine causes for her obesity and discuss ways to tackle her weight problem.

You have 14 min until the patient leaves the room, followed by 1 min for reflection, before the discussion with the examiners.

Subject/patient/relative information

Miss Beagle is a 30-year-old secretary who is having problems with her weight. She has always been a little overweight but she has noticed over the last 2 years that, despite trying simple dietary advice, her weight is still increasing. She has noticed her mobility is more laboured and she feels much less fit than before. The weight has led to a decline in her self-esteem and she would feel intimidated if she were to join a gym or go swimming. Recently, a colleague had a similar weight problem and was found to be hypothyroid and, after starting thyroxine, this colleague lost a considerable amount of weight. All investigations including thyroid function, glucose, FSH, LH and testosterone are normal. Her GP has suggested the possibility of tablets for her obesity but some have side-effects and many have negligible long-term safety profiles. She is convinced that there is a gland problem which is causing her increasing weight and is sure that treating this problem would cure her obesity. She wants to try some form of therapy, even thyroxine, to lose weight.

Examiner information

1 Communication skills—conduct of interview

- Introduce yourself to the patient.
- Ask her what she knows and what the previous doctor has told her.
- Explain that all the endocrine tests are normal, that this is good, and that there is no suggestion of a gland problem as a cause of her increasing weight.
- Allow her to express her feelings on this sensitive matter.
- She may become upset (offer a box of tissues if she cries) and explain that despite trying a diet she has been unable to lose weight. Appreciate any loss of self-esteem in such patients.
- Take a dietary history and ask about the diet which she tried. Make simple suggestions on fat intake if she is unaware of this.
- Avoid focusing purely on the weight in terms of numbers (kg), etc.—the patient knows she is overweight and she will know her exact weight as the clinic nurse will have just weighed her.
- Ask her openly about lifestyle issues: why does she think she has failed with her diet, how does she feel about joining a gym or going swimming. She may feel intimidated by this but encourage her that many gyms have sessions for overweight people and maybe by meeting such people she could share her lack of confidence. Suggest attending 'weight-watchers' groups.
- She may enquire about the possibility of thyroxine therapy to lose weight like her colleague. Tell her this is not advisable in the presence of normal thyroid function.
- She may ask you about weight-reducing therapies. Explain that these are given as adjuncts and not instead of dietary plans.
- Encourage her to keep a diary in which she should document what she eats as she eats it and not at a later date.

2 Communication skills—exploration and problem negotiation

The candidate should be able to:

- convey the normal results and explain that there is no endocrine reason for her weight problem
- discuss a management plan to tackle the obesity
- show empathy and total understanding for the sensitivity that surrounds this case

Ethics and the law and other discussion points

- Explaining normal results should be carried out in a positive manner, emphasizing that this is good news and not bad. The patient may be hoping for an abnormal result in order to explain and legitimize her obesity with the hope of a simple straightforward treatment.
- The candidate should be empathic with respect to the difficulties of losing weight but should clearly emphasize that treatment with active hormones, particularly thyroid hormones, should not be given where a deficiency cannot be shown to exist.
- The vast majority of obese people have increased leptin levels but do not have mutations of either leptin or its receptor; they may have functional leptin resistance. Data looking at the exact role of leptin is contradictory and unsettled. The mechanism for leptin resistance, and whether it can be overcome by raising leptin levels, is not yet established.
- Discussion of the management of obesity should be centred on diet, exercise and, possibly, drug therapy. Despite short-term benefits, medication-induced weight loss is often associated with rebound weight gain after the cessation of drug use, there are side-effects from the medication and there is potential for drug abuse. The old appetite suppressants, such as fenfluramine, have been withdrawn because of their side-effects (e.g. pulmonary hypertension, valvular heart disease, etc.).
- Recently, the National Institute of Clinical Excellence (NICE) has approved the use of two new drugs (orlistat and sibutramine) for use in obesity as adjuncts to good dietary management. For example, both NICE and the pharmaceutical company that markets orlistat (an intestinal lipase inhibitor) advise giving this drug only if a patient has managed to lose weight (2.5 kg) with dieting and increasing activity in the preceding 4 weeks prior to the first prescription. Sibutramine is a reuptake inhibitor of serotonin and noradrenaline and it promotes a feeling of satiety after smaller meals. NICE recommends the use of orlistat in patients with a BMI of 28 kg/m^2 with the presence of comorbidities (e.g. diabetes mellitus, ischaemic heart disease, hypertension, obstructive sleep apnoea, etc.) or 30 kg/m^2 without comorbidities and as part of an overall management plan for obesity. Therapy should continue for more than 3 months only if the patient has lost at least 5% of her body weight from the start of drug treatment, and similarly it should only continue for more than 6 months if weight loss has been at least 10% of

body weight. Treatment should not usually continue beyond 12 months.

- For sibutramine, NICE recommends using it for a BMI of $27 \, kg/m^2$ with comorbidities and $30 \, kg/m^2$ without. People taking sibutramine should only continue with treatment for more than 4 weeks if they have lost 2 kg in weight. People should only continue on this treatment beyond 3 months if they have lost at least 5% of their body weight from the start of the drug treatment. Sibutramine should be stopped if patients do not lose weight as described. Treatment is not recommended for more than 12 months. Because sibutramine can lead to an increase in blood pressure, people taking it should have their blood pressure checked regularly. An increase in blood pressure should be considered carefully and may be a reason to stop treatment. Sibutramine is not recommended for patients who already have high blood pressure (145/90 or above).

Comments on the case

This case illustrates how a patient may blame a separate illness for causing their obesity. The candidate will have to be prepared to disappoint the patient on that account but be supportive in encouraging her to follow a sensible dietary and exercise programme.

Case 30 | Obtaining consent for a lumbar puncture

Candidate information

You are the medical SHO in the emergency admission unit
Please read this summary (it should take no more than 2 min) and then continue with the consultation.

> **Re: Miss Bridget Harvey, aged 31**
>
> Miss Harvey has been admitted with blurred vision. On admission, it was noticed that she has bilateral papilloedema and a subsequent enhanced CT scan of the head is found to be normal. The most likely diagnosis is benign intracranial hypertension and the consultant neurologist has asked for a lumbar puncture with measurement of the cerebrospinal fluid (CSF) pressure and, if raised, for therapeutic aspiration.

Your tasks are to: explain what benign intracranial hypertension (BIH) is and get her consent for a lumbar puncture.

You have 14 min until the patient leaves the room, followed by 1 min for reflection, before the discussion with the examiners.

Subject/patient/relative information

Miss Bridget Harvey has had a 3-week history of blurred vision. She came to casualty and one of the SHOs detected bilateral blurring of the optic discs (papilloedema). She has just had a CT scan but is unaware of the findings. The medical SHO (the candidate) is about to see her to give her the result, to explain the most likely reason for her symptoms and to discuss the need for a lumbar puncture. She is worried that she may lose her vision and is anxious about having needles in her back.

Examiner information

1 Communication skills — conduct of interview

- Introduce yourself to Miss Harvey. Ask how she is.
- Explain the findings of the CT scan of her head. Reassure her that there is no evidence of a tumour.
- Explain that the most likely diagnosis for the blurred vision is a condition called benign intracranial hypertension. Describe this briefly, explaining that there is increased pressure in the brain and spinal canal and that this is putting pressure on the back of the eyes, hence the blurred vision: use a simple diagram to explain.
- Say that the best way to treat the condition is to have a lumbar puncture which allows, through a needle in the back, for the pressure to be relieved by taking away some of the spinal fluid: the same diagram will help to explain this.
- Reassure her that with treatment the outcome is good but it is important to have regular eye checks and spinal fluid pressure checks to minimize the risk of progressive visual problems.
- Ask her if she knows what a lumbar puncture is.
- Explain she has to lie on her left side, keeping very still, and that a needle is inserted into the back after giving local anaesthetic which numbs the skin. The needle is inserted between two vertebral bones and into the

spinal canal. A certain volume of cerebrospinal fluid (CSF) is removed and the needle is then taken out. Reassure her that she will feel no pain after the initial needle-prick and sting. Explain that she must then lie on her back for at least 4 h to minimize any risk of headache. Reassure her that the procedure is performed under strict aseptic conditions to minimize any risk of introducing infection. Reassure her that she will be conscious throughout with a nurse present to assess any discomfort. Explain that she will need the procedure repeating every few days until the CSF pressure is back to normal and that she may need further CSF pressure assessments in the future. Make sure that she understands this last point.

- Ask her how she feels about this and give her time to allow all the information to be considered.
- If she agrees, check that she is not on aspirin or anticoagulants and that she does not have any back problems, including any previous history of spinal problems.
- Ask if she has any queries or worries.

2 Communication skills — exploration and problem negotiation

The candidate should be able to:

- reassure the patient that the CT scan of the head is normal
- explain the likely diagnosis
- reassure that treatment for BIH is available
- explain the lumbar puncture procedure
- provide an opportunity for her to consider the proposal and return at a later stage if she wishes

3 Ethics and the law and other discussion points

- Performing a lumbar puncture is a common occurrence in clinical practice. Normal CSF pressure is usually less than 20 cm CSF. CSF protein is usually less than 0.4 g/L and there should be no more than 5 lymphocytes/mL CSF.
- The most common complication is a headache, usually resulting from continuing CSF leakage through a dural hole. The risk of this headache can be reduced by using a smaller needle. Very rarely, transtentorial herniation may occur if the lumbar puncture is carried out in the presence of high obstructed CSF pressures, e.g. intracranial mass lesion or obstructive hydrocephalus. Infection and spinal haemorrhage are also rare.
- Patients have a right to information about their condition and the treatment options available to them. The amount of information you give each patient will vary

according to factors such as the nature of the condition, the complexity of the treatment, the risks associated with the treatment or procedure and the patient's own wishes. For example, patients may need more information to make an informed decision about a procedure which carries a high risk of failure or adverse side-effects; or about an investigation for a condition which, if present, could have serious implications for the patient's employment and social or personal life.

- The information that patients want, or ought, to know before deciding whether to consent to treatment or an investigation may include:

  (a) details of the diagnosis, prognosis and the likely prognosis if the condition is left untreated

  (b) uncertainties about the diagnosis, including options for further investigation before treatment

  (c) options for treatment or management of the condition, including the option of not to treat

  (d) the purpose of a proposed investigation or treatment; details of the procedures or therapies involved, including subsidiary treatment such as methods of pain relief; how the patient should prepare for the procedure; and details of what the patient might experience during or after the procedure including the common and the serious side-effects

  (e) for each option there should be an explanation of the likely benefits and the probabilities of success; and discussion of any serious or frequently occurring risks, and of any lifestyle changes which may be caused, or necessitated, by the treatment

  (f) advice about whether a proposed treatment is experimental

  (g) how and when the patient's condition and any side-effects will be monitored or reassessed

  (h) the name of the doctor who will have overall responsibility for the treatment and, where appropriate, names of the senior members of his or her team

  (i) whether doctors in training will be involved, and the extent to which students may be involved in an investigation or treatment

  (j) a reminder that patients can change their minds about a decision at any time

  (k) a reminder that patients have a right to seek a second opinion

  (l) where applicable, details of costs or charges which the patient may have to meet

General Medical Council. *Seeking Patient's Consent: the Ethical Considerations*, Section 4–5. Consenting to investigation and treatment. November 1998.

Comments on the case

This case highlights the important principles that apply to patients undergoing an investigative procedure. It is essential that patients are as fully informed as they wish to be and do not feel that they have been railroaded into making a decision. Such principles, as highlighted by the GMC, can apply to any other procedure, e.g. endoscopy, bronchoscopy, angiogram, etc., and for treatments such as radiotherapy or chemotherapy.

Case 31 | Postponing an investigation

Candidate information

You are the medical SHO

Please read this summary (it should take no more than 2 min) and then continue with the consultation.

Re: Mr Malcolm Hatton, aged 69

Mr Hatton has a solitary, left-sided peripheral lung shadow of unknown cause. He has smoked in the past and the consultant is keen to rule out a neoplastic lesion. He has come to the day unit today to have a fine needle percutaneous lung biopsy performed by the consultant radiologist. However, he is on warfarin for a deep vein thrombosis (DVT) diagnosed 6 weeks ago and, at the last clinic appointment, he was told by the consultant to stop his warfarin for 48 h, have the clotting checked on the day of the biopsy and only proceed if the international normalized ratio (INR) was less than 1.5. Normally, he takes 4 mg/day warfarin and his INR has been steady at 2.8. Unfortunately, he has not stopped his warfarin (because the instructions by the consultant were not clear) and in view of this the radiologist judges it to be unsafe to proceed with the biopsy.

Your tasks are to: apologise for any misunderstanding and the resultant delay, explain why it would be unsafe for him to have his biopsy carried out today and to come to some compromise which is acceptable to the patient.

You have 14 min until the patient leaves the room, followed by 1 min for reflection, before the discussion with the examiners.

Subject/patient/relative information

Mr Malcolm Hatton is a 69-year-old man with a solitary left-sided peripheral lung shadow of unknown cause. As he has smoked in the past, the consultant physician is keen to rule out a neoplastic lesion by a fine needle percutaneous lung biopsy. Mr Hatton was diagnosed as having a DVT 6 weeks ago and was started on warfarin. At the last outpatient clinic, the consultant asked him to stop his warfarin for 48 h before the biopsy, come to the day unit and have his INR checked and, if this was less than 1.5, then he would be able to have the biopsy. Unfortunately, Mr Hatton was unclear about the instruction at his last consultation to stop his warfarin and continued to take it. In light of this today the radiologist is not prepared to carry out the biopsy. Mr Hatton is unhappy that the biopsy has been postponed. He is unsure as to why it was necessary to stop the warfarin, and he is worried that the lung shadow might be a cancer. He is therefore concerned that he may have to wait a while for his next biopsy appointment. He is about to see the medical SHO (the candidate) for an explanation. After the consultation, Mr Hatton understands the reason for the postponement and is clear and confident about the proposed compromise.

Examiner information

1 Communication skills — conduct of interview

- Introduce yourself and appologise that the radiologist is unable to carry out the biopsy today and that you hope he will give you an opportunity to explain the reason and come up with and acceptable plan.
- Allow him to express his reasons for his unhappiness.
- Ask why he did not stop the warfarin (instructions not clear, fear of developing another DVT, forgetfulness?).
- Explain the reasons for the postponement, with emphasis on the risk of bleeding if the biopsy is carried out while on warfarin.
- Explain that the warfarin must be stopped for at least 48 h before the procedure to allow its effect to wear off. Say that there is only a minimal risk of developing DVT if the warfarin is stopped for 48 h. Say that usually an INR would be checked before the biopsy to ensure that the blood is not too thin.
- He tells you that he is aware that he might have cancer and he does not want to wait too long for the next biopsy appointment.
- Say that the consultant is unclear if the lung shadow is a cancer or not; which is why they want to carry out the biopsy. Appreciate his concerns and say that you will speak to the consultant radiologist straight away to book another appointment at the earliest possible time. Say to Mr Hatton that you will give him the date before he leaves.
- Again apologize for the inconvenience and any misunderstandings that have led to today's postponement. Ask if he has any other queries or grievances about the postponement of the biopsy.
- Offer him an early opportunity to speak to the consultant about the misunderstanding if he wishes.
- Ask how he travelled to the hospital; if he came by ambulance, say you will let the ambulance desk know that he will be going home soon.
- Let your consultant and the histology department know of the postponement and rearrange the next outpatient appointment to fit around the rearranged biopsy.
- Discuss diplomatically with your consultant the patient's lack of clarity about the instruction given to him by the consultant at the last appointment.

2 Communication skills — exploration and problem negotiation

The candidate should be able to:

- understand the frustration encountered by the patient; that the procedure is being delayed when he might have cancer
- apologise for any misunderstanding that has caused today's postponement
- explain to the patient that there is a safety issue regarding having a lung biopsy with concomitant warfarin therapy
- reassure the patient and ensure that another biopsy appointment is made before the patient leaves the clinic

3 Ethics and the law and other discussion points

The physician should not undertake a procedure if there is a safety issue. Although the patient may show his frustration towards the doctor, the physician is advised to inform him clearly of the reasons for the postponement and to go ahead with delaying the biopsy.

Comments on the case

This case tests the negotiating ability of the candidate with a patient who is understandably unhappy in the delay of a crucial test. Many scenarios occur where decisions (e.g. postponement of procedures) must be made in the best interest of the patient, despite the resulting wrath. It is important to explain clearly and fully the reasons for the postponement.

Where the patient perceives that previously given information either did not contain or clarify instructions that the patient must follow in order to enable a procedure to be carried out, apologising for any resultant misunderstanding and it's consequence is simple courtesy.

Case 32 | Pregnancy and pharmacy

Candidate information

You are the medical SHO in a chest clinic

Please read this summary (it should take no more than 2 min) and then continue with the consultation.

> **Re: Mrs Fatima Bibi, aged 26**
>
> Mrs Bibi is a patient with pulmonary tuberculosis who has been on rifampicin and isoniazid therapy for 4 months and pyrazinamide and ethambutol for the first 2 months. She tells you that she is 14 weeks pregnant (with her third child) and she also tells you that she stopped her medication 2 weeks ago. She has concerns regarding any harmful effects on the baby. She is about to see you in clinic.

Your tasks are to: explore the fears Mrs Bibi has and reassure her about the safety of rifampicin and isoniazid in pregnancy.

You have 14 min until the patient leaves the room, followed by 1 min for reflection, before the discussion with the examiners.

Subject/patient/relative information

Mrs Bibi is a 26-year-old lady who presented with pulmonary tuberculosis 4 months ago having had a cough and fever. She was started on antituberculous therapy and has made excellent progress, with a reduction in her symptoms and gain in weight. She has had no problems with side-effects. However, she discovered 2 weeks ago that she is 12 weeks pregnant with her third child. She was concerned about the possible effects of the antituberculous therapy on her child and so has stopped taking this medication. She is particularly concerned about the possible effects during the first trimester and is not keen on restarting therapy. She is about to see the medical SHO (the candidate).

Examiner information

1 Communication skills—conduct of interview

- Introduce yourself to Mrs Bibi.
- Ask her how she is with regard to the tuberculosis.
- She tells you that she is 14 weeks pregnant with her third child—congratulate her.
- She tells you that she has stopped taking the antituberculous therapy for fear of teratogenic effects on the fetus.

- Explain and reassure her that the antituberculous therapy she is taking is perfectly safe in pregnancy, and that there is no evidence of any teratogenic effects from these products.
- Tell her that by stopping therapy she may in fact cause the tuberculosis to reactivate, which may be more detrimental to the child.
- Reassure her again and ask if she still feels unsure about the relevance of the treatment.
- Tell Mrs Bibi that you will let the TB health visitor know and she can visit her at home to support her and help

with any anxieties she has in relation to the drug therapy.

2 Communication skills—exploration and problem negotiation

The candidate should be able to:

- assess the present state of the tuberculosis
- explore the reasons for stopping the antituberculous therapy
- reassure that the first-line drugs for tuberculosis are safe in pregnancy
- inform the TB health visitor

3 Ethics and the law and other discussion points

- When patients are started on rifampicin, they should be informed about the possible reduced effectiveness of the oral oestrogen-based contraceptive pill if this is what they take for contraception. It is obligatory that the physician should provide contraceptive advice in such circumstances.
- First-line antituberculous medication (e.g. rifampicin, isoniazid, pyrazinamide and ethambutol) are safe in pregnancy and there is no evidence of any teratogenic effects.
- Ethionamide and prothionamide, which are occasionally used in second-line therapy, may be teratogenic and are best avoided. Streptomycin may be ototoxic to the fetus and so should also be avoided.
- Patients can breastfeed normally while taking antituberculous drugs.
- The physician must be seen to reassure the patient in this case and inform her of the potential harm of *not* taking the medication.

Comments on the case

Seeing pregnant patients with medical illnesses is common and usually the issue whether to continue certain necessary medications (and weighing up the risks to the fetus) causes the most dilemmas for the physician. An informed decision made by the mother is important. Another example would be an epileptic lady on phenytoin, carbamazepine and/or valproate (increased risk of neural tube defects) who must receive specialized advice in order to weigh up the risks to the child vs. rebound fits, especially in the third trimester. A further example is the asthmatic lady who has an exacerbation and warrants steroids. In most cases the risk to the mother and fetus (from hypoxia) is greater if steroids are not offered and so the majority of such patients do go on to have a course of prednisolone.

It may be helpful to utilize specialist support for patients from other cultures in order to be able to re-enforce information and to encourage compliance.

Case 33 | Refusal to have effective analgesia

Candidate information

You are the SHO in the medical clinic

Please read this summary (it should take no more than 2 min) and then continue with the consultation.

Re: Mr Donald Murphy, aged 74

You are about to see Mr Murphy in clinic. He had a right apical bronchial carcinoma (Pancoast's tumour) diagnosed 8 months ago. He had radiotherapy for a bony metastasis to the right clavicle. However, his pain has been worse over the last 4 weeks and he was started on morphine sulphate tablets (MST) and is presently on 30 mg b.d., in addition to the Voltarol he was already taking. However, the hospital nurse specialist tells you, before the consultation, that she believes that he may not be taking his analgesia and, as a result, he is suffering greatly from the pain. Mr Murphy is fully aware that he has a terminal illness.

Your tasks are to: analyse the patient's pain control and explore the possible reasons for non-compliance.

You have 14 min until the patient leaves the room, followed by 1 min for reflection, before the discussion with the examiners.

Subject/patient/relative information

Mr Murphy is a 74-year-old man who was diagnosed as having a right apical bronchial carcinoma 8 months ago. At that time, a bony metastasis was discovered in the right clavicle and radiotherapy was given with some relief. However, for the last 4 weeks his pain has recurred in the same area and it keeps him awake during the night. The GP, in conjunction with the local Macmillan nurse, started him on morphine sulphate tablets (MST) in addition to the Voltarol and this has been slowly increased to 30 mg b.d. However, over the last week Mr Murphy has not taken any of the morphine tablets and only takes his Voltarol when he feels like it, which is rarely. He is concerned that he is becoming addicted to them and he has never liked taking tablets; he would rather put up with the pain. Deep down behind a jolly 'what will happen, will happen' exterior is a fear of dying. Because the morphine tablets make him slightly drowsy, he is worried he may never wake up when he goes to sleep. There is also a problem with constipation. His diet has never been very good and the morphine has not helped his bowels at all. So, because of a combination of these factors, he has decided not to take the morphine tablets. He has no family and lives alone. He is about to see the medical SHO (the candidate).

Examiner information

1 Communication skills — conduct of interview

- Introduce yourself to Mr Murphy.
- Ask how he is (open question).
- If he tells you that all is fine, explain that the specialist cancer nurse is worried about the pain he has.
- Ask him about the pain relief (open question). Ask him what he is taking.
- Explore the pain more deeply: where is it, where does it radiate to, is it constant or intermittent, does it keep him awake, exacerbating features, e.g. movement, do the tablets relieve the pain, etc.
- Explain to him that sometimes people on morphine have symptoms which they do not like, or worries about taking the medication. Tell him that this is perfectly normal and that the team can help him if he has any such concerns.
- Approach the subject gently by saying that the team is worried that he may not be taking the tablets regularly or at all.
- If he tells you he is taking tablets and he has no pain then there is not much else you can do apart from believing him. However, you can still remind him of the benefits of treatment with information on the possible side-effects.
- If he tells you he does not like taking the tablets, explore why. Is it a fear of the drugs (e.g. addiction) or side-effects from the morphine (e.g. constipation)? What is his mental state like — confusion (as a result of the drugs). Is there any influence from the other members of the family? Is he in denial about the cancer or is it a fear of the cancer? He may feel that taking morphine equates with dying.
- Find out what the patient's understanding of the pain is.
- What fears does he have about the disease? Has it resulted in depression? Has he any other symptoms of vomiting, poor nutrition, weight loss, etc?
- What are his opinions on the other analgesics he has tried.
- Explain the nature of the pain he has, describe the experiences of other patients with morphine, explain the likely side-effects and, if other members of family are present, discuss future or alternative treatment plans.

- Explain that you would like to carry out an X-ray to look for any bony deposits and if this is suspicious then explain that you would like to proceed to an isotope bone scan. Ask whether he would consider further local radiotherapy if another metastatic deposit is detected.
- He may not agree to restart medication straight away but, in conjunction with the specialist nurse, further meetings fairly soon would be useful to discuss the situation — he may change his mind at the next visit.

2 Communication skills — exploration and problem negotiation

The candidate should be able to:

- take the full history of pain, drugs used and their side-effects
- sensitively explore the possible non-compliance to morphine tablets and reasons why
- explore any fears he may have about his disease
- suggest he speaks to the specialist nurse about this issue in order to produce a positive change in the patient's attitude towards his treatment
- consider investigations looking for further metastatic deposits with the possible consideration of radiotherapy

3 Ethics and the law and other discussion points

- Fears about the disease, the pain and the medication need to be explored compassionately.
- Declining treatment raises difficult dilemmas. Effective communication from the outset between staff, patient and family can allay much of the possible fear and anger. It is unprofessional to suggest to relatives (if present) that they should try concealing the medication in the food and drink, as this would heighten any mistrust if discovered. Working with the patient to understand why they are not taking medication, and giving truthful accurate information and support is far more likely to result in a decision to try or continue with the medication.
- As far as opioids are concerned, psychological dependence (addiction) does not occur when used for terminal pain and so a fear of addiction is unwarranted.

Comments on the case

This case tests the ability of the candidate to explore deeply into the feelings of terminally ill patients, their fears and their beliefs. The candidate should show compassion and understanding rather than dismissing simple misconstrued beliefs as 'nothing'.

The clinician, staff and relatives, no matter how well intentioned, are not the person who has the cancer or has to take the medication. Whilst the patient's position may make no sense to them, it is vital they work alongside the patient in a spirit of openness and do not embark on a campaign of coercion or deceit.

Case 34 | Resuscitation status in a terminally ill patient

Candidate information

You are the SHO on call

Please read this summary (it should take no more than 2 min) and then continue with the consultation.

> ### Re: Mr Wallace Freeman, aged 72
>
> You have just admitted Mr Freeman to the emergency admission ward. He is known to have bronchial carcinoma with liver and brain metastases. You have seen the old notes and the last clinic letter 2 weeks ago from the oncologist confirms that the patient's disease is now so far advanced that neither chemotherapy nor radiotherapy is appropriate and only palliative care for symptom control is advised. The patient is unrousable and his breathing is shallow. A chest X-ray shows complete collapse of the left lung. You have spoken to your registrar and you both feel that resuscitation is not in the best interests of the patient. The patient lives alone and his daughter (Mrs Janice Walker), who lives 200 miles away and has not seen her father for 2 months, has travelled up and would like to speak to you. You are about to meet her.

Your tasks are to: inform the daughter of her father's grave prognosis and discuss with her the resuscitation issues.

You have 14 min until the patient's relative leaves the room, followed by 1 min for reflection, before the discussion with the examiners.

Subject/patient/relative information

Mrs Janice Walker is the daughter of Mr Wallace Freeman, a 72-year-old man who is known to have lung cancer which has spread to the liver and brain. His daughter lives 200 miles away and has not seen him for 2 months. He lives alone. She travelled over when she was informed, by her father's neighbour, of his deteriorating condition. A chest X-ray has shown complete collapse of the left lung and, at this moment, her father is in a coma with shallow breathing. Death is expected in the next few hours and the sudden deterioration has taken her by surprise. She feels guilty that she has not seen her father recently. She cannot understand why he has deteriorated so quickly; she spoke to him on the phone just 3 days ago and he sounded fine. She has never thought about the issues of resuscitation but firmly believes that everything possible should be done for her father. She is about to see the medical SHO (the candidate) to discuss his poor prognosis.

Examiner information

1 Communication skills—conduct of interview

- Confirm who it is you are about to see.
- Introduce yourself to her explaining who you are and that you are looking after her father (as always, make sure you know the patient's name and refer to him by name).
- Make sure the room is quiet with no one there except for a nurse (probably not available in the exam).
- Start off by asking how much she knows already; 'Thank you for coming. How much do you know about your father's condition?' She may say that she only knows what her father's neighbour has said, that her father is more poorly but with no more specific details.
- Tell the daughter, showing empathy, 'I'm very sorry, but your father is very ill' and then pause. Use the pause to let the message sink in.
- Acknowledge that this must be a very difficult time for her. When the time seems right, give more information about her father's cancer, how it has spread to the brain and liver, how the lung has collapsed as shown on the X-ray and that at the moment he is unrousable. Tell her that, as a consequence of this, his outlook is very poor and that neither chemotherapy nor radiotherapy would help. Say that this decision was made 2 weeks ago by an oncologist. Pause again.
- Explain that death is most likely in the next few hours.
- Gently come onto the issue of resuscitation. Ask what she understands by resuscitation (explain in simple language if she requests more information). Ask if her father had shown any opinion on this issue when he was well and ask her if she has any thoughts on this matter.
- Then try to explain why, in the event of cardiorespiratory arrest, resuscitation is likely to be unsuccessful. The prognosis is poor and you feel that active resuscitation would cause more harm, and that it is extremely unlikely to be successful.
- Pause, and ask what she thinks of this.
- Explain your belief that he should be kept comfortable with dignity and self-esteem. Explain that you feel this decision is made in the best interests of her father. Pause again. Hopefully, she will understand your explanation.
- If she starts crying, allow her to express her emotions and sadness. Comfort her and offer her a box of tissues if handy. She may feel upset that her father has deteriorated so suddenly while she was away. Explain the reasons for this sudden deterioration and reassure her that she could not have prevented this. She may feel guilty for not having visited him for 2 months. Reassure her that she could not have prevented his inevitable deterioration.
- Tell her that you will try to arrange a side-room for privacy. Explain about the subcutaneous diamorphine pump which will keep him comfortable and pain-free and that you will continue to give fluids and oxygen in order to keep him as comfortable as possible.
- Ask if there are any other members of the family or offer her the services of the hospital chaplain; give her the telephone number of the ward if she needs it.
- If the daughter says she feels that her father should still be considered for resuscitation, ask her why she feels this way. Do respect her views but you may want the consultant involved to help in the matter. If the family have strong spiritual beliefs, then utilizing an appropriate spiritual guide may be useful.
- Otherwise enquire if she has any further questions.

2 Communication skills—exploration and problem negotiation

The candidate should be able to:
- convey the grave prognosis and the reasons why this is so
- clearly discuss the issue of resuscitation, asking what the relative understands by it, explain why resuscitation is inappropriate and why a 'do not resuscitate' decision is being made
- convey that the resuscitation decision is being made by the appropriate health professionals and not by the daughter, but her cooperation is valued
- describe a clear plan of palliative management
- address all the concerns that the relative has

Ethics and the law and other discussion points

Decisions relating to cardiopulmonary resuscitation (as recommended by the Resuscitation Council (UK) are as follows.
- It is essential to identify those patients for whom cardiopulmonary arrest represents an appropriate terminal event and in whom cardiopulmonary resuscitation (CPR) is inappropriate.
- All hospitals should have an active 'Not for CPR' or 'Do Not Resuscitate' (DNR) policy. A decision about whether to initiate CPR or not involves careful clinical consideration, including the ethical and emotional issues. National guidelines from the British Medical Association, the Resuscitation Council (UK) and the

Royal College of Nursing are available which provide the basic framework on which local policies may be formulated (make sure these are known).

- Where a DNR decision has not been made and the wishes of the patient are unknown, then resuscitation should be initiated if a cardiac or respiratory arrest occurs. However, a 'Not for CPR' decision may be appropriate in the following circumstances:

  (a) where the patient's condition is such that effective CPR is unlikely to be successful

  (b) where CPR is not in accord with the recorded, sustained wishes of the patient who is mentally competent

  (c) where CPR is not in accord with an applicable advance directive ('Living Will'). Such directives are legally binding upon doctors

  (d) where successful CPR is likely to be followed by a length and quality of life which is not in the best interests of the patient to sustain.

- The overall responsibility for a DNR decision rests with the doctor in charge of the patient's care. However, the opinions of other members of the medical and nursing team, the patient and the patient's relatives should be considered when making the decision.

- The most senior available member of the medical team should enter the DNR decision, and the reasons for it, in the medical records. It should also be documented that the relatives have been informed and their comments noted.

- The DNR decision should be communicated effectively to all members of the multidisciplinary team involved in the patient's care. It should be reviewed regularly in the light of changes in the patient's condition. The decision should be documented in the nursing notes and handed on at each change of shift.

- Following the implementation on 2 October 2000 of the Human Rights Act 1998, health professionals must be able to show that their decisions are compatible with the Act as laid out in the Articles of the Convention. Provisions particularly relevant to decisions about attempted CPR include the right to life (Article 2), the right to be free from inhuman or degrading treatment (Article 3), the respect for privacy and family life (Article 8), the freedom of expression which includes the right to hold opinions and to receive information (Article 10), and to be free from discriminatory practices in respect of these rights (Article 14).

Adapted from: *A Joint Statement from the British Medical Association, the Resuscitation Council (UK) and the Royal College of Nursing: Decisions Relating to Cardiopulmonary Resuscitation.* February 2001.

Comments on the case

The candidate should be prepared for the relative to be very emotional. It should become obvious early in the discussion that the daughter has been taken by surprise at the sudden deterioration in her father's condition. It will be important to establish early on what she has previously been told about her father's condition—it may be that the oncologists spoke mainly with the patient and they have not relayed the full picture to his daughter. Active resuscitation would not be indicated on the grounds of futility, but how this issue is explained to the daughter will depend on the views which she herself expresses about his current management plan. Her decision may be related to her concern for his comfort and prevention of any suffering; alternatively her feelings of guilt may translate into a situation where she wants to 'make up for lost time and opportunity', and she may insist that everything possible is done to prolong his life. The guilt issue should be addressed early in the consultation. The emphasis should be on keeping the situation calm while empathizing with the daughter and planning how the events of the next few hours are to be handled.

Case 35 | Screening for prostate cancer

Candidate information

You are the SHO in a general medical clinic

Please read this summary (it should take no more than 2 min) and then continue with the consultation.

> **Re: Mr Eric Spicer, aged 67**
>
> Mr Spicer attends the clinic for hypertension and his blood pressure today is 158/78 mmHg. He tells you that he has read in a newspaper that a blood test now exists that detects prostate cancer (prostatic surface antigen (PSA) test). He asks you if it is worthwhile screening him for prostate cancer using this test.

Your tasks are to: discuss the pros and cons of screening for prostate cancer with Mr Spicer.

You have 14 min until the patient leaves the room, followed by 1 min for reflection, before the discussion with the examiners.

Subject/patient/relative information

Mr Spicer is a 67-year-old retired electrician who comes to clinic for the management of hypertension and he is on amlodipine, ramipril and doxazosin. Recently, his blood pressure has been reasonably well controlled. He has been reading in the paper about a new 'magical' blood test that can decide instantly whether someone has prostate cancer or not. There have been a few scares about prostate cancer in the media, and so he is keen to know if he has prostate cancer. He has read that this is the most common cancer in men and that one may be symptom-free and still have this illness. Admittedly, there has also been some pressure from his wife to have the test. Mr Spicer is relatively well with no prostatic symptoms. After discussion with the SHO (the candidate) he stills decides that he wants to go ahead with the PSA blood test.

Examiner information

1 Communication skills—conduct of interview

- Ask if he has any prostatic symptoms such as poor starting, poor stream, postmicturition dribbling, nocturia, dysuria or haematuria.
- Ask what he knows about prostate cancer.
- Ask why he wants to be screened for prostate cancer. Is

he worried that he may have prostate cancer? Is there a family history? Is he being pressurized by a relative?

- Discover what he has read in the paper with regard to screening for prostate cancer.
- What are his worries? He tells you that prostate cancer is very common in men and that one can be asymptomatic and still have the cancer.
- First, explain briefly what the prostate gland is.
- Reassure him that in the absence of symptoms, it is un-

likely that he will have prostate cancer. Agree with him that prostate cancer is the most common cancer in men *but* it does not cause the largest number of cancer deaths (in contrast to lung cancer in men).

- Describe the ways to investigate the possibility of prostate cancer; digital rectal examination, with a PSA test and, if these are abnormal, a prostatic biopsy.
- Explain that for a screening process to be effective, there are a number of important factors that have to be met. Explain that there are a number of reasons other than prostate cancer for why a PSA test result may be raised, e.g. prostatic infection, recent urinary tract infection and benign prostatic hyperplasia. Say that it is not uncommon to have false positive results. Therefore, there is a chance of having a false positive result and thereby undergoing an unnecessary surgical procedure (prostatic biopsy). Meanwhile, there is a risk of the PSA test being negative when in fact he does have prostate cancer. Reiterate that such screening tests are not 100% guaranteed to detect or dismiss the presence of prostate cancer.
- However, if he did have a prostatic biopsy after finding an abnormal PSA and/or prostate gland (on palpation), and it did turn out to be a prostate cancer, then it could mean that the cancer is detected early and so curative therapy can be undertaken.
- Ask if he wants to have a digital rectal examination and the PSA blood test. He says 'yes'.
- Make sure that there is a follow-up appointment to discuss the results.

2 Communication skills — exploration and problem negotiation

The candidate should be able to:
- decide the reasoning for his request for a PSA screening test
- explain the pros and cons of the screening test
- ensure follow-up plans are arranged

3 Ethics and the law and other discussion points

- For a screening programme to work efficiently, there are a number of criteria which should be met:
(a) importance of the disease (or rarity of the disease)
(b) the natural history of the disease must be known (to allow the identification of potential screening points and to enable the effect of any intervention)
(c) the availability and acceptability of any treatment
(d) the characteristics of the test to be used (false positives or false negatives)

(e) the acceptability and safety of the test
(f) the characteristics of the population to be screened
(g) the resources available to the screening programme.

Ethical considerations which need to be considered when undertaking screening

- Screening (which may involve testing) healthy or asymptomatic people to detect genetic predispositions, or early signs of debilitating or life-threatening conditions can be an important tool in providing effective care. However, the uncertainties involved in screening may be great, e.g. the risk of false positive or false negative results. Some findings may potentially have serious medical, social or financial consequences, not only for the individuals but also for their relatives. In some cases, the fact of having been screened may itself have serious implications.
- You must ensure that anyone considering whether to consent to screening can make a properly informed decision. As far as possible, you should ensure that screening would not be contrary to the individual's best interests. You must pay particular attention to ensure that the information the person wants, or ought to have, is identified and provided. You should be careful to explain clearly:
(a) the purpose of the screening
(b) the likelihood of positive/negative findings and the possibility of false positive or false negative results
(c) the uncertainties and risks attached to the screening process
(d) any significant medical, social or financial implications of screening for the particular condition or predisposition
(e) follow-up plans, including availability of counselling and support services.
- Controversy surrounds the effectiveness of screening for prostate cancer. Although early detection can lead to curative therapy, many individuals with incidental findings will undergo treatment when in fact the tumour would have been so slow-growing that it would not have influenced the length of life for the individual. Prostate cancer therapy has complications including incontinence and impotence.
- It is reasonable to search for prostate cancer in the male patient who is having difficulty voiding (slow stream, urgency) or haematuria, or who has signs and symptoms of metastatic cancer (bone spread resulting in an elevated alkaline phosphatase level and progressive back pain, sciatica or lower extremity neurological im-

pairment). Either curative treatment for cancers confined to the prostate (radical prostatectomy or radiotherapy) or palliative treatments for metastatic disease (orchidectomy to eliminate androgen stimulation of the tumour) are likely to decrease symptoms and improve quality of life.

- The decision to offer prostate cancer screening must be made on an individual basis, depending on the patient's age, health status, family history, risk of prostate cancer and personal beliefs.
- Once a patient undergoes screening and is found not to have prostate cancer, should the patient undergo further annual screening? Guidelines for annual screening do exist but are not necessarily evidence-based.

General Medical Council. *Seeking Patients' Consent: the Ethical Considerations*, Sections 33–34. Consent to screening. November 1998.

Comments on the case

Screening is a topical subject and patients will regularly read in the press of a wonder test to decide whether or not they have disease 'X'. Enabling the patient to make an informed decision, with the consideration that the screening is not contrary to the patient's interests, is paramount.

Case 36 | Self-discharge

Candidate information

You are the medical SHO

Please read this summary (it should take no more than 2 min) and then continue with the consultation.

> ### Re: Miss Stella Newman, aged 19
>
> Miss Newman was admitted 7 days ago with a stiff neck and reduced consciousness. Meningitis was diagnosed and *Listeria monocytogenes* was isolated, although the exact source was unknown. She has been treated with intravenous amoxicillin and the consultant microbiologist has recommended 3 weeks of intravenous therapy. Miss Newman has made an excellent recovery and is now mobilizing off the ward, usually to smoke. Unfortunately, Miss Newman now wants to discharge herself. Her reasons are that she has two young children at home being looked after by her sister, she does not like the attitude of some of the nursing staff towards her—particularly about the smoking issue—and she finds hospital food unpalatable. You have been asked by the ward sister to speak to her to persuade her to stay.

Your tasks are to: ascertain why Miss Newman wants to discharge herself, discuss why it would be best for her to stay and offer alternatives if she refuses.

You have 14 min until the patient leaves the room, followed by 1 min for reflection, before the discussion with the examiners.

Subject/patient/relative information

Miss Stella Newman is a 19-year-old single mother who was admitted 7 days ago with neck stiffness and reduced consciousness. Meningitis was diagnosed and *Listeria monocytogenes* was isolated. She has been treated with intravenous antibiotics. She has made an excellent recovery and is now well enough to go off the ward to smoke. She has never settled on the ward; she has two young children at home being looked after by her sister, she cannot understand why she has to stay when she feels better, she does not like the attitude of the nursing staff towards her—particularly regarding the smoking—and she finds the hospital food totally unacceptable. She is also finding the intravenous cannulae particularly irritating, especially as she has poor venous access and it takes a minimum of three attempts to insert one. She has frankly had enough and now wants to discharge herself. The ward sister has asked her to speak to the medical SHO (the candidate) who is to try and persuade her to stay. Despite the candidate's persuasion to stay and continue intravenous antibiotics, she is still keen to go. She is happy to compromise by continuing oral antibiotics at home but at the same time appreciates that the decision to self-discharge is her own and that she takes responsibility for it.

Examiner information

1 Communication skills — conduct of interview

- Introduce yourself to her and explain why you are here.
- Ask her what her concerns are and show an understanding of the problems.
- Give her the opportunity to tell you if anything else is troubling her and making her keen to leave.
- Explain why it is wise to stay — maybe she is not aware of the importance of continued intravenous antibiotics. Explain all the risks so that she is fully informed about her actions.
- Aim to address her grievances, e.g. ask someone to bring food in for her, suggest that someone more experienced such as yourself will put in any further cannulae and that you will speak to the nursing staff about the situation.
- She may say she is still determined to go.
- Remind her that the hospital would ask her to take responsibility of her own care in this situation and that she will be advised to sign a legal document stating that.
- If she still insists on going you should discuss a compromise. Say you will speak to the consultant microbiologist to discuss the possibility of changing her to oral antibiotics.
- Document everything in the notes.
- Inform your consultant.
- Ensure an early follow-up in the first available clinic.

2 Communication skills — exploration and problem negotiation

The candidate should be able to:

- sit down and discuss the patient's grievances showing understanding and empathy
- aim to persuade the patient to stay
- inform her of the responsibility issue
- provide an alternative antibiotic regimen as a compromise

3 Ethics and the law and other discussion points

- Exploring the reasons for self-discharge is vital in case there is poor understanding of the medical condition.

- Patients cannot be kept against their will, particularly if they do not show signs of psychiatric illness. It is the doctor's responsibility to inform them fully of the importance of staying and that they will be taking full responsibility for the self-discharge against the advice of the medical practitioner. If the patient is still keen to go, it is important at least to make a compromise, e.g. suggesting a course of oral antibiotics. Continued intravenous antibiotics would not be feasible in this case.

> **Comments on the case**
>
> It is possible that the stated reason for wanting to self-discharge is not the main issue. Disrupted sleep, worries about domestic arrangements or fear generated by other patient's behaviour can all contribute toward an overwhelming desire to leave.
>
> It is not uncommon to have patients resenting a no-smoking rule in hospital and likewise some patients are not prepared to compromise with medical staff on any issue. Physicians will find that despite all the considerations provided by them, some patients will not comply with any medical advice and so when it comes to leaving against medical advice, it is not surprising that any persuasive dialogue breaks down. In this type of situation, it is important for the physician to inform the patient fully of the reasons why it is best to stay, that self-discharge is taken against medical advice and that the patient is taking responsibility for their own care. It is advisable to inform a senior colleague and the patient's GP. If the patient falls ill again, at least the GP will be aware of the prior situation.

Case 37 | Smoking cessation advice

Candidate information

You are the medical SHO in a general medical clinic

Please read this summary (it should take no more than 2 min) and then continue with the consultation.

> **Re: Mr Morris Little, aged 58**
>
> Mr Little has come to your clinic for investigation of progressive breathlessness. After full lung function testing a diagnosis of severe emphysema is made. Unfortunately, he smokes 40 cigarettes a day. You feel he would benefit from stopping smoking and you want to try and convince him to do so.

Your tasks are to: explain the hazards of smoking, the beneficial reasons for stopping and make suggestions on how to stop.

You have 14 min until the patient leaves the room, followed by 1 min for reflection, before the discussion with the examiners.

Subject/patient/relative information

Mr Morris Little is a 58-year-old man who has been referred to the clinic because of increasing breathlessness on exertion. He has a chronic cough with sputum. He has found getting out of the house to visit friends more difficult in the last 2 years. He has smoked 40 cigarettes a day since he was 12. His father smoked until his death from an MI at the age of 50. He lives on his own as his wife died 4 years ago and he regards smoking as his only pastime. Every Monday, when he collects his pension, he goes straight to the local tobacconist to buy the week's supply. He has never thought of stopping as he believes his breathing problems are caused by occupational exposure to coal furnaces rather than to his smoking. He always reminds doctors about the 1950s smog which is another reason for his bad health—and not necessarily smoking. He is about to see the SHO (the candidate) who will try and convince him to stop smoking. He appreciates the advice and will think about it before he comes back to clinic next time.

Examiner information

1 Communication skills—conduct of interview

- Explain the diagnosis of emphysema and the implications of this disease with regard to prognosis.
- Explain that smoking has contributed to him developing emphysema and that this will worsen rapidly if he continues to smoke.
- Acknowledge that smoking is habit-forming and difficult to stop.
- Ask him why he smokes and whether he has ever considered stopping.
- Ask him if he has tried to stop before and what happened. If he has a family, explain the effect of smoking on his family.
- Ask about family history. Any smokers in the family and what is their health like?

- Tell him that it is never too late to stop smoking and reiterate that stopping smoking now will help to slow down the rate at which his emphysema will deteriorate.
- Tell him that smoking causes premature death and a number of other cardiovascular and respiratory diseases. If he stops, then his risk of developing lung cancer will also start to fall.
- Tell him he will notice a difference with his breathing soon after stopping and he will also be financially better off.
- Encourage him by saying that many people have successfully stopped smoking.
- Tell him, however, that to have a better chance of succeeding, he must have the will to stop.
- Explore any fears of nicotine withdrawal symptoms.
- Tell him that there are ways to prevent nicotine withdrawal. Describe the types of nicotine replacement therapy (gum vs. patches vs. inhalator).
- Describe other forms of smoking cessation therapy, such as Bupropion (Zyban).
- If he sounds interested in Bupropion, enquire about possible contraindications such as a current seizure disorder, severe hepatic cirrhosis, bipolar disorder, bulimia/anorexia nervosa, known CNS tumour, abrupt withdrawal of alcohol or benzodiazepine withdrawal, concomitant usage of monoamine oxidase inhibitors (MAOIs), antimalarials, tramadol, quinolones, sedating antihistamines.
- Deal with any fears of weight gain.
- Tell him you will provide smoking cessation leaflets and a 'quit-smoking' helpline.
- If he is unsure about quitting, see him in 2 weeks time to reinforce the issues discussed now.
- You may be lucky enough to have a smoking cessation specialist nurse in your trust who you can refer him to.

2 Communication skills—exploration and problem negotiation

The candidate should be able to:
- explain the patient's condition and how it is related to smoking
- explain clearly the benefits of stopping smoking and the health risks of continuing to smoke
- offer suggestions on how to stop
- make sure that follow-up is arranged to reinforce the issue

3 Ethics and the law and other discussion points

About 13 million adults in the UK smoke cigarettes— 28% of men and 26% of women. In 1974, 51% of men and 41% of women smoked cigarettes—nearly half the adult population of the UK. Now just over one-quarter smoke, but the decline in recent years has been heavily concentrated in the older age groups; so almost as many young people are taking up smoking as more established smokers are quitting.

Advice on stopping smoking (adapted from the Action on Smoking and Health [ASH])

- Provide numbers for professional helplines (Freephone 0800 002200 for information and advice is just one example).
- Tell the patient that he or she must prepare mentally to quit smoking.
- Dispel smoking myths.
- Explain about nicotine withdrawal (restlessness, irritability, lack of sleep).
- Make a list of reasons why the individual should want to stop, e.g. health, setting a good example to others (children), financial, social, e.g. smell, managing without a smoke in public places.
- Set a date, which will help mental preparation.
- Involve family or friends—it is easier to quit if the partner wants to quit as well.
- Deal with nicotine withdrawal—nicotine products include Nicorette, NiQuitin CQ and Nicotinell. The strength of gum or patches will depend on how heavily he has smoked.
- Other treatments may help. Hypnosis, acupuncture or other treatments may help some people, but there is little formal evidence supporting their effectiveness. ASH advice is to use them with caution but, even if they help mental preparation, then they will have had some value. Herbal cigarettes are pointless—the individual gets all the tar, but nothing to help deal with the nicotine withdrawal.
- Deal with any weight gain worries.
- Avoid temptation. In the difficult first few days you can change your routine to avoid situations where you would usually smoke.
- Stop completely. Although it might seem like a good idea to cut down and then stop, this is very difficult to do in practice. If the individual cuts down, the likely response is that he or she will smoke each cigarette more intensely. The best approach is to go for a complete break and use nicotine replacement products to help to take the edge off the withdrawal symptoms.
- Watch out for a relapse.

Comments on the case

All medical practitioners should have a sense of duty to offer smoking cessation advice to all patients they see. Unfortunately, the management of smoking cessation can be done badly but the above points should help to provide a basis for advice. Candidates should be able to discuss the types of replacement therapy available as well as the use of Bupropion.

Case 38 | Starting insulin therapy

Candidate information

You are the SHO in a diabetic clinic

Please read this summary (it should take no more than 2 min) and then continue with the consultation.

Re: Mrs Kathleen Hayden, aged 45

Mrs Kathleen Hayden is a lady with poorly controlled diabetes mellitus, despite maximum therapy with oral hypoglycaemic agents and apparent compliance with a diet. Home glucose monitoring has revealed continued levels between 10 and 15 mmol/L. She tried a thiazolidinedione (rosiglitazone) but the glucose levels rose even further when she stopped her glicazide to start this new preparation. The diabetic nurse has informed you that Mrs Hayden has been having more osmotic symptoms during the last 6 months and wonders if it is time to change her to insulin. Her last HbA1c taken 6 weeks ago was 13.4%. Mrs Hayden is not keen on changing to insulin.

Your tasks are to: discuss her present glycaemic control, recommend insulin as the means of improving her diabetic control and ascertain her opinion on this matter.

You have 14 min until the patient leaves the room, followed by 1 min for reflection, before the discussion with the examiners.

Subject/patient/relative information

Mrs Hayden is a 45-year-old lady who has had diabetes for 5 years. She has been on oral hypoglycaemic therapy and, despite adhering to a diabetic diet, her glucose levels remain around 10–15 mmol/L. She has, over the last 6 months, been developing more osmotic symptoms, particularly polydipsia with a feeling of tiredness during the day. She is aware that many diabetics eventually need to be transferred over to insulin but this idea is totally abhorrent to her. She has a needle phobia and she used to witness her mother, who had diabetes, self-inject with subsequent bruising, pain and skin lumps. Her mother used to have hypoglycaemic episodes and she remembers, when young, that her mother had an episode where she could not rouse her from the hypoglycaemia attack and she had to call an ambulance. Her mother later had a CVA and Mrs Hayden had to administer the insulin to her herself. She remembers the needles being long as well as the trouble of storing the needles in disinfectant. She is about to see the medical SHO (the candidate) to discuss the present state of her diabetes and she is aware that the SHO may discuss the possibility of changing over to insulin. Mrs Hayden is determined to defer the change over for as long as she can.

Examiner information

1 Communication skills — conduct of interview

- Introduce yourself to the patient.
- Ask if she knows why she is here.
- Ask how her diabetes is and whether she is having any osmotic symptoms.
- Tell her that the diabetic team is worried that the glycaemic control is not very good and that her HbA1c is very high. Say that it is common for such patients to be changed over to insulin. Ask how she feels about this.
- If she is not keen then explore, with empathy, why this may be so.
- Say how much you appreciate her concerns but that you feel that insulin is in her best interests, particularly with the increased risk of complications. Explain that insulin treatment has improved over the last few years to minimize the difficulties that patients face.
- Try to reassure her that some patients do have a needle phobia and that there are ways to overcome this. Persuade her to come to the diabetic centre to have one of the nursing staff demonstrate the new equipment and techniques available. Also explain that even if she feels totally incapable of self-administering insulin, a district nurse can do that for her or even a relative can be taught to do it.
- Explain that there are a lot more support staff available these days and she can get advice and help whenever she needs it.
- Emphasize with delicacy that changing to insulin is inevitable but she can defer it for a couple of months while she attends the diabetic centre.
- Discuss any other concerns not already addressed.

2 Communication skills — exploration and problem negotiation

The candidate should be able to:

- discuss the importance of converting to insulin
- explore any fears of insulin therapy
- provide suggestions on how to overcome any fears

3 Ethics and the law and other discussion points

- Although this patient cannot be forced to take insulin, it is important that in her best interests she is fully informed of the risks of progressive disease. It is important to explore the real reasons for rejecting therapy and to address these in a positive and sensitive way.
- This lady's view on insulin therapy has been influenced by her previous experiences with her mother and so it is important to educate her about the new therapies available.
- Even when the patient absolutely refuses insulin therapy the first time, it is important to review them regularly in case they decide to change their mind — which they usually do.

Comments on the case

This case is influenced by previous psychological experiences and it is a test for the candidate to address these in order to convince her that the therapy recommended is in her best interest.

Case 39 | Submitting an audit project

Candidate information

You are the medical SHO about to see the audit department manager

Please read this summary (it should take no more than 2 min) and then continue with the consultation.

Re: An audit of the mortality rate for disease 'A'

Disease 'A' is a common acute illness which comprises nearly 5% of all acute medical admissions at your hospital. Your hospital has approximately 40 acute medical admissions a day. The average national inpatient mortality rate is 10%. You would like to know whether patients with disease 'A' at your hospital have a better inpatient mortality rate when they are admitted under the care of the physician with an interest in this disease, compared to other physicians. There is also some suggestion from a recent survey undertaken by the Royal College that the mortality rate is better when the patient is under the care of the physician with an interest in disease 'A'. In order to undertake this project, you decide to embark on a retrospective casenotes survey of all admissions of disease 'A' over a 6-month period. You are about to see the head of the audit department, Mrs Norma Hunter, to discuss this project and to obtain permission to have the notes retrieved. The secretary has agreed to put the notes in one of the offices in the department.

Your tasks are to: discuss the audit project with the audit manager.

You have 14 min until the audit manager leaves the room, followed by 1 min for reflection, before the discussion with the examiners.

Subject/patient/relative information

Mrs Norma Hunter is the audit manager. She is about to see the medical SHO (the candidate) who would like to submit an audit project looking at whether the inpatient mortality rate for disease 'A' is better when such patients are admitted under the care of the physicians with a specific interest in disease 'A' compared to when they are admitted under the care of physicians without a special interest in disease 'A'. Like all other audit submissions, she is keen that the medical SHO has a proper understanding of the principles of audit, with particular reference to:

- setting the standards (e.g. from data elsewhere)
- observing the practice (i.e. the audit)
- comparing the practice with the standards
- implementing change and then reauditing to detect any improvement in the standard of care

Examiner information

1 Communication skills — conduct of interview

- Introduce yourself to Mrs Hunter.
- Tell her you would like to discuss an audit project which you would like to carry out.
- Start off by telling her what the aims of your audit are.
- She asks you how common disease 'A' is in the hospital. Tell her that 5% of acute medical admissions are a result of disease 'A' and therefore over a month the average number of admissions is approximately 60.
- Tell her that the evidence from the Royal College suggests that the mortality rate may depend on who looks after these patients.
- Explain how you would undertake the audit and over how long a period the audit should cover (6 months). Say you would like the coding department to give you a list of the names of patients admitted with disease 'A'. Ask if you can then get the audit department to retrieve the notes. Suggest where the notes should be sent.
- She asks you what you will do with the results. Say you will present them at the local audit meeting.
- She asks you what changes you will implement and when you plan to reaudit.
- Say this depends very much on the findings and that this will be discussed at the medical meeting. If changes are implemented then say that you hope your department would reaudit 1 year after implementation of the changes.
- When finished, thank her and say you will give her regular updates.

2 Communication skills — exploration and problem negotiation

The candidate should be able to:
- understand the basic principles of audit
- understand how to set the standards
- know how to carry out the audit (notes survey)
- appreciate that observed practice should be compared with the standards
- decide how to implement change
- appreciate that an audit is not complete unless the subject is reaudited

3 Ethics and the law and other discussion points

Audit can be regarded as the systematic and critical analysis of the quality of clinical care, including the procedures used for the diagnosis and treatment, the associated use of resources and the resulting outcome and quality of life for the patient.

Audit departments provide general advice and support to professionals on any aspect of clinical audit and help plan and design audit projects. They offer assistance to collect and analyse data and produce reports and presentations. They help to identify ways in which quality improvements can be made and to assist with the implementation of change identified by the audit. The above audit project is a typical project undertaken by a medical SHO.

Key principles

- Maintaining and enhancing continual professional education and development.
- Collaborative audit programmes to enhance integration across professions.
- Incorporating audit into the quality strategy and involving general managers.

Important features of audit

- Success and effectiveness is variable.
- Audit is better established in a well-managed supportive organization with good communication.
- Developing clinical audit is a long-term commitment requiring real support from managers.
- Costs of audit must be measured and justified as a large resource commitment has been made by the Department of Health.
- Audit demands skills in teamwork, process analysis, data collection and problem solving.

Practical problems faced by the SHO

- Coding is never 100% accurate and so some patients will have been wrongly given the diagnosis of disease 'A', or some patients who had disease 'A' will not have had this diagnosis registered by the coding department (coding should be checked by the relevant physician on a weekly basis).
- Notes retrieval is never 100% successful as some notes are always missing. Having a notes retrieval of over 60% is excellent; therefore straight away up to 40% of the data are missing, which may skew the results.
- Data from the notes are often unavailable, poorly documented or inaccurate.
- Patients often change consultants, which may obscure the data collection.
- Collecting and storing notes can be a problem if space is unavailable. Confidentiality must be guaranteed —

are notes going to be kept in the departmental corridor where other patients may come and go?

- Data collection must be robust—using a computer database and not proforma sheets of paper.
- Comparing audit results with results in peer-reviewed journals can sometimes be difficult as study designs differ.
- Implementing change may not be easy—if a difference in mortality rate is found, does the medical director insist that all future admissions with disease 'A' be transferred immediately to the physicians with an interest in disease 'A'? Will these teams be able to accommodate a further 60 admissions a month?

- Completing the return audit loop is not always successful. For example, the junior doctor may move on and sometimes no changes are implemented, so the audit cycle has broken down even before the reauditing stage.

Comments on the case

This case highlights the principles of audit and points out the common problems which affect audit projects undertaken by junior doctors.

Case 40 | The improper doctor

Candidate information

You are the medical SHO and Dr Richard Morgan is your house officer

Please read this summary (it should take no more than 2 min) and then continue with the consultation.

> ### Re: Dr Richard Morgan
>
> Sister on the High Dependency Unit (HDU) has complained to you that your house officer, Dr Richard Morgan, while on call last night, refused to take an urgent U/E sample on an anuric patient. The Sister also tells you that he was rude on the phone and that his excuse was that the phlebotomists would be coming round routinely later that morning anyway. Dr Morgan is a bright young man who has settled reasonably well into his job, but you do appreciate that support for him has been minimal. Your consultant is rarely seen except for one business ward round per week, there is no regular registrar available, and you are rushed off your feet doing clinics (which are on a different site), compiling discharge letters, seeing referrals and, at present, covering for another SHO who has taken indefinite compassionate leave for depression. You and your house officer are never on call together because of the shift rota system that the house officers follow and so it is impossible to have any 'firm' bonding. You approach the house officer to obtain his version of the complaint while appreciating that you ought to do more for him.

Your tasks are to: obtain from your house officer his version of the events, explain that there has been a complaint against him and generally counsel him to avoid any further similar occurrences.

You have 14 min until the house officer leaves the room, followed by 1 min for reflection, before the discussion with the examiners.

Subject/patient/relative information

Dr Richard Morgan is a bright young house officer 4 weeks into his first post. He has settled into this job reasonably well but, unfortunately, support from senior staff is minimal. The consultant is rarely seen except for one business ward round a week, there is no registrar regularly available, and the SHO (the candidate) is too busy doing clinics (which are on a different site), compiling discharge letters, seeing referrals and covering for another SHO who has taken indefinite compassionate leave for depression. There is never any time to ask for advice and quite simply he feels as if he is running the show single-handedly. He is never on call with the SHO because the shift rota system that the house officers follow does not allow this. He has to review sick patients on the HDU for which he feels totally out of his depth, and in the early hours of this morning he had an altercation with one of the night sisters who is notorious for insisting that everything has to be done by the book. The patient concerned was an elderly man with worsening heart failure who had become anuric late in the evening, probably as a result of hypotension and sepsis. The urea and electrolytes were deranged and the on-call registrar (who started the patient on intravenous dobutamine) wanted the tests repeated at 6 a.m. so that the results would be available for the 9.30 a.m. ward round. Dr Morgan was up all night doing ward cover and when he was rung by the Sister at 6 a.m. to take blood samples, he felt quite exasperated because these could be taken by the phlebotomists in 2 h time and still be available for the ward round at 9.30 a.m. He felt that if blood was taken at 6 a.m., the registrar on call was not going to alter his management as he was quite happily asleep in bed. So he felt that doing the blood test was inappropriate at that time, although he admits to losing patience with the Sister for not using her common sense.

Examiner information

1 Communication skills—conduct of interview

- When speaking to the house officer show empathy, understanding and sensitivity, so that he feels you are on his side as a colleague.
- Tell him that you have received a complaint from one of the Sisters on the HDU.
- Tell him what the complaint is about and the Sister's version of the event.
- Ascertain his version of the story, acknowledging his feelings with empathy. Get the facts right.
- Make sure you appear to be listening with an open mind.
- Have there been any other clashes with other members of staff? Does he feel he is being targeted for criticism?
- Is he having difficulty in coping with his duties? Does he feel he needs more support when he is on call? Admit that support has not been adequate and show an appreciation of his hard work.
- Explain the broader picture by explaining that if a specific management plan for that patient has been set, then it is important that it should be followed. There might have been a chance that the phlebotomist would not have arrived and so no blood would have been taken, leading to a delay in management decisions.
- Tell him that in these situations, politeness to other members of staff is very important to allow everyone to work as a team.
- Tell him that you will speak again to the Sister but encourage your house officer to speak to her directly if she is willing and apologize to her for any offence caused.

- Reassure him that if there are any other incidents similar to this or if he ever feels he is under any particular pressure then he should not be afraid to speak to you personally.
- Explain that you will try to be more supportive and you will mention the problem with regard to support to the consultant.

2 Communication skills—exploration and problem negotiation

The candidate should be able to:
- be diplomatic in the consultation without appearing to take sides
- demonstrate objectivity and take on board both sides of the story
- explain that medical practice is team-work and that losing patience with nursing staff can be detrimental to team-building
- be supportive of the house officer, showing appreciation of the difficult job he has to do and say that you will strive to achieve a better supportive role on the wards with improved supervision

3 Ethics and the law and other discussion points

- The improper colleague tends to be clinically competent but rude and offensive to staff, often with poor time-keeping as well. In contrast, the difficult colleague is clinically competent, fine with patients and staff but often uncooperative and obstructive, especially with managers, perhaps with unorthodox ways of practising clinical medicine.

- One must get the facts right, particularly if there is an allegation of rudeness.
- Remain diplomatic without taking sides and always aim for an informal resolution speaking to both parties involved.
- Aim to prevent a recurrence, e.g. by altering practice (in this case ensuring better support and making the house officer feel that you are approachable with any problems).
- Seek advice from senior colleagues.

Comments on the case

The circumstances surrounding this case may sound ill-fated but, unfortunately, are all too common in modern medicine. The candidate will encounter situations like this whatever his or her seniority and the importance of being able to handle them as a diplomatic manager cannot be overstated.

Case 41 | The incompetent doctor

Candidate information

You are the medical SHO and Dr Andrew Stanton is your house officer

Please read this summary (it should take no more than 2 min) and then continue with the consultation.

> ### Re: Dr Andrew Stanton
>
> Dr Stanton has been your house officer for the last 4 weeks. He has had a difficult start to his first job as his mother died 7 weeks ago with breast cancer and he is going through a stormy divorce after only 18 months of marriage. You have got to know him reasonably well and he is generally keen and career-minded. However, Sister Francis from your ward is not happy with his clinical performance. Dr Stanton is making numerous mistakes when writing up dosage of drugs, he is often unable to obtain intravenous access on the first attempt and when taking blood he has left needles on the bedside cabinet. Last week he put the wrong patient label on the biochemistry form. Sister Francis is becoming increasingly concerned about these incidents and wants to speak to you about them.

Your tasks are to: discuss these incidents with Sister Francis and provide suggestions on how the problems can be tackled.

You have 14 min until the house officer leaves the room, followed by 1 min for reflection, before the discussion with the examiners.

Subject/patient/relative information

Sister Francis is a senior nurse on the medical ward. She has seen house officers come and go for over 20 years. She is quite a good judge of clinical competence and she does not think highly of Dr Stanton. He is very nervous with patients, his general medical knowledge is low and he is constantly making silly errors with drug dosage on the drug charts. The house officer on call ends up rewriting the drug chart on most evenings. Changing venflons is an agonizing event; repeated attempts are the rule, leading to patients becoming quite distressed. When taking blood, he has left needles on the bedside cabinet and last week he wrongly labelled a biochemistry form (using a different patient's identification sticker) but thankfully one of the nurses spotted this mistake. Sister feels that his performance must improve and she wants to speak to the SHO (the candidate) to discuss a clear plan of action. She also wants the SHO to speak to the consultant.

Examiner information

1 Communication skills — conduct of interview

- Discuss with Sister what her main concerns are, with examples. Listen intently and with interest. She must have confidence in you otherwise she would not have asked for your advice.
- Be diplomatic and say that you are saddened to hear about these incidents and that you will speak to Dr Stanton about them to try and establish what has been happening and what can be done to help him improve his practice.
- Thank Sister Francis for bringing the matter to your attention.
- Be supportive of Dr Stanton (the last thing Dr Stanton wants is for everybody to take sides against him). Explain that the last few months have been unsettling for him but you agree that good standards of clinical competence have to be maintained whatever his background plights (you are not allowed to reveal the problems with regard to his mother or the divorce as this may be strictly confidential).
- Explain to Sister Francis that you will speak to the consultant as he or she ought to know.
- Offer a constructive plan for future training and say that you will try to improve matters by supervising his ward work more closely, constructively correcting any mistakes, improving his general medical education with regular one-to-one hourly teachings and guarantee regular appraisals of his work with the consultant.
- Reassure the Sister that you will explore other alternatives after discussion with Dr Stanton and the consultant, such as leave of absence for a brief period for personal circumstances.

2 Communication skills — exploration and problem negotiation

The candidate should be able to:
- listen to what the Sister has to say, respecting her concerns
- maintain objectivity, and agree to speak to the house officer personally to get his side of the story
- have a plan of management to improve the house officer's clinical performance

- reassure the Sister that the consultant will be informed and all alternatives will be considered

3 Ethics and the law and other discussion points

- Doctors are not perfect and their clinical skills and human relations may be suboptimal. However, some are so bad as to be dangerous and if the quality of medical care is to improve, these doctors need to be identified and given further training and re-education.
- To improve such doctors, it is important that they have insight to understand that they need further retraining and re-education.
- Those aspects of clinical ability that need improving have to be identified.
- A plan of further retraining and re-education has to be contrived in a structured and systematic way after consultation with the consultant and the postgraduate dean — it is no good sending such individuals to more lunchtime grand rounds or audit meetings and in the end achieve nothing. A training programme has to be tailored to the individual's needs.
- The individual will need to be reappraised and reassessed regularly to see if clinical performance has improved.
- Seek advice from senior colleagues.

Comments on the case

Underperforming doctors must be identified and any changes or support negotiated in the proper manner. There must be a sense of responsibility for these individuals and they should not be left to languish in this and subsequent jobs. Doctors are not immune from bereavement and personal distress and there is no reason to think that they are any less likely to be affected by it. Candidates must be able to recognize such individuals and have a plan of action that will support such colleagues practically and compassionately.

Case 42 | The sick doctor

Candidate information

You are the medical SHO and Dr Stuart Pemberton is your house officer

Please read this summary (it should take no more than 2 min) and then continue with the consultation.

Re: Dr Stuart Pemberton

You suspect that your house officer has an alcohol problem. Rumours are rife that, when on call, he disappears to have a drink in the on-call room. Recently, he had a car accident in which he drove his car onto a motorway embankment without any other cars involved. You have noticed the smell of alcohol on his breath on a number of occasions. You are worried that his decision making may be sub-standard and that he has been forgetting to carry out certain jobs he has promised to do. You feel he may pose a risk to patients so you decide to speak to him privately about the matter.

Your tasks are to: determine if Dr Pemberton has a drink problem and suggest ways of providing help.

You have 14 min until the house officer leaves the room, followed by 1 min for reflection, before the discussion with the examiners.

Subject/patient/relative information

Dr Stuart Pemberton has been a house officer for 8 weeks. He has always had a reputation of being a 'lad who can take his ale' but, behind this exterior, he is quite an insecure young man who lacks confidence and finds being a doctor extremely stressful. He is finding the hours particularly punishing and the on-calls very demanding. He was criticized by his consultant as being the laziest house officer ever — this was particularly hurtful especially as he works as hard as anybody else. Often on ward rounds the consultant has ridiculed him in front of students with unprofessional foul-mouthed ripostes to sensible suggestions. He has not found anyone to confide in and as a result has turned to drink. On-calls are especially hard because of the fear of failure and escaping to 'the bottle' in the on-call room is the only way to achieve some form of relief. He has been drinking quite heavily over the last few weeks and recently was involved in a car crash when he drove off a motorway onto the embankment. The police breathalysed him and he was found to be positive, so he is expecting a court summons. He does not believe he has a problem and probably lacks insight. He is not in a relationship at the moment and has not previously suffered from depression, although current events are resulting in a low mood and poor self-esteem. He does not take any other illicit drugs.

Examiner information

1 Communication skills — conduct of interview

- When speaking to him be open without being threatening. Develop a good rapport.
- Explain that you are concerned that he may be drinking heavily.
- Explore if there is a reason behind the alcohol intake, e.g. break up of a relationship, stress at work.
- Has he ever been off sick as a result of alcohol, e.g. because of a hangover?
- Ask if he feels he has a problem.
- If he denies there is a problem, give him the evidence why you and others may suspect that there is a problem.
- Say you have heard that he was in a car crash. Ask if he had any injuries and if the crash was alcohol related. Were the police involved?
- Ask about the alcohol drinking, including the CAGE questionnaire (see p. 67).
- Ask if anyone else has hinted that there may be a problem or if he thinks he should reduce his drinking.
- Ask if there is a drug problem.
- Explore any evidence of depression.
- Explain that you are concerned as continuing in this way may be putting patients at risk and you feel that he should seek help.
- Explain that you are obliged to speak to the consultant. If he objects, he may agree to you speaking to someone else with authority, e.g. the medical director, but ensuring that confidentiality will be maintained throughout.
- Ask if he is registered with a local GP. The GP should also be involved.
- You can also suggest the BMA helpline for sick doctors (telephone number 08459 200169). The Sick Doctors Trust (0870 4445163) is a confidential service for doctors which provides early intervention in chemical dependency and the Doctors Support Network (07071 223372) is a self-help group for doctors with mental health problems.

2 Communication skills — exploration and problem negotiation

The candidate should be able to:

- recognize and assess the problem
- determine if the individual has insight into the problem
- offer help
- explain the importance of the situation (the risk to him and to patients)
- seek advice from senior colleagues

3 Ethics and the law and other discussion points

- You must protect patients from any risk of harm posed by another doctor's, or other healthcare professional's conduct, performance or health, including problems arising from alcohol or other substance abuse. The safety of patients must come first at all times. Where there are serious concerns about a colleague's performance, health or conduct, it is essential that steps are taken *without delay* to investigate the concerns to establish whether they are well-founded and to protect patients.
- If you have grounds to believe that a doctor, or other healthcare professional, may be putting patients at risk, you must give an honest explanation of your concerns to an appropriate person from the employing authority, such as the medical director, nursing director, chief executive, director of public health or an officer of your local medical committee, following any procedures set by the employer. If there are no appropriate local systems, or local systems cannot resolve the problem, and you remain concerned about the safety of patients, you should then discuss your concerns with an impartial colleague or contact your defence body, a professional organization or the GMC for advice.

General Medical Council. *Good Medical Practice*, Sections 26–28. Conduct or performance of colleagues. May 2001.

Comments on the case

Contrary to popular beliefs, doctors do become sick and these individuals must be attended to. Dr Pemberton's case can, unfortunately, be a real one in your own hospital and so the capability for recognizing a sick doctor and instigating appropriate management must be acquired by all doctors in training. Doctors who are sick tend to deny their illness, fail to seek advice early, self-diagnose, self-medicate and obtain informal and non-specific advice from colleagues who most likely possess no insight into the real problem. They resist the slightest contemplation of taking time off work.

Sick doctors may be driven to continue working and fail to seek help because of the culture of doctors being superhuman. Encouraging and promoting a culture where seeking help and support to survive in an environment fraught with emotional trauma that impacts on doctors who, after all, are human beings too, may go some way to lessen the reduction in confidence and self-esteem that may lead to alcohol and drug misuse.

Case 43 | Third party confidentiality

Candidate information
You are the SHO in the HIV clinic

Please read this summary (it should take no more than 2 min) and then continue with the consultation.

> ### Re: Mr Andrew McDonald, aged 24
>
> You are about to see Mr McDonald who is known to be HIV positive. He is reasonably well on his antiretroviral therapy. However, the HIV nurse specialist has told you that she suspects he is not practising safe sex with his new partner. She believes the partner is unaware of Mr McDonald's HIV status and is worried that the partner may be put at risk. Mr McDonald, however, believes he has the right of confidentiality.

Your tasks are to: establish a rapport which will enable you to discuss with Mr McDonald whether his partner is aware of his HIV status, determine if they are practising safe sex and discuss the issue of confidentiality.

You have 14 min until the patient leaves the room, followed by 1 min for reflection, before the discussion with the examiners.

Subject/patient/relative information
Mr McDonald is a 24-year-old bisexual man who has been under the care of the HIV clinic for 2 years. He is reasonably well on combination antiretroviral therapy which was started after a low CD4 count. He is working as a journalist and has recently met a new lady who he is now dating. He is having sex with her without using condoms and is worried that if he reveals his HIV status she will leave him. For this reason he is not keen to tell her. He believes that his HIV status should remain confidential and expects the doctor to respect his views. He has mentioned his new partner to the nurse specialist and she has told the SHO (the candidate) he is about to see. The SHO is going to try to persuade Mr McDonald to inform his partner but he remains adamant that confidentiality should be preserved. At the end of the consultation he agrees to think about telling his partner.

Examiner information

1 Communication skills — conduct of interview
- Introduce yourself to Mr McDonald followed up by a general 'What's happening in your life at the moment?'
- He may volunteer that he has a new partner. Express an interest in her.
- Ask if he is practising safe sex with her (using condoms); the patient says he is not. Ask why.
- Ask if he has had an opportunity to tell her about his HIV status, if he says 'No, not yet', tell him that you appreciate it must be difficult and ask whether he has thought about how he might do this.
- If he does not want to pass on this information tell him,

without sounding patronizing, that he is putting his partner at risk of HIV infection.
- Mr McDonald may give an excuse such as the partner may not want to date him if she knew that he is HIV positive.
- Reaffirm that she needs to know as she is being put at risk.
- Discuss whether Mr McDonald would consider using a condom.
- Explain that you are faced with a decision about breaking confidentiality in order to safeguard the partner from acquiring this infection.
- He informs you that he has the right to preserve confidentiality. You reply by saying that you appreciate the confidentiality issue but, because of the risk of infection, a medical practitioner is allowed to inform the sexual partner.
- Ask him if he wants time to think about telling his partner himself and, if so, tell him to come back to clinic in 2 days for an update, not forgetting to refrain from sexual intercourse without protection. (It is to be hoped that Mr McDonald agrees.)
- Inform Mr McDonald that you will be letting the nurse specialist know if she was not already present at the consultation.

2 Communication skills — exploration and problem negotiation

The candidate should be able to:
- establish a rapport with the patient
- discuss, in a non-confrontational manner, the sexual practices of the patient with the new partner
- ascertain whether the patient has told the partner about his HIV status and, if not, why not
- explain the importance of informing the sexual partner and particularly the importance of safe sex
- discuss the confidentiality issues with the patient
- allow the patient to have a short time to think about the issue

3 Ethics and the law and other discussion points

- Where HIV infection or AIDS has been diagnosed, any difficulties concerning confidentiality will usually be overcome if doctors are prepared to discuss this openly and honestly with patients. Such issues include the implications of their condition, the need to secure the safety of others, and the importance for continuing medical care by ensuring that those who will be involved in their care know the nature of their condition and the particular needs which they will have.

- With regard to informing other healthcare professionals (e.g. the GP), the specialist diagnosing the HIV, or continuing the HIV care, should explain to the patient that the GP cannot be expected to provide adequate clinical management and care without full knowledge of the patient's condition.
- If the patient refuses consent for the GP to be told, the specialist should counsel the patient about the difficulties which his condition may pose for the team responsible for providing continuing healthcare. For example, if a practice nurse wishes to take a routine non-HIV related blood test (e.g. cholesterol) then she may be put at risk if she gets a needlestick injury. If the patient continues to refuse to allow the GP to know, then the specialist should respect this decision but he or she is allowed to disclose such information if the need for information arises in order to protect this person from the risk of serious harm. In such a circumstance the doctor should tell the patient before the disclosure with the preparation of justifying this decision.
- With regard to informing a third party other than another healthcare professional (e.g. the patient's spouse or sexual partner), there are grounds for disclosure only when there is a serious and identifiable risk to a specific individual who, if not informed, would be exposed to infection. Most patients agree to disclose the information themselves, but in circumstances where this is not the case, the doctor should consider it a legal duty to ensure that any sexual partner is informed, in order to safeguard that individual from infection.

General Medical Council. *HIV and AIDS: the ethical considerations.* October 1995.

Comments on the case

It is vitally important for the candidate to be honest and open about the possible risks which may then persuade the patient to do the honourable thing and inform the partner. Taking care at this stage to be non-confrontational, and to avoid appearing intrusive or dictatorial, is more likely to gain the patient's trust and respect. Being judgemental will dash any hopes of them informing their partner and will make the situation worse. As a golden rule, avoid being judgemental whenever you are counselling or taking a history.

Case 44 | To ventilate or not to ventilate?

Candidate information

You are the medical SHO on-call

Please read this summary (it should take no more than 2 min) and then continue with the consultation.

Re: Mr Roger Barnes, aged 74

Mr Barnes has just been admitted to casualty complaining of breathlessness and confusion. He has a long history of COPD although his past notes are not available for any further information (including any previous arterial blood gases). The GP's letter states that Mr Barnes is on nebulizer treatment and smokes 30 cigarettes a day. He has been treated by the GP for a 'chest infection' using oral erythromycin over the last 6 days. However, his condition has progressively worsened and now he is drowsy and pyrexial. The chest X-ray reveals a left lower lobe pneumonia. Arterial gases are pH7.0, Po_2 7.7 kPa and Pco_2 12.5 kPa. He is clearly in need of urgent intervention. You call the intensivist who, on reading the GP's letter, feels that assisted ventilation is inappropriate because of his established COPD. You tell the senior nurse looking after him that you are going to obtain more information from the eldest son (Mr Geoff Barnes) who is waiting to see you in the visitors' room.

Your tasks are to: tell the son how ill his father is, get an idea of the father's general pre-morbid condition and discuss whether ventilation should be offered.

You have 14 min until the son leaves the room, followed by 1 min for reflection, before the discussion with the examiners.

Subject/patient/relative information

Mr Roger Barnes is a 74-year-old retired welder who has a long history of COPD. Nowadays, he rarely gets out of the house but does manage to get to the bottom of his garden most days. He has to stop twice when going up stairs. He has a chronic cough with sputum and still smokes over 30 cigarettes a day. He has a nebulizer which he uses in the morning only. He also has an oxygen cylinder which he uses on a *pro renata* basis. He is aware that he must not smoke at the same time as having the oxygen. Otherwise, he takes ipratropium and salbutamol inhalers. Apart from regular visits to the chest clinic in the centre of town, he has never been in hospital for an exacerbation of his COPD. He has no other comorbidities such as ischaemic heart disease. Over the last 2 weeks his symptoms have worsened; his sputum is purulent with some haemoptysis. He was given a course of erythromycin but this caused a gastrointestinal upset so he did not finish the course. He has deteriorated and now is breathless at rest, drowsy and pyrexial. A chest X-ray reveals a pneumonia but his condition is now so critical that a decision about whether to support him with a ventilator must be taken as soon as possible. The anaesthetist has reviewed him and feels that Mr Barnes would not be an appropriate candidate for ventilation because of the high morbidity and mortality risk, plus a high chance of difficulty in coming off a ventilator. The son, Mr Geoff Barnes, is the next of kin. He is waiting see the medical SHO (the candidate) with regard to the issue of ventilation. The medical SHO is keen to obtain an idea of the previous quality of life and whether Mr Barnes has ever wished not to be considered for ventilation. As far as the son knows, his father seems to enjoy life very much despite his limitations and is sure he would not object to trying ventilation. This is a view echoed by the rest of the family.

Examiner information

1 Communication skills — conduct of interview

- Introduce yourself to the patient's son, Mr Geoff Barnes.
- Explain how poorly his father is from the pneumonia and that his previous history of COPD is contributing to his present ill-health.
- Explain that his father is in a casualty bay being looked after by a senior nurse but that a decision will have to made very quickly with regard to his management.
- Tell him that in his present state he may not live and the only other option is artificially ventilating his lungs to give them a rest and that would mean being looked after in the ITU.
- Get an idea of his father's normal state: exercise ability, social life, general quality of life, treatment regimens, e.g. nebulizers, home oxygen (cylinder or long-term oxygen therapy machine), previous illnesses, previous response to treatment, previous admissions to ITU and, if so, length of ventilation, difficulty in weaning off and the need for a tracheostomy.
- Explain what ventilation in the ITU involves: a tube passed into the windpipe connected to a machine which will help to rest his lungs while treatment is given for his pneumonia; tubes in the arm and neck to give antibiotics and fluids and other treatment; sedation to overcome the discomfort of the tube.
- Tell him the risks of ventilation and ITU admission: further infection and sepsis, difficulty in weaning off the ventilator, psychosis and sometimes death.
- Ask if his father has shown any previous objections to ITU admission and ventilation.
- How does the rest of the family feel?
- Ask if there are any queries.

2 Communication skills — exploration and problem negotiation

The candidate should be able to:
- obtain an idea of the everyday activities of the patient
- decide on the severity of the COPD
- decide whether the patient would be a candidate for ventilation
- discuss with the son if there are any advanced views on ventilation by the patient and family

3 Ethics and the law and other discussion points

- If you feel that ventilation should be offered you should speak to your next senior colleague and then the consultant. If the intensivist disagrees with the decision, get your consultant to speak to the intensivists to come to an agreed plan of action. Conflicting opinions should not be expressed in front of relatives.
- If *you* feel that ventilation should not be offered then think to yourself 'Have I made the right decision or not?' Never make such a life or death decision on your own — always speak to your seniors.
- There are guidelines that may help to decide if ventilation is appropriate; however, these are only guidelines. For example, the British Thoracic Society 1997 guidelines on the decision to ventilate states:
  (a) factors encouraging the use of invasive positive pressure ventilation (IPPV) include: a demonstrable remedial reason for current decline, e.g. pneumonia, first episode of failure, acceptable quality of life or habitual level of activity
  (b) factors likely to discourage use of IPPV include: previously documented severe COPD that has been fully assessed and found to be unresponsive to relevant therapy, a poor quality of life, e.g. housebound despite maximal appropriate therapy, severe comorbidities, e.g. cor pulmonale, neoplasia.

The COPD Guidelines Group of the Standards of Care Committee of the British Thoracic Society. BTS guidelines for the management of chronic obstructive pulmonary disease. 1997. *Thorax* 52, Supplement 5, S19.

- Each case must be assessed carefully. Do not be put off by the patient using home oxygen and home nebulizers. Get an idea of exactly what this means, e.g. long-term oxygen therapy vs. *pro renata* cylinder or *pro renata* nebulizer vs. 6 times/day nebulizer.
- Obtain an idea of what 'housebound' means exactly. The patient and/or the candidate may consider that the inability to get to the local shops equates to being housebound, when in fact the patient may manage to get to the bottom of the garden. If he does go to the shops, how he get there — by car or on foot.
- Consider a patient with COPD for invasive ventilation if there is an obvious reversible illness (e.g. bronchoconstriction, pulmonary oedema, pneumonia) if the patient has no other organ failure, if this presentation of respiratory failure is the first ever, or if the patient has made an informed wish for ventilation.
- Do not let misconceptions about the difficulty in weaning off a ventilator or poor outcome deny a patient ventilation unless that patient is in end-stage failure with a high premorbid arterial $P\text{CO}_2$.

Comments on the case

Not an easy case but very common in everyday medical practice. Most candidates have probably never appreciated the immense complexities that come with deciding on whether to ventilate or not. Never allow a single person to make a 'not for ventilation' decision. There will always be a case for 'yes' and for 'no'.

The issue of quality of life should always be explored from the patient's values and perspectives which will not necessarily reflect those of the clinicians. These may vary even from one clinician to another.

Case 45 | Treating a prisoner

Candidate information

You are the medical SHO in a chest clinic

Please read this summary (it should take no more than 2 min) and then continue with the consultation.

> ### Re: Mr Tony Garrett, aged 27
>
> Mr Garrett is a prisoner at the local high security HM prison. He has been attending the chest clinic for the last 3 months for multidrug-resistant pulmonary tuberculosis. He is always accompanied by two prison officers and handcuffed to one of them. You are aware that the clinic staff are alarmed by this, believing that if this is necessary he may be dangerous. His treatment is progressing reasonably well and he is due to come back in 6 weeks. The clinic sister, Sister Rollinson, wants to speak to you concerning this patient. She feels it is inappropriate to have him treated in the chest clinic and wants him to be discharged back to the care of the prison doctor.

Your tasks are to: talk to Sister Rollinson to ascertain her worries and to remind her of the importance of continued care at the chest clinic.

You have 14 min until the Sister leaves the room, followed by 1 min for reflection, before the discussion with the examiners.

Subject/patient/relative information

Mr Tony Garrett is a prisoner at the local high security prison. He was diagnosed as having multidrug-resistant pulmonary tuberculosis and he visits the clinic every 4–6 weeks. When he comes he is handcuffed to one prison officer and closely watched by another. His presence makes all the staff very uncomfortable and none of them wants to undertake the routine clinic measurements such as his weight. Sister Rollinson is the senior nurse at the clinic and feels that the patient should have his tuberculosis managed by the prison doctor. She is keen to speak to the medical SHO (the candidate) to discuss the possibility of discharge for security and safety reasons.

Examiner information

1 Communication skills — conduct of interview

- Ask Sister Rollinson what her concerns are.
- Tell her that you understand how she and the other staff feel but remind her that as professionals you all share a duty of care which means that he is entitled to the same treatment as any other patient.
- She asks why he cannot be managed at the prison by the prison doctor.
- Explain that as he has complicated multidrug-resistant tuberculosis, he has to be followed-up closely by a physician with expertise in tuberculosis.
- Reassure and explain that the risk of escape or threat to others has been assessed and that is the reason for the presence of two prison officers.
- Say that next time you will discuss with her and the

prison officers the current risk of escape or violence and decide how best to conduct the consultation.
- Reassure her that her concerns will be relayed to the consultant.

2 Communication skills—exploration and problem negotiation

The candidate should be able to:
- ascertain why Sister Rollinson is not happy
- explain why the patient should continue to be managed at the clinic
- reassure that security and safety for all staff and patients are of paramount importance, hence the presence of the prison officers

3 Ethics and the law and other discussion points (guidelines by the BMA)

- Doctors have a duty to provide the best possible care for each of their patients. This includes respect for the patient's dignity and privacy. These issues are equally as important when treating those detained in prison, whether convicted or on remand, as when treating any other patient. Prisoners must have access to the same standards of healthcare as are available to the rest of the society.
- When prisoners are taken outside the prison grounds for medical care, the duty of the healthcare team to provide optimal care can often conflict with the prison authorities' duty to ensure that appropriate levels of security are maintained. Any measures which sought to remove all possibility of escape or violence would be so draconian as to lead to an unacceptable loss of the patient's dignity and basic human rights. It is therefore necessary to reach a balance between the dignity of the patient and the security needs. Where there is a serious risk of escape or the prisoner represents a threat to themselves, the health team or others then safeguards are required. However, these safeguards should be commensurate with the actual or perceived risk and should respect the patient's right to privacy to the maximum extent possible.
- There should be a presumption that prisoners will be examined and treated without restraints and without prison officers present, unless there is a high risk of escape or it is considered that the prisoner represents a threat to himself, the health professionals or others. It is important to assess the level of risk in each individual case and to tailor the safeguards to suit the circumstances. Where the level of risk is considered to be low then the prisoner should be treated accordingly.

- In cases where there is a high risk of escape or where there is a threat of violence, the safeguards should nevertheless respect the prisoner's right to privacy to the maximum extent possible. For example, where there is a risk of escape, but no likelihood of violence, it should be possible for a prison officer to be stationed outside the consulting or treatment room with another in the grounds immediately outside. These precautions will allow the patient some degree of privacy, dignity and confidentiality while also ensuring that security is maintained. Occasionally, where there is a serious threat of violence or where the prisoner is considered to be dangerous, it will be necessary to use restraints and it may also be necessary to have a prison officer inside the consulting room.

> **Comments on the case**
>
> It is not uncommon to have prisoners as patients and, despite any prejudice the physician may harbour, these patients still have the right to confidentiality, privacy and dignity as does any other patient. Delivering these rights is influenced by the potential risk of escape, self-harm and threat to staff and so an assessment of these risks must be made between the doctor and prison officer before the consultation.
>
> It is important to ensure that you are up to date with any Home Office and professional guidance regarding the treatment and care of prisoners in a public hospital setting. Following the death of a cancer patient at a Welsh Hospice, who had remained handcuffed to the bed, comprehensive guidelines have been developed. Be mindful that prisoners who are receiving inpatient care should have a regular risk assessment carried out by a senior member of the prison service. Special contingencies should be discussed and agreed verbally and in writing in advance. For example, if a patient is physically too ill to get off a bed then what justification is there for keeping him handcuffed? If a patient is at risk of a cardiac arrest, how quickly can the handcuffs be removed to enable safe defibrillation?

Case 46 | Unrelated live organ donation

Candidate information

You are the SHO in a diabetes clinic

Please read this summary (it should take no more than 2 min) and then continue with the consultation.

> **Re: Mr and Mrs Bowman**
>
> Mr Bowman is a 42-year-old man who has diabetic nephropathy and is now on the renal transplant list. His wife, who is genetically unrelated, has been wondering whether or not to donate one of her kidneys. She has come to see you for more advice.

Your tasks are to: discuss the pros and cons of live organ donation.

You have 14 min until the patient's wife leaves the room, followed by 1 min for reflection, before the discussion with the examiners.

Subject/patient/relative information

Mr Bowman is a 42-year-old man with a long history of insulin-dependent diabetes mellitus. He has diabetic nephropathy and has been on the waiting list for a renal transplant for 4 years. He has not had any calls for a kidney and, despite being fairly stable on dialysis, his concerns are increasing that he may never find a donor. Mrs Bowman, for the sake of her husband, has been considering whether or not she should donate one of her kidneys as she has read that unrelated donations are often successful nowadays. Her concerns are about the risks to her and her husband and so she has come to see one of the specialists (the candidate) for further information.

Examiner information

1 Communication skills—conduct of interview

- Ideally, the husband and wife should both be present at the consultation.
- Ask what the husband and wife know about organ donation so that you have some idea as to what level of knowledge the counselling should be directed at.
- Explain that live organ donation has a better outcome than donation from a deceased person and that matching will be assessed. Matching may not need to be perfect and it is not vital that the donor should be a close relative of the receiver.

- Explain that while on the organ waiting list, it is difficult to know when a suitable organ will be available. A non-related organ donation will take him off the list and will remove the need for continuing dialysis and will minimize his deteriorating health.
- Kidneys from living donors do not need to be transported from one site to another so the kidney is in a better condition when it is transplanted.
- Mrs Bowman will gain psychological satisfaction from helping her husband in this way.
- Although small, there are peri- and postoperative risks to organ donation and the long-term risks of living with only one kidney. There is also a small risk of developing hypertension.

- Kidney donation is a major surgical operation and requires about a week in hospital to recover and a few weeks postoperatively to recover fully.
- The psychological impact of donating a kidney, and having only one kidney left, must be highlighted, although one can live perfectly normally with one kidney.
- Explain to Mrs Bowman that she will have to undertake several preoperative assessments including compatibility tests which may reveal an illness that may have psychological and medical implications (such as hepatitis B).
- Explain that recuperation will mean time off work and possibly lost earnings.
- Mrs Bowman should check the implications of a donation with her insurance agency.
- Make sure there are no third party interests involved.
- Relay the possible risk of the transplantation not being successful as a result of rejection.
- The recipient will have to be on life-long medication to prevent rejection which may increase the risk of further infections.
- Tell her that if they decide to go ahead, both of them will be assessed formally by a transplant team.

2 Communication skills — exploration and problem negotiation

The candidate should be able to:
- ascertain what the couple know already about live organ transplantation
- discuss the pros and cons of live organ transplantation
- fully inform the couple of the risks involved

3 Ethics and the law and other discussion points

- A donation may be obtained from a non-genetically related person provided no payment has been made or is to be made. Historically, live non-related donors of kidneys were rarely considered because of the medical difficulties involved: that the kidney obtained has no better chance of survival as a graft than an equally tissue-matched cadaveric organ. Advances in immunosuppression now mean that grafts which are less well tissue-matched may survive. Thus, non-genetically related individuals are now increasingly acceptable as donors.
- The Human Organ Transplants Act 1989 restricts transplants between persons who are not genetically related. A person is guilty of an offence if he removes from a living person an organ intended to be trans-

planted into another person or transplants an organ removed from a living person into another person to whom they are not genetically related *unless* the approval of the Unrelated Live Transplant Regulatory Authority (ULTRA) has been obtained. The extent of genetic relationships for the purposes of the Act is specified in Section 2(2) and the regulations specify the tests which must be carried out to establish the fact of a genetic relationship. In every case where the transplant of an organ is proposed between a living donor and a recipient who is not genetically related, the proposal must be referred to ULTRA. As an independent authority, its function is to consider cases where no genetic relationship exists or where such a claimed relationship cannot be established. When an organ becomes available the Authority will have to be satisfied that no payments have been made or are proposed.
- ULTRA was set up under the Human Organ Transplants Act 1989 to approve all transplant operations involving a living donor who is not a close blood relative of the recipient. However, the Act does not apply to transplants of regenerative tissues such as bone marrow, so these do not need ULTRA approval. The chairman and members of ULTRA are appointed by the Secretary of State for Health. The chairman is a doctor not involved in transplantation and the members include doctors, nurses, scientists and others with knowledge about transplant ethics.
- Living donor kidney transplantation should only be undertaken once the following criteria have been met:
  (a) the risk to the donor must be low
  (b) the donor must be fully informed
  (c) the consent must be fully and freely given
  (d) the donor must understand that he or she is entitled to withdraw his or her consent at any time before the operation
  (e) the offer of the organ must be totally voluntary and not made through inducements
  (f) the transplant procedure must have a good chance of a successful outcome for the recipient.

Department of Health. *Unrelated Live Transplant Regulatory Authority.* 2001.

> **Comments on the case**
>
> The candidate must understand the basic concepts of organ transplantation, particularly the advantages of live over cadaveric donation.

Case 47 | Unwanted drug reactions

Candidate information

You are the medical SHO in a cardiology clinic

Please read this summary (it should take no more than 2 min) and then continue with the consultation.

Re: Mr Bill Teale, aged 77

Mr Teale has been attending the clinic for 4 years after having had a myocardial infarction complicated by left ventricular failure and ventricular tachycardia (VT). He is on treatment with amiodarone 200 mg o.d. which resulted in thyrotoxicosis and for which he is now on carbimazole 5 mg o.d. He also takes aspirin 75 mg o.d., lisinopril 10 mg o.d., Imdur 60 mg o.d. and frusemide (furosemide) 80 mg o.d. He is reasonably well with some breathlessness on walking and minimal ankle oedema. The amiodarone has been particularly effective in preventing any more episodes of ventricular tachycardia. He has mild chronic renal impairment and has had two strokes 17 and 19 years ago which have left him with a residual left-sided weakness. He is able to walk with a stick and, apart from a carer who does the shopping and housework, he is fiercely independent. However, Mr Teale is fed up with having to take so many tablets and he finds the amiodarone particularly irksome because of its photosensitivity. He loves his cricket, and sitting in the sun watching his local side is his main pastime. He wants to speak to you about whether he can stop some of his tablets.

Your tasks are to: ascertain the patient's concerns and explain the relative merits of each medication.

You have 14 min until the patient leaves the room, followed by 1 min for reflection, before the discussion with the examiners.

Subject/patient/relative information

Mr Teale is a 77-year-old former army man who had a large myocardial infarction 4 years ago followed by numerous bouts of ventricular tachycardia and resulting left ventricular failure. He was started on amiodarone for the ventricular tachycardia and this has been particularly effective in suppressing any further episodes. At present, he is reasonably well with dyspnoea after about 300 m on the flat but no orthopnoea and only mild ankle swelling. A few months after starting the amiodarone he began to notice that he was feeling hot, agitated and shaky and a thyroid function test showed him to be hyperthyroid. He was started on carbimazole which returned him to a euthyroid state. He also takes aspirin 75 mg o.d., lisinopril 10 mg o.d., Imdur 60 mg o.d. and frusemide 80 mg o.d. He has noticed that when he sits in the sun, particularly while watching his local cricket team, he develops a sore rash on his arms and face (the exposed areas). His past medical history includes two strokes 17 and 19 years ago and mild renal impairment. He walks with a stick and is independent although he has a private carer to do the cleaning and shopping. His main source of discontent is that he is fed up with so many tablets which cause unwanted reactions. He argues that he has been really well and so cannot see the need for taking them any longer. The frusemide stops him from going out anywhere first thing in the morning, the photosensitivity is particularly unpleasant and to stop his cricketing pastime would be unwelcome as he has just been made chief scorer at the club.

Examiner information

1 Communication skills—conduct of interview

- Introduce yourself to the patient.
- Ask him how he is.
- Approach the subject of the medication by making sure exactly what he is on, for how long and when he takes these during the day.
- Ask if he knows why he takes these—there may be a lack of understanding.
- Ask about side-effects. Take a detailed history of the amiodarone side-effects. Ask about other side-effects, e.g. pulmonary fibrosis, jaundice, corneal microdeposits, peripheral neuropathy. Ask about side-effects from his other medication.
- Listen to his concerns about the tablets.
- Explain the importance of each medication in turn: frusemide and lisinopril for the heart failure, Imdur for angina, amiodarone to prevent dysrhythmias and carbimazole for the amiodarone-induced thyrotoxicosis.
- Discuss the pros and cons of stopping the amiodarone: reappearance of the dysrhythmia if stopped and the possibility of other antidysrhythmics not being as effective vs. avoiding the side-effects of the amiodarone and removing the need for carbimazole.
- Explain that the reason he is feeling so well is probably because of his adequate treatment regimen.
- Discuss the possibility of wearing a hat, using sun cream and sitting in the shade.

2 Communication skills—exploration and problem negotiation

The candidate should be able to:

- ascertain the full drug history, its complications and explain why the carbimazole is needed
- discuss the wishes of the patient
- discuss the pros and cons of stopping any or all of the medications

- have a plan to determine his risk of further dysrhythmias: ECG, 24-h ECG tape and, possibly, an exercise ECG

3 Ethics and the law and other discussion points

- All drugs may cause adverse effects. The two types of adverse drug reactions that are described are dose-dependent and dose-independent. The former is characterized by an increasing pharmacological effect as the dosage is increased. As a rule such reactions are less serious and rapidly resolve on stopping the drug. Dose-independent reactions are usually more serious with a large variability between individuals in their susceptibility to an adverse effect.
- Preventing adverse reactions can be accomplished by not using a drug unless there is a good indication, avoiding drug interactions, prescribing the correct dosage in patients with altered metabolism (e.g. the elderly, those with renal or hepatic disease), prescribing as few drugs as possible and, where possible, using drugs that are familiar.
- Unwanted drug reactions are common in the elderly, particularly when drugs of a narrow therapeutic index are given. Multiple factors can lead to morbidity, such as multiple pathology, concurrent drug use and subsequent drug interactions, patient's perceptions of their illness and drug taking. Poor compliance in the elderly can be because of poor motivation, lack of understanding and the practicalities of taking tablets. Most elderly patients would like a simplified regimen with simple instructions, positive involvement of carers, use of memory aids and, most importantly, evidence of a clear-cut benefit from taking the medicine.
- Amiodarone is structurally related to thyroid-hormone-containing iodine and so, even at a dosage of 200 mg/day, there will be a very high iodine intake. As a result the following thyroid effects are possible:
  (a) acute, transient changes in thyroid function

(b) hypothyroidism in patients susceptible to the inhibitory effects of a high iodine load

(c) thyrotoxicosis that may be caused by at least three mechanisms—from the iodine load in the setting of a multinodular goitre (Jod-Basedow phenomenon), a thyroiditis-like condition and, possibly, induction of autoimmune Graves' disease.

Ideally, in amiodarone-induced thyrotoxicosis the drug should be stopped, if possible, although this is often impractical because of the underlying cardiac disorder. Discontinuation of amiodarone will not have an acute effect because of its storage and prolonged half-life so, even after stopping the amiodarone, the carbimazole will need to be continued for at least 6 months. Amiodarone-induced thyrotoxicosis may also exacerbate coronary artery disease and dysrhythmias.

- Possible management plans to investigate whether the patient is still at risk of dysrhythmias are to consider reducing the dosage of amiodarone to 100 mg/day, review the thyroid status, realize that radioiodine is not an effective means of countering thyrotoxicosis in this case and that surgical thyroidectomy would be a risky anaesthetic procedure.

Case 48 | Violent and abusive patients

Candidate information

You are the medical SHO on call and you are asked to see the senior Sister of your ward regarding Mr Thomas Jenkins

Please read this summary (it should take no more than 2 min) and then continue with the consultation.

Re: Mr Thomas Jenkins, aged 43

Mr Jenkins is a 43-year-old man with insulin-dependent diabetes mellitus who was admitted under your consultant's care yesterday with pneumonia, poorly controlled diabetes and confusion. As a consequence of his confusion, he has assaulted one nurse and verbally abused another on the ward about half-an-hour ago. The security staff are with him at the moment trying to calm the situation. However, the senior sister (Sister James) wants to talk to you about the situation. She wants him removed from the hospital and threatens to call the police. However, Mr Jenkins is clinically unfit to leave hospital.

Your tasks are to: discuss the recent incidents with Sister James, acquire full details of what has happened and discuss how to manage the situation.

You have 14 min until the Sister leaves the room, followed by 1 min for reflection, before the discussion with the examiners.

Subject/patient/relative information

Sister James has been a well-respected member of the nursing staff for many years and she works on your consultant's ward. Mr Jenkins is a 43-year-old man with insulin-dependent diabetes mellitus who was admitted yesterday with pneumonia, poorly controlled diabetes and confusion. From the start of the admission, he has been quite agitated with constant wandering around the ward despite being told by the staff to stay in bed. There are no other obvious causes for the confusion such as toxic/alcohol, pharmacological, head injury, postictal, etc., and no reason for the acute escalation of misbehaviour. He pulled out all his drips including his intravenous insulin, shouted expletives at the student nurse, and punched in the face a male nurse who had come to the aid of the student nurse. The male nurse has a suspected broken nose. There are four security men by the bedside but they are not physically holding Mr Jenkins down. Sister James is utterly disgusted by Mr Jenkins' behaviour and she wants to call the police to evict him from the ward despite his illness. He has an oxygen saturation of 91% on air and his blood sugar test results are still over 15 mmol/L. He has not been on any benzodiazepines or opioids and there is no evidence of any head injury.

Examiner information

1 Communication skills—conduct of interview

- Sit down with the Sister and ask for the full details of what has happened, who has been attacked and what injuries have been caused. Make sure all details are officially written on an incident report form. Ask if any of the other patients have been harmed or distressed by the incidence.
- Ask how Mr Jenkins has been since admission.
- Determine if there has been any particular reason for Mr Jenkins to be more unsettled.
- Ask if Mr Jenkins has a particular dislike towards the two staff affected by this incident.
- Get an idea of how Mr Jenkins has been medically: oxygenation, blood sugars, temperature, etc.
- Ask if any benzodiazepines or opioids have been given and enquire about any history/evidence of a head injury.
- Ask if hospital security has been called and what are they doing now (restraining).
- Show that you fully understand Sister's concerns for the safety of her staff.
- Remind her that Mr Jenkins is ill and such patients have a right for their medical treatment to be continued despite their lack of cooperation.
- Explain that you feel that Mr Jenkins cannot be removed from the ward by the police as he is unfit to leave the ward.
- Reassure Sister that you will see Mr Jenkins and make an attempt to calm him and to determine any particular reason for the bad behaviour.
- Explain that you will ask advice from the on-call psychiatrist with regard to controlling his violent behaviour.
- Ask the Sister if it would be helpful to request specialist nursing help whilst Mr Jenkins is agitated and offer to talk to the on-call senior nurse for the hospital about arranging this.
- Explain that you will inform your own consultant immediately and that you will report the matter as a critical incident.

2 Communication skills—exploration and problem negotiation

The candidate should be able to:
- listen to Sister's concerns

- take a careful account of what has happened and who has been involved
- determine if there are any medical causes for the worsening behaviour
- reassure Sister that advice and practical support from senior colleagues will be sought
- persuade Sister into understanding that the patient remains ill and that he cannot be removed from a hospital ward by the police and that it would result in a risk of further medical deterioration
- have a clear plan of management that Sister can agree with

3 Ethics and the law and other discussion points

- Such patients cannot be left without treatment.
- Hostility may be directed against a particular healthcare professional, in which case he or she must not be further involved in the patient's care.
- Sedation may be considered if the violence is a symptom of the illness and when, in the interest of the patient, this is needed to prevent injury to themselves or others.
- Advice from a psychiatrist should be sought. He or she may be able to give advice on sedation and provide a nurse experienced in violent behaviour.
- An experienced and appropriately trained senior male nurse should be allocated to care for the patient, preferably isolated away from other patients.
- Antipsychotics should not be used to facilitate easier management.
- If the patient is physically violent then security must be called at once.
- It is not an acceptable request that a patient be removed by the police solely because he or she has behaved badly and when the patient needs medical care.
- Restraining measures may be required to prevent violent patients from hurting themselves or others, but restraint must always be the minimum necessary or required.
- Early communication with the relatives to explain reasons for restraint is prudent.
- Every case of restraint should be fully documented and reported as a critical incident (usually to the clinical risk department).
- Restraint should not be routinely used as an excuse for insufficient staffing.
- Junior nurses or doctors should not make decisions regarding medical care and the consultant and hospital management must be informed.

Comments on the case

Unfortunately, this type of case is becoming more and more common. It is important that all doctors working in the NHS have some knowledge of how to deal with difficult patients, avoiding the temptation of taking the law into their own hands, and appreciating that there may be medical reasons to explain the bad behaviour.

You can support nursing colleagues by demonstrating empathy and practical support in these circumstances.

Case 49 | Withdrawing treatment (1)

Candidate information

You are the SHO in intensive care medicine

Please read this summary (it should take no more than 2 min) and then continue with the consultation.

> ### Re: Mr Alfred Swallow, aged 80
>
> Mr Swallow, an 80-year-old man, has cardiorespiratory and renal failure following an emergency aortic aneurysm repair 2 weeks ago. He remains intubated and sedated on the ITU and has been on maximum support including inotropes and haemofiltration for the last 8 days. You feel strongly that the patient will not recover despite continuing with maximum therapy and you have been asked by the vascular surgeons for an opinion on withdrawing treatment. You approach the senior sister (Sister Green) to discuss the possibility of withdrawing treatment.

Your tasks are to: discuss with Sister Green the present medical condition of Mr Swallow, his most likely outcome and the possibility of withdrawing treatment.

You have 14 min until Sister Green leaves the room, followed by 1 min for reflection, before the discussion with the examiners.

Subject/patient/relative information

Sister Green is the nurse in charge of the ITU today and she and her other colleagues have been looking after Mr Swallow for the last 8 days. He was admitted to the unit after an emergency repair to a ruptured abdominal aortic aneurysm. His past medical history includes ischaemic heart disease and COPD. Since his admission, Mr Swallow is intubated and sedated, requires inotropes (dobutamine and adrenaline) to maintain a decent cardiac output and 4 days ago he became anuric and acidotic which necessitated haemofiltration. He continues to be acidotic (base excess of -15), with a poor cardiac output (3.5 L/min) and needing a high F_iO_2 (60%). There is one daughter who has been very supportive and understanding of the whole situation. She has been aware of the risks involved from the outset and visits every day. The SHO (the candidate) has been asked by the surgeons whether a plan should be made to withdraw treatment and whether he or she would like to discuss this with the ITU Sister. Sister Green does feel that a decision ought to be made regarding withdrawal of treatment as the patient now has multiorgan failure and the outlook is very poor.

Examiner information

1 Communication skills — conduct of interview

- Explain to Sister Green that you need to discuss Mr Swallow's condition.
- Confirm that there has been no improvement in the patient's condition over the last 8 days and obtain some objective evidence for this, e.g. physiology, etc.
- Is there any family visiting the patient and how much interest they have expressed?
- Has the family expressed any views about the patient's management and condition?
- Ask if she is aware of any wishes with regard to withdrawing treatment expressed by the patient (prior to illness) or the family.
- What is the Sister's opinion about whether continuing active treatment would be in the best interests of the patient?
- Ask what Sister Green's opinion is on withdrawing treatment.
- Ask if there is any member of staff known to her who would object to withdrawing treatment.
- Explain to Sister that you will be speaking to your consultant who will make the final decision.
- Ask Sister to call you when the family comes to visit the patient so that you can discuss the possibility of withdrawing treatment with them.
- Discuss with Sister which method of withdrawing treatment she feels is best for the patient and the family (withdrawing everything at once or gradually).

2 Communication skills — exploration and problem negotiation

The candidate should be able to:
- acknowledge that withdrawing treatment is a team decision and not based purely on one individual's perspective
- appreciate the viewpoints of staff and family, including that of the patient before this illness
- recognize that the nursing staff are more aware of the present condition of an ITU patient as they are the ones who are looking after the patient on a 24-h basis
- recognize that when a patient is in multiorgan failure and the outlook is poor, continuing treatment is not in the best interests of the patient

3 Ethics and the law and other discussion points

- The primary goal of medical treatment is to benefit the patient by restoring or maintaining the patient's health as far as possible, maximizing benefit and minimizing harm. If treatment fails or ceases to give a net benefit to the patient, that goal cannot be realized and the justification for providing the treatment is removed. Unless some other justification can be demonstrated, treatment that does not provide net benefit to the patient (ethically and legally) may be withheld or withdrawn and the goal of medical care should shift to the palliation of symptoms.
- Prolonging a patient's life usually, but not always, provides a health benefit to that patient. It is not an appropriate goal of medicine to prolong life at all costs with no regard to its quality or the burdens of treatment. Although emotionally it may be easier to withhold treatment than to withdraw that which has been started, there are no legal, or morally relevant, differences between the two actions. Even so, this is not to say that emotionally and psychologically the two are equivalent. Many health professionals, as well as patients, feel an emotional difference between withholding and withdrawing treatment. This is likely to be linked to the largely negative impression attached to a decision to withdraw treatment which can be interpreted as abandonment or 'giving up on the patient'. The BMA considers that where a particular treatment is no longer benefiting the patient, continuing to provide it would not be in the patient's best interests and, indeed, might be thought to be morally wrong. Greater emphasis on the reasons for providing treatment (including artificial nutrition and hydration), rather than the justification for withholding it may challenge this perceived difference. Treatment should never be withheld when there is a possibility that it will benefit the patient, simply because withholding is considered to be easier than withdrawing treatment.
- Developments in technology have led to a misperception in society that death can almost always be postponed. There needs to be a recognition that there comes a point in all lives where no more can reasonably or helpfully be done to benefit patients other than keeping them comfortable and free from pain.

British Medical Association. *Withholding and withdrawing life-prolonging medical treatment: guidance for decision making.* 1999.

Comments on the case

This case illustrates how important it is to make a team decision on the further management of the patient. Do not forget that the patient and their family constitute an important and integral part of the process. In a high-tech environment where the emphasis is on striving to maintain life, clinical and nursing staff often also experience a strong sense of dismay when the withdrawing or withholding of treatment has to be faced. Remember to look after yourself and colleagues as well. Withdrawing and withholding treatment decisions involve many ethical issues, of which the candidate must be aware.

Case 50 | Withdrawing treatment (2)

Candidate information
You are the SHO in intensive care medicine

Please read this summary (it should take no more than 2 min) and then continue with the consultation.

> ### Re: Mr Alfred Swallow, aged 80
>
> You have spoken to Sister Green and both of you decide that withdrawing treatment is in the best interests of the patient. The consultant agrees and the team looking after the patient feels this should begin by tailing down the inotropes first. This, in the opinion of the consultant, will probably lead to eventual death within an hour as Mr Swallow has been dependent on high doses of inotropes for a while. Mr Swallow is well sedated with opioids and benzodiazepines and shows no signs of distress, pain or discomfort. Sister Green has also just told you that his daughter (Mrs Wild) is waiting in the relatives' room to be briefed on the decision.

Your tasks are to: break the bad news regarding Mr Swallow's condition, explain that the ITU team feel that withdrawing treatment is in the best interests of the patient and explain how this will be done and answer any queries.

You have 14 min until the patient's daughter leaves the room, followed by 1 min for reflection, before the discussion with the examiners.

Subject/patient/relative information
Mrs Wild is the only daughter of Mr Swallow. Mrs Swallow has severe Alzheimer's disease and has been in a nursing home for over 3 years. She is not aware of Mr Swallow's present condition and Mrs Wild does not feel it would be appropriate to bring her over to the unit. Mrs Wild has been aware of her father's poor prognosis, particularly with the past comorbid history, and she has noticed how her father has been deteriorating over the last 4 days. Her personal opinion is that her father will not survive this event but she is unsure about how the withdrawal of treatment would be carried out. She has no objections in principle but wants reassurance that her father will be comfortable and in no distress.

Examiner information

1 Communication skills — conduct of interview
- Introduce yourself to the patient's daughter (make sure she is his daughter). In a real situation you would

have a member of the nursing staff present who knows Mr Swallow and the daughter.
- Ask her what she knows about her father's condition and what she has already been told (she will hopefully say that she knows her father remains very ill).
- Say how sorry you are that Mr Swallow remains very

poorly and that, despite all efforts, he has not improved. Allow a pause for the daughter to take all this in.

- Explain that you want to share with her some thoughts about the next step. Say that despite being on the active treatment, the ITU team looking after him feels his outlook is poor and that he is going to die. Then pause.
- Explain that your team feels that continuing active treatment will not achieve the desired result (restoring her father back to how he was previously) and introduce the concept of withdrawing treatment.
- Obtain an idea of who makes up the family and ask if she, or any other member of the family, has already expressed any views on this matter.
- Ask if she knows of any opinions expressed by her father when he was well as to how he would like this situation managed.
- Ask if there is any member of the family who is unaware of the situation who might not have expressed an opinion on the patient's condition and management.
- Explain that her father is well sedated, not in pain and that he is not aware of what is happening.
- Explain that if the family allows the withdrawal of treatment, he may deteriorate quickly and die soon after. Again reinforce the fact that he will be comfortable, in no pain and unaware of what is happening.
- Point out politely that the final decision of withdrawing treatment does *not* reside with her or the family but with the ITU staff, so they must not feel as if they are actively causing the death of their father.
- Describe how the withdrawal will be undertaken (tailing down the inotropes) and give an estimate of how long Mr Swallow may survive after this (explain this is only a guess). This will at least give her an idea of how long the process will last, particularly if she has to inform family who live far away.
- Reassure the daughter that her father will be comfortable and free from pain and distress; her father's heart will probably slow down and eventually stop but explain that the ventilator will be doing the breathing for him. The haemodialysis machine will also be disconnected when the inotropes are being tailed down.
- Explain that a decision is not needed right away and that she should speak to the other members of the family and that you should meet again later in the day to answer any questions she has.
- Ask if she has any queries now.
- Once again empathize with her and ask Sister if she has anything else to add to the discussion (if Sister is present during the consultation).

2 Communication skills — exploration and problem negotiation

The candidate should be able to:

- know in detail the situation concerning the patient
- explain, with understanding and empathy, the reasons why the team feel that withdrawing treatment is in the best interests of the patient
- appreciate that withdrawing treatment is not a subject the daughter may be familiar with
- share her grief and say that withdrawing treatment is as sad an undertaking for medical staff as it is for the relatives
- describe how withdrawal will take place and what are the events most likely to occur after this

3 Ethics and the law and other discussion points

General considerations

- The primary goal of medicine is to benefit the patient's health with minimal harm and this should be explained to those close to them so that they can understand why treatment is given, and why a decision to withhold or withdraw further life-prolonging treatment may need to be considered.
- The approach of the doctor in these difficult and sometimes highly charged circumstances must always accord with the ethical principles of medical practice, and with the interests of the patient first and foremost.

Benefits

- Benefits to the patient can result either from treatment or non-treatment, depending on the clinical context. Clearly, if there is a possibility of the patient receiving benefit from treatment then it should be continued, unless the competent patient has refused treatment at the time or in advance of becoming incompetent. Wherever there is any doubt about this, the balance must be in the direction of treatment. Effective palliation, as distinct from life-prolonging treatment, should never be withdrawn. On the other hand, there are clinical situations where treatment is not beneficial and only prolongs suffering. There may be the concern that a course of treatment, once started, may be hard to stop if found to be ineffective. This difficulty can be avoided by the construction of a management plan specifying time-limited goals, drawn up in discussion with the patient (if possible), the relatives and with the clinical team.

- Whatever decisions are taken, it is important to stress that the autonomy of the patient must be respected. In this context an advance statement, if available, will be helpful, particularly if the patient subsequently becomes incapable of consenting to a proposed course of action. However, there is no absolute right to a treatment that a responsible professional opinion considers as inappropriate.

Harm

A further ethical consideration relates to the need to do no harm (part of the Hippocratic oath). It is in this area that there is particular controversy. The bulk of opinion holds to the view that painful, invasive procedures or drugs that have unpleasant side-effects should be avoided in situations where they will confer no material benefit. However, questions remain regarding the withdrawal of measures such as tube feeding from those who are either unconscious, or suffering from a persistent vegetative state with no chance of recovery, where such measures may do no more than prolong life. It has been argued that thirst distresses patients and witnessing the patient 'starving to death' when nutrition is withdrawn may certainly add to the distress of the attendants. The rule to be applied, as ever, is that the welfare of the patient comes first, so nothing should be done that could add to their discomfort without benefit.

Equity

There is a further ethical matter which, in these days of healthcare rationing, needs to be acknowledged. With regard to the allocation of treatment, whether or not it is definitive or life-prolonging, it is unethical to deny a subject access to treatment or withdraw treatment (e.g. in ITU) in order to make it available to another individual. This is particularly relevant in the case of the elderly.

Advance statements

In relation to life-prolonging treatment, there are advantages in people recording their wishes in a formal manner while they are competent to do so. There is no requirement for doctors to obey a request for any particular treatment, but they are under an obligation to withhold or withdraw treatment if that is the competent patient's expressed desire given at the time of treatment or, if incompetent, given as a valid advanced refusal, even though the doctor may disagree.

Legal aspects

There are circumstances where the issues are unclear or the decisions of the doctors are challenged. In such cases there may be a recourse to the courts. A situation where this has been specifically recommended by law is when there is a move to withdraw artificial nutrition and hydration from a patient deemed to be suffering from a persistent vegetative state. Despite all the power of the Courts, the law itself still looks to authoritative medical opinion for guidance.

D.R. London. Withdrawing and withholding life-prolonging medical treatment from adult patients. *Journal of Royal College of Physicians, London* **34**, March/April 2000.

Comments on the case

As more and more patients are treated in the ITU, circumstances such as these are becoming common. The candidate must have the ability to discuss these ethical issues as part of a team and this case illustrates how all angles have to be carefully covered.
Never make a decision to withdraw or withhold treatment on your own; someone will challenge you!

Section F
Experiences, Anecdotes, Tips, Quotations

'I know 'coz I was there'*

* Max Boyce — referring to the victory of the Welsh rugby team in the 1970's over the All Blacks

This section starts with MRCP short-case *experiences* of recent candidates from the first three PACES examinations. We have reported here 26 complete PACES accounts written in the first person. We start off with those that are most detailed to give you the greatest insight into the type of experience that may lie ahead for you. Gradually we move to shorter versions, the aim being to give a greater flavour of the types of combinations of cases that occur. Following this we give further Station 2 and Station 4 *experiences* written in the first person. Obviously, all these accounts represent the candidate's unchecked view of what the case was and what happened. Also they have not necessarily always remembered, or bothered to record the exact wording of the written instruction, often preferring to just give us the basic 'Examine this patient. . . .'

This is followed by the majority of the experiences from the second edition of *An Aid to the MRCP Short Cases*, which are from the old style examination. They span the last 10–20 years and, although the examination has changed from the 'short cases' which involved seeing six or more varied cases in 30 minutes with just two examiners, the later surveys have indicated that the same cases are still appearing for the new format. We have amended the older experiences so that cases are described individually. However, we have included a series of complete experiences but hope that you can imagine seeing these cases individually with different examiners at the appropriate Stations (1, 3 and 5). The tragedies and triumphs do not seem to change with time.

We have placed the older extracts into specific groups. If an examiner spots a weakness, such as poor observation or examination technique, he or she is likely to explore this further before deciding whether to pass or fail a candidate. Consequently, some of the experiences are grouped according to which aspect of the candidate's clinical competence the examiner might have been probing most. A miscellaneous group of *anecdotes* follows the experiences. Although the outcome was not necessarily decided by the particular short case described, for additional information we have usually indicated whether the candidate passed or failed.

A list of useful *tips* is given, and then the section finishes with a selection of *quotations* from successful MRCP candidates. At the end of the questionnaire, the candidates in our survey were asked if there were any comments they would like passed on to the candidates of the future. We felt that the consistencies and occasional discrepancies in the advice of such a large number of 'authorities' might be of interest to some candidates and so we present here a selection from the large number received. In order not to distort the force and intentions contained in these advisory comments, we have tended to offer them verbatim. Inevitably, some of the quotations are contradictory in their opinions — as with all examinations, individuals have different experiences and offer differing advice. Our views on these discrepancies are reflected throughout the book as far as they could be dealt with.* Ultimately, you will have to come to your own conclusion depending upon the circumstances of a particular case.

* For example, the discrepancies of quotations under the heading: 'Listen, obey and do not stray'—in general we support extending the examination beyond the examiner's instruction, whenever necessary, so long as this is done with intelligence and discrimination.

Full PACES experiences in the first person

1 *I said that the brachio-radialus was weak and this was met with utter astonishment and 'What! Where is brachio-radialus? Which nerve is damaged?' I wasn't sure.*

Station 1

Examine this patient's respiratory system and comment on the positive findings as you go.

The clinical findings were of finger clubbing, nicotine staining of the fingers and fine, inspiratory crackles at both bases.

I was stopped at the hands and asked for my thoughts. I suggested that the differential diagnosis would be between a bronchial malignancy, suppurative lung disease and fibrosis unrelated to the nicotine staining. After suggesting these possibilities I was asked about the causes of pulmonary fibrosis. I mentioned occupational dust exposure, extrinsic allergic alveolitis and drugs, but was not allowed to go on. They asked about investigations and I said pulmonary function tests which would reveal a reduced FEV and FEV_1 but with a normal $FEV_1 : FVC$ ratio, high-resolution CT scan and possibly bronchoscopy but they interrupted by saying that this was not often done now!

For occupational dust exposure I was pressed further so I said asbestos exposure, coal dust and beryllium. I was then stopped and the examiner said, 'Why did you say that—it just slipped out, didn't it?' I agreed that I had not meant to say this but maybe I should have stuck to my guns as I knew that beryllium is used in the aerospace industry and does cause fibrosis. At the end, after asking about investigations, they smiled and said, 'And having diagnosed cryptogenic fibrosing alveolitis you can now go', just as the bell rang. I had never even mentioned this!

Examine this man's abdomen commenting on what you are doing.

He had hepatosplenomegaly. I was not allowed (I was actually stopped when I tried) to examine for lymphadenopathy. There were no peripheral stigmata *at all* of chronic liver disease. I said he probably had a lymphoproliferative or a myeloproliferative condition and possibly portal hypertension but I pointed out that this was highly unlikely in view of the *large* spleen and the absence of any peripheral stigmata.

They went on to ask why it was not a kidney on the left

and for some reason I do not think I answered this terribly well. I mentioned the inability to get above it, dullness to percussion and the splenic notch and they pushed me for more. They prompted me with, 'What about movement?' to which I replied that the spleen moves with respiration. They pressed on with, 'Does the kidney?' I said, 'Yes, but less so'. They then asked for that other causes of left upper quadrant masses and I said that other than the kidney it could be pancreatic but it was more likely to be gastric or adrenal. They looked happy and asked if I had ever felt an adrenal mass. One of the examiners said, pointing to his colleague, 'Dr X here sometimes feels them!'.

Station 2

This is a 36-year-old lady who has been diabetic for 2 years and is on insulin. She has recently been treated for a foot ulcer and wants to be more involved with her treatment and her diabetic control. Discuss her treatment with her.

She had had an ulcer on her right big toe for the last 3 months. It had healed once but had broken down again and for this second time she had needed intravenous antibiotics. The doctors had been worried about osteomyelitis but this had not actually occurred. The ulcer had now healed again. She had had three hypoglycaemic episodes in the past which had led to near unconsciousness but she had not been to the hospital. She had had laser treatment to the eyes and now had no visual symptoms. She complained of tingling in the right foot but of no weakness. She was a bank clerk and her place of work knew that she was diabetic. She only checked her BMs about 3–4 times a week and they normally ran between 8 and 15 mm/L. She was taking Human Mixtard 20 units b.d. using a syringe and needle. Her diet was poor. She ate anything and everything and had failed to attend her dietitian's appointment. She confessed to liking chocolate. In addition she had never seen a chiropodist. I suggested there was a need for more home monitoring for a while until we had established a better pattern. I also suggested modification of the administration of insulin to using a pen (in fact she asked for this) and that she should attend a chiropody and dietetic appointment. Overall, she appeared to be a woman who had not really taken on board the seriousness of her condition. She probably had not realized that the ulcer and the eye problems were caused by the diabetes and that tighter control was needed. I think this is what I failed to address with her. I discussed treatment and management with her including more intensive BM monitoring so that we could modify her treatment. She did not like the testing and said it was painful so I asked how she did it and she told me that she pricked the finger pulps. I had read something specifically about this which said that the side of the finger was better as it had fewer nerve endings and I explained this to her.

The examiners asked me whether I thought she would be amenable to a more intensive regimen but I thought that she probably would not, given her dislike of needles. However, I pointed out that she may find the pen device more acceptable. (Unfortunately it was *she* who brought this up, not me.) The examiners also asked me how much chocolate she ate. I did not know because I had not asked. In the heat of the exam I thought I might run out of time so I chose to move on to other things, although I would certainly have asked this in outpatients (and would probably have run well over the 14 min!).

I think the time limitation is difficult at this station. I failed this section during a mock exam because I did not get round to discussing the management side of the case. I thought I had taken a good history but did not feel I handled or even fully uncovered her concerns. At the end she started asking me about different types of diabetes. She plainly wanted to know more and at this point the bell rang. I think that I should have asked earlier on what she knew about the disease and the case would have fallen into my lap.

Station 3

This gentleman came in on the medical intake 2 days ago and he was breathless. Examine his cardiovascular system.
He had an irregular pulse and mitral regurgitation. There were no splinter haemorrhages. The apex beat was not displaced and by this stage he was no longer breathless.

The examiners wanted to know what I thought might be the cause of his breathlessness. I said that he could have a superimposed infection or he could have had a myocardial infarction, but I was told that his troponin levels were normal and that his ECG was OK. I mentioned the possibility of a pulmonary embolus but they said that he had no chest pain. I got stuck at this stage and the examiner said, 'I know you know this — forget it's the MRCP exam. What else did you say you had found?' I then remembered the irregular pulse and said the atrial fibrillation might be acute. They asked what I would have done so I said I would have given him

diuretics, controlled his rate with digoxin or amiodarone and that DC cardioversion would probably not be an option as the exact time of onset was not known. They asked for another drug and I foolishly did *not* think of warfarin!

Examine this lady's nervous system but concentrate on the legs.
She looked fairly normal and her gait also looked normal to me. There was no wasting or fasciculation and she certainly did not have champagne-bottle legs. She had pes cavus but I hedged a bit on that, saying I was not sure but I thought in the end that she did. Her tone was normal as was her power but she had mild weakness of ankle dorsiflexion on the right. (They pressed me for other power abnormalities but I insisted that that was it.) There were absent ankle jerks, normal knee jerks and they would not let me check the plantar reflex or for sensation. Coordination, according to them, was normal.

The examiners asked me for my findings. I said that I had found pes cavus and distal weakness which led me to think about a hereditary sensory and motor neuropathy. Also I said that pes cavus occurs in Friedreich's ataxia but I said that, as her coordination was normal, this was unlikely. They did not press me for other causes of a peripheral neuropathy but they asked why pes cavus occurs and I tried to come up with something sensible but could not really explain the pathophysiology other than that the flexors must be stronger than the extensors. They requested that I ask the lady a question and so I asked about family history, which was positive. They asked me to examine her hands which had no wasting but there was mild weakness of the abductors of the fingers. Their final question was, 'We call this Charcot–Marie–Tooth but do you know any new terms?' I just said, 'Hereditary sensory and motor neuropathy'. I think they were fairly happy it was not an easy case.

Station 4

You are asked to see the son of Mr JK who has metastatic carcinoma of the lung and has presented with shortness of breath and pain in his leg. It is thought that he could have a deep venous thrombosis (DVT) and a pulmonary embolus (PE). However, the patient does not want to be treated. The son agrees that he does not want his father to suffer and thought that 'he was on the way out'. The patient is very cachectic and unwell. Please discuss treatment, prognosis and resuscitation status.
The son was very aware that the cancer had spread, that we suspected a blood clot and that the outlook was poor.

He wanted to know what we could do to treat him and I explained that we would need to confirm a clot and then give him blood-thinning injections which were not excessively painful but rather uncomfortable. I said that the treatment might prolong his life a little but that the prognosis was poor and that he would die sooner or later from the lung malignancy. I emphasized that I did not want to guess how long he might live. I said that if his father did not want treatment we would respect his wishes. The son wanted to know if he might get home following treatment of the DVT/PE and I said it might be possible. Then the son said, 'My mother would never cope with him—she would have another heart attack and it would kill her'. I talked about pain relief and palliative care. He asked if we could give him something to end it all quicker to which I replied, 'We cannot deliberately end his life'. I said that we would discuss the resuscitation status with his father and the son thought he would almost certainly say 'No' to resuscitation. I said that 'My team would consider it appropriate not to resuscitate'.

The examiners asked me about how one would decide whether a patient is competent to give consent. At this point it occurred to me that I did not know if the patient was *compos mentis* or not. I had rather assumed that he was but this was probably a fatal error. I wondered if they were giving me a chance to salvage things by asking what I would do if I thought he might be depressed and I mentioned that there should be a formal psychiatric review. I think this station was tricky because in real life I would have known the patient and would have already assessed whether he was confused/depressed or not. They also asked what I would have done if I discussed resuscitation with the patient and he had wanted to be resuscitated. I ran out of time on this but pointed out that the medical team can override his wishes but should discuss it fully and try to persuade them to agree.

Station 5

This man has a rash on his face. Please examine him.
There was a confluent, maculopapular, erythematous, lightly scaling rash over the whole face extending to the back of his neck and scalp. There were plaques on the anterior surfaces of the lower legs with thicker scales. Over the elbows there was some dry scaling but no erythema. There were no nail changes and the mouth and eyes were normal. There were no lymph nodes.

I said that this might be an atypical presentation of psoriasis and they looked pleased and asked why it was atypical. I said it was not on the knees/elbows and that

there were no nail changes. I ventured that I would also consider a drug eruption. They asked the patient what it was and he said, 'Psoriasis'. I know I got a clear pass for this one—I saw the mark-sheet!

Look at this man's face and examine whatever else you think is necessary.
I found scant facial hair. There was no visual field defect and he looked normal in all other respects. In addition, his hands were normal.

This was a disaster! I said he had evidence of pituitary failure or gonadal failure and they asked why. I cannot remember what happened next but I found myself looking at his teeth and tongue in a vain hunt for acromegaly which clearly was not there. They said, 'Ask him to stand'. He was very tall as well as having what I thought was an odd-shaped chest but he was fully clothed in a room full of people! I am not sure why Klinefelter's syndrome popped out of my mouth but as everything I knew about this escaped me I retracted it and, after much prompting, I figured out that growth hormone lack causes failure of epiphyseal fusion and therefore tall stature. I am sure this is all wrong. It is a gonadal failure that does it.

Examine this lady's eye movements.
There was no ptosis and the left eye was slightly down and out. There was some reasonable movement in the left eye but she had diplopia throughout except when looking down and out. She had a poor pupillary response.

The examiners asked me about pupillary sparing. I got this right but I was a bit flustered following the endocrine case and launched badly into my presentation saying, 'The eye is deviated down and out' and did not even say which one was affected!

This man had an operation which is unrelated to the case and then woke up with a weak left arm. Why?
He had weak dorsiflexion of the wrist, weak finger extension and numbness and paraesthesiae over the first dorsal interosseus. I said he had a radial nerve palsy secondary to compression at a mid-humeral level.

The examiner asked me if any of the other muscles were weak and, 'Would you like to check elbow flexion again'. I did so and there was mild weakness. I was asked why and I said that the brachioradialis was weak and this was met with utter astonishment and 'What! Where is brachioradialis? Which nerve is damaged?' I was not sure. I knew I had got it all wrong and I still do not know what the examiner actually wanted.

2 I gave a differential diagnosis of firstly pyoderma gangrenosum and they asked why it wasn't, and finally they told me he was diabetic so I suggested necrobiosis diabeticorum. They then asked me why it wasn't typical!

Station 1

This man has become increasingly breathless over the past 2 years. He is a non-smoker. Please examine his respiratory system to determine a cause.

I only found a small area of bronchial breathing over the right upper lobe posteriorly. There were no peripheral signs of respiratory disease and I have to emphasize that the clinical signs of the bronchial breathing were very slight. There was no asymmetry of chest expansion, no scars and I did not detect any dullness on percussion or any increase in tactile focal fremitus. I wrongly reached a diagnosis of cryptogenic fibrosing alveolitis because there were some mild, bi-basal, fine, inspiratory crepitations. The examiner asked, 'What was not in keeping with that diagnosis?' and I said that there was no clubbing and no cyanosis. He asked me to examine the chest again. I was not swayed about the percussion note or the tactile focal fremitus but had to agree with the bronchial breathing. He asked me for a differential diagnosis for the cause of the bronchial breathing. I said, 'Consolidation', but at that point the bell went.

The case was an absolute nightmare. I had never been asked to re-examine a chest in all my practice teachings and I died inside when I was directed back. However, I was determined not to shrivel up and I just kept to being honest, I looked the examiner in the eye and carried on. I kept thinking that one nightmare does not fail the exam and tried to keep going. I also made a concerted effort to forget the respiratory fiasco as I was led to the abdominal case.

This 43-year-old man failed a routine medical examination for insurance purposes. Please examine the abdomen and suggest if you can find a reason why.

I found numerous spider naevi and lone hepatomegaly at about 4 finger-breadths.

The examiner asked, 'What might be the underlying diagnosis; how would you investigate this man; what would an abdominal ultrasound scan show and what would his liver biopsy show?'

Station 2

This 54-year-old man with a history of haemochromatosis, hypopituitarism and diabetes mellitus is now troubled with arthritis. He has previously been on voltarol but he had a perforated duodenal ulcer. He is now on meloxicam, testosterone injections and insulin. His HbA1c is 9.8%. His haemoglobin is about 14g with a ferritin of 40mg/mL. Please see and advise him regarding the painful joints.

I asked the patient to tell me what problems he was experiencing and he said impotence. He did not mention his joints and I was a wee bit thrown here! However, I kept going and gained some history of his main problems which were: (a) impotence; (b) his joints—in particular his hands were painful as a result of his part-time work as a fisherman; (c) heavy drinking of about 140 units/week; (d) marital disharmony secondary to (a) and (b)—he was unable to do any heavy work at home; and (e) poor diabetic control with lack of home monitoring.

We went through the whole standard history including past medical history, drug history, social history, family history, system review, etc. and then just ran out of time! I was feeding back to the patient a plan of action when the bell went. The examiner did agree with me that this was quite a complicated history so I think/hope that I was OK for not getting the whole plan over to the patient. I was asked what I was going to say and to summarize the main problems. We discussed the impotence, which was possibly secondary to his alcohol intake or to the poor diabetic control; the arthritis, and I was asked how to rule out other types of arthritis so I suggested by X-raying his hands and requesting a rheumatoid factor, antinuclear antibodies (ANA) and an erythrocyte sedimentation rate (ESR) test. We discussed whether he was a candidate for a Cox 2 inhibitor and we discussed the role of physiotherapy, occupational therapy and joint protection. With regard to the alcohol, we discussed coping strategies and access to a counsellor, and for the diabetes I said that I would encourage him to keep a monitoring booklet and that we would need to review him fairly soon.

Station 3

This woman, who is about 60 years of age, is becoming increasingly breathless. Would you examine her cardiovascular system and see if you can find a reason for this.

There was a malar flush. There were no scars and she was comfortable at rest. The pulse was irregularly irregular at a rate of about 92/min, it was not collapsing and was of variable volume. The jugular venous pressure (JVP) was not elevated. The apex beat was in the fifth intercostal space in the mid-clavicular line but she was very overweight so it was hard to find. The heart sounds were loud and I thought I could hear a pansystolic murmur at the apex.

I found this really hard because of the atrial fibrillation and the fast rate and the patient's habitus. However, I presented the findings of mitral stenosis! The examiner raised his eyebrows and asked how that could cause breathlessness. I struggled through a discussion including uncontrolled fast atrial fibrillation, right ventricular hypertrophy, pulmonary hypertension, etc. I was asked what investigations I would do and I suggested a chest X-ray, ECG and echo and they asked what I would ex-

pect to see. I am haunted by the thought that she may have had a systolic murmur at the left sternal edge which could have been pulmonary stenosis. It was all very difficult.

This 84-year-old lady has been having difficulty walking and with her balance. Would you examine her neurologically to find out why.

I asked if I could see her walk and they said, 'No—just examine her neurologically on the bed'. My findings were of bilateral weakness of about grade 4/5 with the left side worse than the right. There was no difference between the distal and proximal muscles. No reflexes were elicited as the lady could *not* relax! I found a peripheral glove and stocking sensory loss to light touch with loss of vibration sense, and equivocal joint position sense. I was stopped because of time constraints and asked to present what I had found.

They asked what I thought could be the cause and I suggested a peripheral neuropathy and mentioned a few tests I would like to do including a blood sugar and also to ask about drug history and then the bell rang.

Station 4

You are the SHO on the ward. A 50-year-old teacher, and mother of two children, has been admitted to your ward with hypercalcaemia and confusion, and a history of back pain. She now has a normal calcium and is lucid. She has a past history of a mastectomy 10 years ago with follow-up radiotherapy. Explain to her that you want to refer her to the oncologist for further treatment, probably chemotherapy and radiotherapy.

I introduced myself and asked the patient if she understood what had been happening in terms of the high calcium, which was now better, and her painful back. I asked about her family and who was at home. I explained the cause of the high calcium and of the back pain, which were both likely to be related to her previous breast cancer. The patient denied all of this by saying, 'I was clear at my check-up 2 months ago'. I explained to her that it was hard to tell if some cells had remained after the surgery and then she became angry and asked, 'Why wasn't I given chemotherapy 10 years ago?' I said that it was impossible to comment on other doctors' treatment but I could get hold of the old notes and discuss it with the specialist. She did not want me to tell her family but I explained that the family could be a source of support and help and they would want to know in order to help her. I also suggested that it would be hard to keep the diagnosis hidden with repeated hospital trips and the side-effects of the treatment. She wanted to know exactly what treatment would be given and I explained the broad principles and said that I would arrange an urgent appointment with the cancer doctors who could answer her more detailed questions. She asked if it would be cured and I had to say, 'No, the treatment would help the symptoms but would not cure the cancer'. I summarized the diagnosis and the plan of action and asked if she had any questions.

At this stage the examiners came over and asked me how I would cope with the patient's anger and what would I do if the daughter cornered me on the ward and asked what was wrong with her mother.

Station 5

This lady has had previous problems with her thyroid. Examine her to determine her thyroid status.
She had a pulse of 80 beats/min which was regular, there was no palmar erythema and no tremor. There were no eye signs but she had a small, smooth goitre. However, there was no water present to watch her swallow. There was no pretibial myxoedema. I said I would like to examine her reflexes to complete the examination. However, I thought that she was euthyroid.

The examiners asked me what her thyroid status was and I confidently said, 'Euthyroid'. There were then lots of complicated questions involving her management and investigations and I think I mentioned thyroid function tests, an ultrasound scan and thyroid uptake scans.

Your House Officer has examined this lady's fundi. She is a 23-year-old nurse. He is concerned and has asked for your opinion.
I found a reduced red reflex in the right eye and myelinated nerve fibres on the right side.

The examiner said to me, 'This lady presents with headaches, what would you say to her?

This 50-year-old lady has problems driving. Examine her arms to find out why.
She had a peripheral symmetrical arthropathy affecting the proximal interphalangeal joints and the metacarpophalangeal joints with a boutonnière deformity. She had a small mouth but there were no other signs of connective tissue disease.

They asked me for a diagnosis and I gave a differential between connective tissue disease and psoriatic arthropathy. I was told that she did not have psoriasis but that she had had a hemicolectomy for ulcerative colitis 10 years ago. What did I think now? I suggested arthritis secondary to ulcerative colitis. They said, 'Can you get this after a complete cure?' Then they asked me what other types of arthritis can occur with ulcerative colitis.

Examine this man's leg.
I found a raised erythematous area over his left shin with old, atrophied scars. There was pigmentation over two of the scars on the inner shin/calf.

I gave a differential diagnosis of first pyoderma gangrenosum and they asked why it was not that, then I suggested discoid lupus erythematosus and again they asked me why it was not. Finally, they told me he was diabetic so I suggested necrobiosis diabeticorum. Then they asked me why it was not typical!

3 *She also did not want a letter to go to her GP until their return in case the GP told her husband.*

Station 1

This gentleman presented with a cough and shortness of breath. Please examine his respiratory system.
He had obvious weight loss and there was very marked asymmetry in his chest expansion with reduced expansion on the right side. There was a small scar from a previous chest drain in his axilla, stony dullness to percussion and a trachea that was deviated away from that side.

The questions centred on, 'What might be the causes of the dullness?' and 'What investigations would you like to do?' We talked about investigations on pleural fluid for quite some time, 'What would you do if you couldn't aspirate any fluid?' and we discussed ultrasound guidance for aspiration or for premarking a specific point for aspiration.

This gentleman has lost weight and is experiencing fullness in his abdomen.
There was hepatosplenomegaly with axillary lymph nodes. There was no ascites but the patient looked very cachectic.

They asked me how I would best investigate this gentleman to make a diagnosis. We discussed lymph node biopsy and histology, and bone marrow examination. This led to a discussion about the Philadelphia chromosome.

Station 2

This 52-year-old lady has chronic active hepatitis initially treated with steroids and she is now quite stable on azathioprine. However, several other problems have emerged and the GP thinks it better if she is followed up by the hospital. You are the SHO in the general medical clinic.
She was a quiet lady who had obviously been told not to volunteer anything unless I specifically asked the right questions. She had had non-insulin-dependent diabetes mellitus but was now on insulin. She had coeliac disease and was on a gluten-free diet. She had hypercholesterolaemia and was on a low cholesterol diet. She had chronic anaemia and had been treated with B_{12} injections and was

now on iron supplements. She had osteoporosis which had been confirmed on a previous scan and she was on cyclical etidronate and calcium. She had had a hysterectomy at quite a young age for heavy and irregular periods. There was a possibility of primary ovarian failure or struma ovarii. She now had paraesthesiae in her fingers which was possibly caused by a peripheral neuropathy secondary to the diabetes. She was depressed, her husband was unemployed and they had financial difficulties. She was the sole carer for her young schizophrenic daughter.

The examiner asked me to summarize her main problems and he wanted to know what else I would have asked if I had had more time. He asked me what she might find most difficult to cope with and wanted a discussion about her dietary restriction of gluten, sugar and cholesterol. I had to outline what dietary advice I would give and the examiner also asked if I thought her diabetes was well controlled and how often I would test her haemoglobin A1c.

Station 3

This young lady presented with increasing shortness of breath on exertion.
I found aortic regurgitation but no stigmata of subacute bacterial endocarditis.

They asked me for the causes of aortic regurgitation and how I would monitor her to determine when, and if, valve replacement was going to be necessary. They asked me what advice I would give her about preventing endocarditis and what prophylaxis would I choose for: (a) dental work; and (b) a colonoscopy.

This elderly lady has had some falls and now has difficulty with mobility. Please examine her upper limbs.
I found dystonia and choreoathetoid movements mainly affecting her left side. However, I felt the need to perform a full upper limb examination and I also examined her gait. I was not interrupted at all.

They asked me for a likely cause and I plumped for the side-effects of anti-Parkinsonian medication. They asked me how I would manage her and they expected a discussion of other therapeutic options. I remembered to say that I would include the patient in the discussion because most patients would prefer to be jerky and switched on than rigid and completely immobile. They asked me what other abnormal movements one might find in drug-induced dystonia and they were expecting me to say facial grimacing and orofacial dyskinesias.

Station 4

This is a young woman in her fifties who has had a non-small-cell lung cancer treated 2 years ago with radio-

therapy. She now has extensive metastases in her spine causing pain down her right leg. You have the bone scan results which she does not yet know. Discuss them with her.
The patient was a very good actress. I asked her what she was worried about and she volunteered that she thought the cancer may have spread and at this stage she became tearful. She did not want her husband to know just yet because they were due to go to France on a holiday with all her family including her grandchildren and she did not want it to spoil the holiday. She promised she would tell him on their return because she appreciated that he needed to be involved as her main carer. She also did not want a letter to go to her GP until their return in case the GP told her husband. She desperately wanted to be able to go on the holiday as she thought it may be the last one she would have. I explained that I needed to see the films myself and to discuss with the radiologist to see if there was any evidence of cord compression, but on the whole I felt the right thing to do was to let her go on her holiday.

They asked me questions about holiday insurance and would the insurance company pay to get her treated abroad if her illness was already known? They asked me if she was legally obliged to tell her insurance company of her deterioration and would a fellow EEC country treat her anyway? Would the insurance company pay to get her back home if she deteriorated rapidly? Are you skating on thin ice if you do not notify the GP straight away?

Station 5

This middle-aged man complains of headaches. Would you like to assess him and tell me why.
He was acromegalic but with inactive disease. They quickly stopped me examining him any further when they were satisfied that I knew the diagnosis.

The questions included, 'How would you confirm the diagnosis?', 'What imaging modalities would you use and why?', 'What typical visual field defect do patients get?' (they did not ask me to demonstrate this).

Examine this man's fundus. Just the right one.
I found dot and blot haemorrhages with a normal macula. He had a bilateral corneal arcus and I said the diagnosis was background diabetic retinopathy.

They asked me why I wanted the light on in the room at the beginning and they said, 'Good for you!', when I answered that I was looking for a ptosis, arcus, pupillary irregularity and xanthelasmas. They then asked why I did not use the green light and suggested that I look again. They laughed when I said I never use it. They said, 'Nobody does, but don't the haemorrhages and aneurysms look much clearer?'

Have a look at this lady's hands and talk me through your examination.

She had rheumatoid hands with no obvious skin thinning or purpura, but she did have a Cushingoid face.

They asked me what treatments she might be taking and I suggested steroids. They asked what other investigations would be appropriate and I replied a DEXA scan. 'Good girl', they said.

Have a look at this lady who presented to the casualty department with acute shortness of breath and tell me why.

The lady had adenoma sebaceum and subungual fibromas, so I diagnosed tuberous sclerosis.

They wanted a spontaneous pneumothorax, caused by lung fibrosis and bleb formation as the cause of the acute shortness of breath. I did not get this!

Examine this man's neck.

He had definite pseudoxanthoma elasticum.

They asked whether this was inherited or acquired and I said, 'Acquired'. They then asked what drugs have been implicated and I said penicillamine. They wanted to know which condition(s) is penicillamine exclusively used for. I mentioned autoimmune 'things' but they specifically wanted Wilson's disease. Looking back, he was a young man with Parkinsonian features.

Comments

I sat the traditional format of the exam in October 2000. This new PACES exam was much fairer. It gave you time to compose yourself and collect your thoughts before moving onto the next case. I started with the history-taking station. This went particularly well and gave me the confidence to proceed. In this sense it tests what you do every day in a more realistic manner than the previous format. Candidates with good English skills definitely have an advantage in the history and ethics stations. The examiners never interrupted me in the main stations. There does seem more time for discussion and I would suggest that candidates need to have thought of the answers before they are asked, as the questions were really quite predictable.

A colleague of mine missed her first murmur so was taken to a second cardiovascular case. She definitely got this one correct and still passed.

4 *She was short in stature and had a large head with a hearing aid, so I immediately looked at her shins. They were a bit prominent so I said Paget's disease and felt very pleased with myself. Unfortunately, the examiners weren't pleased at all.*

Station 1

This gentleman is breathless on climbing stairs. Examine his respiratory system.

I found diminished chest expansion with intercostal retraction and the use of accessory muscles, the lung fields were hyperresonant with no audible wheeze and the liver dullness was obliterated. I completed my examination by saying that I would like to examine his sputum pot and look at his peak flow chart.

I was asked, 'What did you notice when you examined this patient from the end of the bed?' 'Intercostal retraction', I replied. I was asked what diagnosis I was considering and I replied that it was most likely chronic obstructive pulmonary disease (COPD). They then asked for the criteria for long-term oxygen therapy.

During my examination of the patient I was interrupted while I was assessing vocal resonance, with the examiner asking me, 'Why are you doing that?' I said that I was looking for consolidation. The examiner said, 'Do you think there is any consolidation?', and my answer was, 'No'.

The moral of this is do not do something for the sake of completion. Instead, show the examiner that you are thinking while you examine.

This gentleman was found collapsed. Examine his abdomen and give a differential as to the cause of his collapse.

I found mild jaundice, spider naevi, dilated veins, hepatomegaly but no splenomegaly and there was definite ascites. There was no flapping tremor or any other stigmata of chronic liver disease.

I was asked for some possible causes for his collapse and I suggested encephalopathy, hypoglycaemia, alcohol intoxication/withdrawal, fits or anaemia. Then they asked me how I would manage the patient and how much fluid I would shift in a day. I said not more than 1 kg in weight with careful monitoring of his kidney function.

Station 2

This patient has a serum cholesterol level of 8 and triglycerides of 2 mmol/L. He has persistent symptoms of claudication despite previous vascular surgery. The surgeons have referred him to you for an opinion regarding the use of a statin.

This gentleman had no other risk factors for ischaemic heart disease or for a stroke apart from being a heavy smoker and the raised cholesterol. He had a previous alcohol problem but this was now under control. He had the classic symptoms of peripheral vascular disease (PVD) which seemed not to have resolved with surgery. I persisted with the idea of a recurrence of the PVD on the grafted vessel.

At the end of the discussion I was asked how I thought the interview went. My response was that I thought it went well (I was trying to seem confident even though I was not). I think I failed to entertain other causes of pain such as neurogenic pain. Consequently, I was failed by one examiner in my interpretation and use of the information but I made up for it with clear passes in obtaining data and in the discussion. I therefore passed the station.

I was also requested to answer the surgeon's question. The answer I gave was, 'Yes', but a more accurate answer would be that he should be on both a statin and a fibrate because of the increased triglycerides and that he needs a complete lipid profile. The triglyceride level of 2 mmol/L is at the top end of the normal range. The initial treatment would be with a statin alone.

Station 3

Examine this patient's cardiovascular system.

I found a regular pulse with good volume and a normal character. There was a displaced apex beat which was heaving. There was a pansystolic murmur at the apex and a mid-diastolic murmur best heard in the left lateral position. There was also an early diastolic murmur at the left sternal border.

The examiner asked for my diagnosis. I answered that there was mixed mitral valve disease and aortic regurgitation and that the predominant lesion was mitral regurgitation. The examiner asked, 'What investigation would you do?' I said, 'Full blood count, urea and electrolytes, liver function tests and a coagulation screen'. The examiner was surprised. He asked me why I would do these. I had to think of reasons to justify what I would ordinarily do in a routine day's work. I said the patient may have infective endocarditis and I may wish to start antibiotics or to anticoagulate. He asked me, 'What is the definitive

test?' I replied, 'An echo'. He asked, 'When would you refer for surgery?'

Examine this lady's central nervous system. She has difficulty in dressing.

There was wasting of the small muscles of the hands with a claw hand. The upper and lower limb muscles were wasted bilaterally. The tone was normal but power was reduced because of the wasting distally. The reflexes were intact.

The examiner asked, 'What is your diagnosis?' I did not have a clue! The examiner then asked what else I had noticed. At this point I saw fasciculation, so I said the patient could have motor neurone disease. While examining the patient, I did the finger–nose test which was normal. I went on to look for dysdiadochokinesis and the examiner stopped me to say, 'Now what does that tell you?' I think he was trying to point out that I had already established that there was no cerebellar lesion so why was I wasting time.

Station 4

A 28-year-old lady with a recurrence of Hodgkin's lymphoma, and who has refused further chemotherapy, presents in casualty with a deep vein thrombosis (DVT). She refuses warfarin and prefers to take herbal medication. Try to convince her to take warfarin.

The patient's point was that she had lost faith in doctors as they had failed to cure her Hodgkin's disease. She had therefore reverted to alternative medicine. She was very tearful as she thought that everyone felt that she was being difficult.

I started the conversation by assuring her that she was not being difficult and that it was perfectly normal to feel apprehensive. She wanted to know for how long, if she took the warfarin, should she continue with it and, once she stopped it, would the clot recur. I said there was no guarantee that it would not recur. To that she said, 'Why should I take something that is not going to cure me?' I explained about the potential risk of further thromboembolic disease to which she said, 'Well, I am dying anyway'. I finally managed to convince her to come back to clinic the next week to speak to me again after she had talked it over with her husband.

I was asked what the ethical issues were and replied that the patient has a right to refuse treatment and that the medical staff must do what is best for that patient. He then went on to ask for my opinion as to what would be the best way to discuss this issue further with the patient. I said that probably it would be best to have a group discussion with her in the presence of her family and with senior members of the medical team and the palliative care team (case conference). I was then asked what I thought about her request to try alternative medicines. I replied that I could not endorse it but that I did not have any problems with it so long as there were no interactions or contraindications of any sort.

Station 5

This lady has had multiple fractures. What is your diagnosis?
She was short in stature and had a large head with a hearing aid so I immediately looked at her shins. They were a bit prominent so I said Paget's disease and felt very pleased with myself. Unfortunately, the examiners were not pleased at all.

I was told to look harder and I still did not have a clue. One examiner took pity on me and said, 'Look at her neck and elbow'. She had so much loose skin on her that I said, 'pseudoxanthoma elasticum', which again was wrong. So I began to think, what has something in the neck and elbow and is short in stature? I started looking at her spine and one examiner cheekily said, 'You won't find anything there'. I took a shot in the dark and rather unconvincingly said, 'Turner's syndrome'. This was followed by, 'So, tell us the complications of Turner's syndrome'.

Examine the patient's fundus.
I found hard exudates and a circinate around the macula.

I was asked the diagnosis so I said, 'There is background diabetic retinopathy with hard exudates'. One examiner passed me and the other one failed me. I should have said, 'There is a circinate maculopathy with background changes as well'. One examiner kept asking me . . . what else? . . . what else? I was too unsure to comment.

Examine the patient's hands.
I found swelling of the metacarpophalangeal joints, proximal and distal interphalangeal joints, ulnar deviation and the surgical scars of previous tendon transplants. There were no psoriatic patches and there was some functional limitation.

I was asked the diagnosis and suggested rheumatoid arthritis. This was wrong! I was asked why I thought this. I said there was a symmetrical polyarthropathy. However, in actual fact there was one joint that was spared which I had failed to notice. And, although there were no psoriatic patches there was minimal nail pitting and onycholysis.

This time I was not so lucky and failed on this case.

Examine the patient's hand.
There was tight skin with minimal telangiectasiae.

I was asked to give the diagnosis so I volunteered scleroderma. I was asked about the major complications, usual causes of death, and treatment options. I was asked about other questions I could ask her. This was to determine the associated features.

Comments

By and large the examiners are very nice.

They are stone-cold in expression and that often makes you feel that you are doing badly but it is not always true.

Do not feel obliged to complete or stick to your routines for the sake of it. Examiners prefer it if you think and show that you are able to change your routines and adapt as necessary. Do not do something for the sake of it when it is obvious that it is not going to yield any positive signs.

Do not lose hope even if you think you are doing badly. That only makes the rest of the stations feel worse.

---

5 *The 'son' was an SpR in medicine who was a dismal actor with no infexion, actions or responses. It was very different from a real 'relative' or actor.*

Station 1

Examine this man's chest from the back.
There was a tender area on the anterior chest wall at about the third or fourth intercostal space just to the right of the midline, together with a deformity of the anterior chest at the apex. I found reduced expansion on the right side with reduced breath sounds and increased vocal resonance at the right apex.

I was asked about the significance of the increased vocal resonance and for the underlying diagnosis. The examiner wanted to know the significance of the tender area which also had a small scar over it. I assumed that there had been a previous biopsy. Both examiners gave me 1/4.

Examine this man's abdomen.
The patient was a middle-aged man who was obese and appeared Cushingoid. He had multiple scars on his right

wrist but there was no arteriovenous fistula. There was a thyroidectomy scar. There were at least six abdominal scars and some deep small scars which looked like healed fistulas or drain sites. There was also fullness in the left iliac fossa.

The examiner asked what else I noticed so I replied that he appeared Cushingoid with muscle wasting. I was asked for a diagnosis so offered the possibility of a relapsing/remitting disease such as Crohn's. 'What else could it be?' he asked. I suggested a renal transplant. The examiner asked what all the scars were for. I thought that one of the scars in the right iliac fossa would be an appendectomy, the other two might be from a renal transplant that was later removed. The scar in the left iliac fossa was probably a later transplant which was still present. The midline scars could have been from peritoneal dialysis, infection, drains, etc. My marks were 1/4 and 2/4.

Station 2

This man has been losing weight. Please take a history.
This was a real patient, a man in his fifties who appeared quite cachectic and had a nasogastric tube in place. He had lost 2 stone in weight over the last year with reduced appetite and he had postprandial vomiting. He had had a partial gastrectomy and proton pump inhibitors (PPIs) had failed to eradicate multiple gastric and duodenal ulcers. His past medical history included alcoholic pancreatitis and a partial pancreatectomy in 1985 which then led to insulin-dependent diabetes. He had also had Henoch–Schönlein purpura. He had not drunk any alcohol since 1985. He had also been a heavy smoker until then and since had cut down to 20 cigarettes/day. He was unsure of his medication and had no known allergies. However, he was on ferrous sulphate which had given him black stools, and creon which had resolved the steatorrhoea. PPIs had had little effect. The family history revealed that his mother had died from cancer at the age of 48 but the primary was unknown. He had retired early from journalism because of ill-health and now lives alone. He was otherwise well and his diarrhoea seemed to be related to medical compliance.

I was asked to present his history and to say what I thought was contributing to his problem. I suggested that his smoking must be irritating any ulcers that are present. 'And his physicians!' was the reply. Then they asked what investigations I would like to do. I mentioned an endoscopy (OGD), biopsy and histology and was told that these were all normal. As he had multiple peptic ulcers which had not healed on high doses of PPI they wanted me to consider the Zollinger–Ellison syndrome and to do a gastrin level. Marks: 4/4, 4/4.

Station 3

You are seeing this elderly lady in the cardiology clinic. She has been attending for some time.
She had a midline sternotomy scar, a displaced apex and a prosthetic first heart sound.

Before I listened, the examiner asked me what I thought, and then afterwards said, 'What's the diagnosis?', 'Is the valve functioning well?', 'How do you know?', 'If you were seeing her in clinic what would you ask her?', 'What causes for anaemia would you think of?' Marks 3/4, 3/4.

Examine this man's legs.
The patient was in his mid-thirties. He had an upper motor neurone weakness in the left leg with a normal right leg and an upper motor neurone facial nerve palsy.

The examiner asked me what else I noticed and I replied that the left arm was also paralysed. He said, 'What would you consider if the left arm had lower motor neurone signs?' He wanted me to say, 'Cervical myelopathy'. 'Why is this not the diagnosis?' He wanted to hear that the weakness was not symmetrical and that there was no fasciculation. 'Demonstrate his facial nerve signs', 'Why is this an upper motor neurone lesion?', 'What do you think has happened to him?' I suggested a differential of embolic disease, a haemorrhagic event and a space-occupying lesion. 'What do *you* think happened?' 'A subarachnoid haemorrhage'. 'Yes!' Marks 3/4, 3/4.

Station 4

You are the SHO on call at night. You have to see the son of a patient who you do not know. She presented yesterday with a fit and the CT scan today shows a large mass consistent with a glioblastoma. She had a transient ischaemic attack (TIA) 4 months ago and the CT scan at that time was reported as normal and she was given aspirin. The son is irritated that he was told by the ward sister on arrival that his mother has a brain tumour.
The 'son' was a specialist registrar in medicine who was a dismal actor with no inflexion, actions or responses. It was very different from a real 'relative' or actor. As an introduction I asked him what he knew already. He was angry at having been told by the ward sister in the corridor. I apologized. 'Don't you have mechanisms for this kind of thing?' Again, I apologized. The son asked me, 'What can we do for her?' I said that this needs to be discussed with the team and with the neurosurgeons but that it was likely to be inoperable. He asked if this had been missed on the CT scan 4 months ago as his mother had never been right since that time. I said that I personally would not know and that the scan needed to be re-

viewed by the neuroradiologists. He wanted to know what might have been if it had been diagnosed 4 months ago. I did not know but explained that we needed to move on from where we were now. I discussed the complaints process.

The examiner asked me what I thought about his grievance that 4 months had made a difference. I answered that we needed to discuss this with the neurosurgeon. There was a possibility that a swelling was visible on the CT scan 4 months ago but even so we still need to discuss it with the neurosurgeon.

'Couldn't you have put him off from complaining? You told him about the complaints procedure.' I replied that, 'It's not my role. I need to set up an appointment for him to discuss with the consultant and his mother to have it explained, but if he wishes to complain he is entitled to do so and trying to put him off will only make things worse.' The examiner went on to ask me, 'What about the way he was told?' 'One needs to apologize unreservedly', I said. 'What should you do next about it?' 'I would next find the ward sister, ask for her side of the story and discuss it with her.'

Station 5

Examine this lady's thyroid status.
She was a middle-aged lady who was euthyroid. There was no lid-lag or exophthalmos. She was in sinus rhythm at 80 beats/min. There was no tremor but there was a small nodule within the large goitre.

The examiner asked me what I thought. I said that she was euthyroid but that I would like to ask her some questions. He asked me what tests I would do to confirm. I said thyroid-stimulating hormone. He then asked me for my differential diagnosis.

Examine this lady's eyes.
Visual acuity was good on the left, even without glasses. On the right she was unable to see the first line of the Snellen chart although she was able to perceive light. On examination of movements, initially I thought there was defective abduction of the right eye but then I thought it was normal. On examining the pupils the right was dilated with no response but I was told that it was 'always like that'. The left pupil had normal direct and consensual responses, normal reaction to light and accommodation. On examining her fields the acuity was poor on the right and on the left there was a nasal field defect. I was stopped before I could examine the fundi. The bell rang just in time as I did not know what the diagnosis was!

One examiner gave me a clear pass on this eye case and the other a fail — I am not sure what to make of this!

Examine this lady's hands.
I found normal nails, elbows and skin. There was a symmetrical, deforming polyarthropathy affecting the metacarpophalangeal and proximal interphalangeal joints.

I was asked for the diagnosis, what else I would like to examine, how to treat her and about the use of first-line disease-modifying drugs.

Examine this lady's skin.
There were lots of red plaques, particularly on the elbows. I felt that they may indicate psoriasis but there was no scaling.

'Where else would you look for psoriasis?' Answer: scalp. 'Go on then.' I found psoriasis on the scalp. 'What else would you like to look for?' Answer: arthropathy. I found an asymmetrical arthropathy involving the distal interphalangeal joints and was asked about treatment — both for the skin and the joints.

6 *What are the RCP guidelines for home oxygen and what is the evidence behind the guidelines?*

Station 1

This gentleman is short of breath, please examine the chest.
The patient was very cachectic and using the accessory muscles for respiration. On further examination I found clubbing and bibasal, fine, end-inspiratory crepitations.

The examiner asked me for my diagnosis and to give some possible causes. 'What investigations would you do?', he asked, 'and what would you expect to find on arterial blood gasses, X-rays and CT scan of the thorax?', 'What is his prognosis, and how can one tell?' The examiner carried on with questions, 'What are the RCP guidelines for home oxygen and what is the evidence behind the guidelines?' and 'How would you counsel the patient and what advice would you give him?'

This lady presents with lethargy, please examine her abdomen.
My clinical findings were of a thin, pale lady with no stigmata of chronic liver disease but I did find hepatosplenomegaly. I thought the diagnosis could be myelofibrosis.

I was asked for a differential diagnosis, how would I investigate the patient, and then what would I expect to find on a full blood count, film, and bone marrow aspiration. He wanted to know what I thought would be the prognosis and how would I counsel the patient, 'What problems can occur with the platelets?' Then there was a discussion about platelet storage disorders and coagulopathies, and finally we touched on the treatment of disseminated intravascular coagulopathy.

Station 2

This 70-year-old gentleman has recently moved to our practice and has noticed worsening of his diarrhoea. He was diagnosed with ulcerative colitis 5 years ago at his local hospital and has been on mesalazine ever since. He has also had two pulmonary emboli in the past. I would welcome your advice.

The patient had concerns that he needed a colectomy as he had recently noticed a deterioration in his vision, and he had been told initially that if he had too many complications that a colectomy would be needed. He had originally been diagnosed following a colonoscopy and biopsy. However, he had been on mesalazine since diagnosis, with no problems. He was having about three bowel actions per day with no blood or mucus and the patient was not concerned about the frequency despite the GP's comments. He had also seen an ophthalmologist who had reassured him regarding the formation of an early cataract which was probably steroid-induced. He had had only three courses of steroids for flare-ups since diagnosis. He could not remember if he was on a calcium supplement but thought he did have 'weak bones'.

The first pulmonary embolus occurred during the initial illness following a deep vein thrombosis (DVT). He was treated with warfarin for 3 months and then it was stopped. Two years later, following a flight back from Australia, he developed another pulmonary embolus. He was aware that he is now on warfarin for life. He is fit and independent and lives with his wife. He visits his son in Sydney every year and has no problems with his bowels when flying.

The examiner asked me about the patient's priorities and concerns, and were they the same as the GP's or mine. They wanted to know what I would do next. I said that I would reassure him, arrange a routine colonoscopy and get his notes from the old hospital. 'Why do you want to scope him?', they asked, 'and what would you do regarding his warfarin if rectal bleeding should become a problem?' They asked me about the eye complications of inflammatory bowel disease and what evidence there is for the need for bone protection with steroid therapy.

Station 3

This gentleman has been more short of breath recently, please examine.

I only found a possible collapsing pulse and the early diastolic murmur of aortic regurgitation.

The examiners asked, 'Why do you think it is aortic regurgitation and not mitral stenosis?', 'What qualities are discriminatory?', 'How would you investigate?', 'What would you look for on the transthoracic echo?', 'What would you tell the patient?' 'If it was aortic stenosis what would you expect to find, what problems would you expect and what would be decisions for surgery, etc.' 'How would you initiate warfarin, and what would you tell the patient about risks, etc.' 'Why don't you think it could be a ventricular septal defect (VSD)?'

This gentleman is having difficulty reading his newspaper. Please examine his hands and proceed accordingly.

It was a Polish chap who was sitting with his wife and was fully clothed. He had a blank expression. I found a fine, resting tremor bilaterally and there was increased tone with lead pipe and cog-wheel rigidity. I was told not to focus on his hands (muscles, power sensation, etc.) as there would be nothing to find. I assessed his gait and it was hesitant and shuffling. I found a gross tremor on finger–nose testing but there was no dysdiadochokinesia. There were no other cerebellar signs and the speech was normal.

I was asked for a differential diagnosis and would I like to ask him some questions. I said that Parkinson's disease was above benign essential tremor in my list of possibilities but after asking how long he had had the tremor for I was invited to revise my order! I was then asked how I would treat both of these conditions and what role does physiotherapy have in the management of Parkinson's disease.

Station 4

You are the medical SHO in clinic and are about to meet Mrs X who is the daughter of the patient, Mr Y, who underwent an endoscopy (OGD) for dyspepsia last week. They have returned to clinic for the results of the investigations. Mr Y is hard of hearing so has asked you to speak to his daughter while he is next door getting changed. The results have come back, surprisingly, as gastric carcinoma. You are expected to inform the daughter of the results and discuss further options.

The conversation flowed easily as the lady was very understanding and calm. She took the diagnosis very well and then progressed to ask some sensible questions. She was obviously upset and asked me questions about how long, how bad, should he cancel his holiday to visit his son and newborn grandson in the USA which was due in 2 weeks' time, should she tell her brother to come over, will her father be admitted, what treatment is there, will he be in pain, how will she tell him, how does she tell her mother, etc.

I addressed each question in turn, clearly explaining those that I could answer and those we would leave on hold until after the CT scan and the combined meeting, etc. We agreed to meet up next week with the CT scan results and the decision about surgical treatment options.

The examiners asked me how I felt the conversation went. They asked if I thought it was too harsh using the word 'cancer'. Then they went on to question me about the first principles of talking to relatives in terms of consent, autonomy, etc. 'What would happen if the family did not want him told or if they didn't want him to have an operation?' 'What would you do if the patient wanted treatment but the family were not happy?

Station 5

This lady has headaches, please examine and proceed accordingly.
I found that the patient had acromegaly with a bitemporal field defect and carpel tunnel syndrome.

The examiner asked me if I thought that the disease was active and how I would investigate and treat. 'What would you tell the patient?' they asked me. 'What does visual field testing involve?'

Please examine this man's fundi.
My clinical findings were of the background changes of diabetic retinopathy with two laser scars visible just below the macula. The eyedrops were wearing off so I was unable to get a full view of the left eye. However, the examiners seemed satisfied that I tried!

They asked me for my diagnosis and would I be concerned if this gentleman was examined in clinic and these findings were detected? What would I suggest regarding follow up? What is the pathophysiology of the lesion requiring coagulation? How would you manage the patient and what is the evidence for such treatment? Should he be driving?

This gentleman keeps dropping things. Please examine him.
He had severe, chronic, rheumatoid arthritis with fusion of the wrists and various joint replacements. There was obvious purpura so the patient was possibly on steroids.

I was asked for my management plan in terms of pharmacological and non-pharmacological methods. He wanted to know how I would assess function and what impact would this have on his quality of life. What could I suggest to help with some of the household chores? He then said, 'Imagine you are a rheumatologist and this pa-

tient has been referred to you with rheumatoid arthritis that is resistant to all first- and second-line disease-modifying agents, what would you suggest, what are the side-effects of using TNF (tumour necrosis factor) and what are the contraindications of using such drugs?'

This lady has had an episode of episaxis, please examine and proceed accordingly.
She had telangiectasiae over her face and around her mouth. There were no peripheral lesions to suggest CRST syndrome.

I was asked for the diagnosis and how I would manage the patient. What would you tell her? What would you expect to find if you were examining other members of the family? What would you do and what is the prognosis?

7 *I thought in my head that the patient had Cushing's syndrome but for some bizarre reason I said the patient had scleroderma!*

Station 1

This man has a cough. Please examine his chest.
He had coarse crackles over the right lower and mid zones but there were no other physical signs. I said that bronchiectasis was the most likely diagnosis.

The examiner asked what my investigation of choice would be. I suggested a chest X-ray, high-resolution CT scan, bronchoscopy and sputum analysis. There was a discussion of all of these.

This man has high blood pressure. Please examine his abdomen.
On examination I found that he had a left arteriovenous fistula with a thrill. There were warts on his hands and he had a midline sternotomy scar. He had a right hernia scar, no organomegaly, and I forgot to auscultate.

I was asked what my concern would be in a patient with high blood pressure when performing an abdominal examination. I said that I would look for polycystic kidney disease and renal artery stenosis. 'Oh!' I said, 'I would have auscultated for bruits'. He asked me about the warts and we discussed immunosuppression but I could not palpate a transplanted kidney and the fistula was active. I was then asked for the causes of a failed transplant and I was shown the medication chart. He was on cyclosporin and prednisolone. Then the examiner said, 'What about the midline sternotomy scar?' I said, 'Has he had a heart transplant?' and they said, 'Yes!'

Station 2

You are in the outpatient clinic. Mr X is a 50-year-old man with a history of alcoholic cirrhosis and variceal bleeding. He presents with abdominal pain. Please review his medications.

The whole experience was awful. He had had about 15 previous hospital admissions with various degrees of cirrhosis and hepatic decompensation. I had no time to review his medications and when I finally did the bell went and the examiner shouted 'Give it back!' at me as I was reading the prescription chart.

The questions I was asked by the examiner included, 'What were the main differential diagnoses?', 'Do you think that he has truly given up drinking?' and 'What precipitated him to give up drinking?'

Station 3

This man has just returned from ITU. Please examine his cardiovascular system.
He had a midline sternotomy scar. There was gynaecomastia and a tracheostomy site which was covered with gauze. He had a right brachial percutaneous transluminal coronary angioplasty (PTCA) scar and there was peripheral oedema. He had prosthetic second heart sounds with no features to suggest a leaking valve. He was in congestive cardiac failure but there were no stigmata of subacute bacterial endocarditis.

The examiner asked me, 'What are the likely causes of gynaecomastia in this man?' I replied that it could be a result of digoxin and spironolactone in a patient with a cardiovascular history. The examiner wanted to know, 'What else causes gynaecomastia on an ITU?' I had no idea!

This man is unable to walk. Examine his legs.
He had an ulcer on the base of his right foot and there was a urinary catheter *in situ*. He had global reduction of tone, power, reflexes, coordination, vibration sense and proprioception and there was a stocking distribution sensory loss.

The first question was, 'Do you think that testing coordination in a patient with 3/5 weakness and who can't walk is helpful?' 'No', I said, feeling very stupid. Then the examiner asked me for a differential diagnosis and I said that he had a sensory motor neuropathy. I was asked why I included a motor element. I replied, 'Because of the weakness'. He asked me what could explain the need for a catheter and I wondered if he had a corda equina lesion. 'What else would you want to do?' In retrospect I should have said, 'Ask about the timing of the onset'. Instead I uttered, 'Examine the remainder of the nervous system!' The last question was, 'Would you expect signs in the arms with a corda equina lesion?' 'No', I said.

Station 4

This is a middle-aged lady who has a top position in cosmetic sales and today she has had her first seizure. You are the SHO on call. She is almost ready to leave the casualty department and you need to instruct her about the implications for driving, about possible treatment options and the need to avoid other dangerous situations.
We discussed the presentation of the seizure and that it may not necessarily be epilepsy. The patient was very concerned about why she had had a fit and what could be done to find the cause. She was extremely upset about the driving implications as driving was her livelihood.

The examiner quizzed me on, 'Would I, and when would I, inform the DVLA, what would I tell her boss if he telephoned, and what might be important to mention about treatment if she requires it?'

Station 5

This lady has uncontrolled hypertension. Please examine her.
I thought in my head that the patient had Cushing's syndrome, but for some bizarre reason (?microstomia) I said the patient had scleroderma! The examiner said, 'No, what are the causes of high blood pressure?' I said that 90% were idiopathic, 10% were a result of endocrine causes such as Cushing's and Conn's syndromes and a small number had renal artery stenosis. The examiner said, 'One of those answers is correct'. Then she asked the patient to stand up and she had obvious proximal myopathy. We discussed the causes of Cushing's syndrome and then she said, 'The patient has a mass in the pituitary on an MRI scan. What would you examine to assess the size?' 'Visual fields', I said. Then she asked me to demonstrate.

This lady has had neurosurgery. Please examine her eyes.
I found a right upper homonymous quadrantanopia but I was not asked any questions as the bell went at this stage.

Examine this lady's hands.
I found a symmetrical deforming arthropathy with scars over the wrists. There were no nail changes. She also had scars over both elbows but there were no nodules and no evidence of psoriasis.

I said the patient had rheumatoid arthritis and the examiner asked if I was sure about this to which I replied, 'Yes'. The examiner asked me if it could be anything else. I replied that, 'If psoriatic plaques had been present then possibly this could be arthritis mutilans as there was evidence of telescoping of the fingers'. He then asked if I thought one had to have psoriatic plaques in order to have psoriatic arthropathy. I replied, 'Probably not!' I was asked what drugs she could be on and I suggested nonsteroidals. The examiner asked me, 'Would you take methotrexate?'

This man has itchy skin. Please examine.
He had thickened skin with diffuse extensive erythema and multiple abrasions.

I said I would be concerned about the drug history. 'What else?', they asked. 'I would consider infections such as herpes zoster but the abnormality is not in a dermatome distribution.' The examiner asked, 'What would give you extensive skin thickening?' I replied, 'Repeated trauma and itching'. 'What diffuse processes?', he asked and I suggested, 'Psoriasis or eczema'. 'Yes', he said, 'This is eczema!'

Comments

The exam was horrible and extremely stressful. I felt like an idiot with things coming out of my mouth that I wished had stayed in.

Afterwards, I was full of *disappointment* that they did not see the real me, *frustration* about what did they really want when they asked a question and *tears* both of relief and a fear of failure.

---

8 *I was asked 'What is the diagnosis and what investigations would you do next?' I said, 'A chest X-ray' and they produced one!*

Station 1

This man complains of shortness of breath. Examine him and found out why.
He had obvious finger clubbing with bibasal, inspiratory, fine crepitations.

I was asked, 'What is the diagnosis and what investigations would you do next?' I said, 'It's pulmonary fibrosis and I would do a chest X-ray'. They produced one! 'Does this support your diagnosis?', 'What further tests would you do?', 'What causes pulmonary fibrosis?', 'Ask him some questions to find a cause'. I asked about his occupation and discovered that he was an electrician so they wanted me to ask about asbestos exposure. Finally the examiner asked, 'How would you treat him?'

This lady has thrombocytopenia. Examine her abdomen and come up with a likely diagnosis.
The lady had purpura on her forearms. I found a small

spleen but I could not feel a liver. She also had a lower midline abdominal scar.

The examiner asked me, 'What is the diagnosis?' I suggested that it was likely to be a lymphoproliferative or myeloproliferative disease. 'Does she have any petechiae?', 'Is the abdominal scar relevant?' I said she may have had a hysterectomy because of menorrhagia and he seemed satisfied with that answer. 'Would you expect hepatomegaly with your diagnoses?', he said.

Station 2

You are the SHO in clinic. This 57-year-old man has had asthma since the age of 7 and was then diagnosed with pulmonary eosinophilia in 1960. Since January he has had recurrent chest infections including Haemophilus influenzae pneumonia. Please see and advise.
The patient had never smoked and had not been treated for the pulmonary eosinophilia. He had been asthmatic most of his life but for the last few months had noticed increasing shortness of breath and a cough with green sputum and this was now associated with sweats. He had had repeated courses of antibiotics from his GP. He had worked as a wood machinist for 20 years. He had used a mask but his symptoms always improved when off work. He was now a manager for a cleaning company. He was on inhaled steroids and had been on oral prednisolone 10 mg/day for the past 10 weeks.

I was asked to give an account of the history. The examiner said, 'What do you think is going on?' I said it could be poorly controlled asthma or pulmonary eosinophilia but he may now have bronchiectasis secondary to allergic bronchopulmonary aspergillosis (ABPA). After offering this diagnosis they asked, 'How do you diagnose ABPA?', 'What blood tests could you do?', 'How do you treat it?' I mentioned postural drainage, etc. 'If the bronchiectasis is localized to the upper lobes how could you treat it?' 'Have you heard of a flutter valve?' I said, 'No!'

Station 3

This man has a heart murmur. Please examine him.
He was in sinus rhythm with a non-displaced apex but with a pansystolic murmur best heard at the apex and radiating to the axilla. There was a midline abdominal scar.

The examiner asked me, 'What is the murmur?', 'What are the features that make you say mitral regurgitation?', 'Can you connect the murmur and the abdominal scar?' I said, 'No', and he said, 'We'll come back to it at the end and I bet you get it!' Then he asked me about the causes of mitral regurgitation and finally he asked about the scar again. I said he may have had mitral regurgitation secondary to ischaemic heart disease and therefore he may have generalized atheromatous disease with an abdominal aortic aneurysm repair. He said, 'Told you so!'

This lady has difficulty walking. Please examine her legs.
She had a broad-based gait but was steady on her feet. There was lower leg wasting but with brisk reflexes and upgoing plantars. I thought that she may also have a stocking distribution sensory loss.

The examiner said to me, 'You have described upper and lower motor neurone signs. What is the diagnosis?', 'How does the sensory component fit in?' I offered a combination of common diseases such as cervical myelopathy and diabetes. The examiner did not seem to be impressed! Thankfully, the bell went before he could grill me any more!

Station 4
A 75-year-old lady who had a stroke 1 year ago, now living alone with social services support, has presented with a gastrointestinal bleed but is stable. You have requested an endoscopy (OGD). There is no organic confusion but the patient has refused the investigation and says she wants to die. Her daughter has come from Scotland. Explain to her what is going on.
The daughter was very upset. She said, 'Mum isn't thinking straight, go ahead with the test, you must do everything. I'll sign the consent form.' I had to explain that her mother was not confused and we had to abide with her wishes. Then the daughter said that her mother had been depressed at home and that she is doing this to spite her as she has had little contact with her mother since moving to Scotland. I explained that I would ask my consultant to see her and that also I would get a psychiatric opinion to exclude depression.

The examiner said, 'What is the essential problem here?' I said, 'A consent problem in someone who is refusing treatment and who is mentally competent and of sound mind'. The examiner said, 'What is the legal term for that?' I didn't know. 'If she became comatosed would you do the OGD then?', 'Do you think the daughter will complain?', 'How would you prepare for this?'

Station 5
This man is followed up in the eye clinic. Have a look at him and tell me why.
I said the patient had exophthalmos.

The examiner said, 'Go on to examine his eyes'. I found he had diplopia but I forgot to mention the lid-lag. I ended up saying I would do fundoscopy. Somehow I then

got confused and started thinking of diabetes. It was all a bit of a mess!

This man has trouble with his vision.
He was wearing yellow, plastic glasses. The right eye looked normal but there were black, pigmented lesions on the temporal part of the retina of the left eye.

The examiner asked, 'What is the diagnosis?' I said, 'Choroidoretinitis', and he replied, 'Where did you see it?' He did not seem impressed and asked what would be my main differential. When I said retinitis pigmentosa he was satisfied. This diagnosis was confirmed by the registrar invigilator afterwards.

This man has had painful hands. Please examine him.
There were obvious rheumatoid changes in the hands with nodules at the elbows and evidence of previous surgery.

I was asked, 'What is the diagnosis? List your findings.' 'What could cause wasting of the small muscles of the hand in this man?' I went through all the neurological causes, e.g. nodules causing ulnar nerve palsy, etc., but he just wanted me to say 'diffuse atrophy'.

This lady has a rash. Examine it.
There was an obvious, deforming arthropathy of the hands with a rash on the dorsum of the upper arms and upper chest, i.e. the sun-exposed areas.

The examiner said, 'What do you think it is?' I said psoriasis at first but he asked, 'Is it the typical distribution, i.e. why is it worst on sun-exposed areas? What else could it be?' I said, 'systemic lupus erythematosus (SLE)'. Then he asked, 'Would SLE cause this degree of arthritis?' We eventually got around to mixed connective tissue disorders, which was the correct diagnosis.

Comments

The 5-min gaps between cases are great if it is a 'talking station' as you have time to prepare the given material. If it is a 'clinical station' it is too long to sit and become more nervous. They did supply us with drinks, though, to combat the xerostomia!

I ended with Station 1. As I was leaving, the examiner said, 'If I were you, I would go and have a good drink now!' I was not sure if this was meant to reassure me or not!

---

9 *The surgical registrar calls you and tells you that his SHO has been found collapsed in her room with syringes around her and with all the signs of diamorphine having been given.*

Station 1

Examine this patient's respiratory system.

The patient had a hoarse voice, a trachea that was central but there was a noticeable scar on the right side posteriorly with no other obvious chest deformity. He had, in fact, had a right-sided lobectomy.

The examiner asked me what I noticed about the voice and to explain my findings. I had to give some possible reasons why the patient had had a lobectomy. They asked me about the different types of lung cancer.

Examine this patient's abdomen.

The patient had bilateral Dupuytren's contractures which were more noticeable on the left side. There were lots of spider naevi on the chest wall and, on abdominal examination, there was hepatosplenomegaly. The examiner told me that he was anaemic and my diagnosis was of alcoholic liver disease.

I was asked for a differential diagnosis for hepatosplenomegaly and the examiner asked me if I thought he was anaemic. Then he changed the subject to questions about lymphadenopathy and hepatosplenomegaly, what investigations would I do and what would be my management plan.

Station 2

There was a GP letter regarding a 54-year-old lady who had moved from America 2 weeks previously. She presented with jaundice and pruritus to her GP who had carried out a blood test which showed abnormal liver function tests with an obstructive picture. She had a recent history of weight loss and had been using herbal medicines. She had now noticed swelling of her abdomen.

The history that evolved just clarified the information given in the GP letter.

I was asked for a differential diagnosis and what further investigations I would do and then what management I would instigate. I was asked for the causes of an obstructive picture in the liver function tests and I forgot to mention the important cause, i.e. gallstones (I was so preoccupied with the history of weight loss). Neither did I mention primary biliary cirrhosis!

Station 3

Look at this patient and describe what you see.* Then listen to the heart.

I found that the patient had a kyphoscoliosis with a wide arm span and a high-arched palate. On auscultation, it was obvious that he had had a mechanical aortic valve replacement but there was no evidence of a paraprosthetic leak.

The examiners first asked me to inspect the patient generally and to describe what I saw. I said he had the features of Marfan's syndrome but there was no obvious lens dislocation. Then they asked me to examine the heart. Next, they wanted to know how I would manage this patient in terms of anticoagulation with warfarin. I was expected to say that I would need to know the rest of the patient's drug history, especially with regard to any non-steroidal anti-inflammatory drugs (NSAID) medication. Finally, they asked me to outline the problems that can occur with valve replacement.

Examine this patient's cranial nerves and check the reflexes in the lower limbs as this patient has had noticeable weakness of both legs.

The patient had obvious nystagmus—internuclear ophthalmoplegia and brisk reflexes. I also checked for clonus, although I was not asked to do so, and found that the patient had noticeable sustained clonus.

The examiners asked for my diagnosis and I suggested demyelination as there was evidence of an internuclear ophthalmoplegia and a spastic paraparesis. They asked me what internuclear ophthalmoplegia is and I named five causes for it. The examiners seemed very happy with this case and they stopped me as soon as I had told them the causes of the ophthalmoplegia.

Station 4

You are the medical SHO on call. The surgical registrar calls you and tells you that his SHO has been found collapsed in her room with syringes around her and with signs of diamorphine having been given, such as pinpoint pupils. She has been given naloxone and has woken up. The surgical registrar would like you to talk to her.

I told her that the surgical registrar was concerned about her and that we suspected that she was abusing diamorphine. I explained to her the risks of hepatitis and HIV by using needles and this included explaining the risk to herself and to her patients. I had to tell her that her consultant would have to be informed. The SHO denied the use of intravenous drugs and said that she was a diabetic and was checking her blood sugars.

---

* A clue to the diagnosis is in the instruction.

The examiners asked me who I would like to inform, and I said the GMC, and would I suspend her from work and I said, 'Yes'.

Station 5

Examine this lady's neck.

She had a multinodular goitre with no bruits. She was euthyroid as she was not anxious or sweaty. There was no tremor, tachycardia or lid lag. I mentioned all of this to the examiner.

He asked me what sort of goitre she had and I responded that it was multinodular. He asked me for the most likely cause and what my further investigations and management would be.

Look at the fundi and describe what you find.

There were bilateral cataracts and bilateral laser therapy scars.

I initially forgot to mention the cataracts but managed to bring it into the conversation when one examiner asked me what else could I see. He asked me about the other complications of diabetes mellitus and about the use of ramipril and the HOPE study.

Examine this patient's gait.

He had a very protuberant abdomen and a kyphosis so I diagnosed ankylosing spondylitis.

The examiner asked me for the possible complications and I listed anterior uveitis, aortitis, apical fibrosis, atlantoaxial subluxation and the risks during anaesthesia.

Look at the hands, look at the face and give the diagnosis.

I found evidence of hypertrophic osteoarthropathy at the wrists and bilateral periorbital xanthelasma. These findings were not connected in any way.

The examiner asked me what X-ray finding I would see in hypertrophic osteoarthropathy and then he asked me what I could see when looking at the patient's face. I mentioned the xanthelasma.

Comments

It is more likely that one will not score as highly in the ethics and history-taking stations but that one can make up for this if one knows the clinical examination routines well.

Read the instructions properly at each station as they usually give vital clues.

Pretend that you are a registrar presenting cases on a ward round.

---

10 *It was unusual to have a Marfan's syndrome as the respiratory case. The patient was not a typical Marfan's because the kyphoscoliosis made him look much shorter and the flexure deformity of the fingers obscured the arachrodactyly.*

Station 1

This is a 56-year-old lady who has been dyspnoeic for a long time. Examine her respiratory system.

I found bilateral, fine, inspiratory basal crackles. I also noted the kyphoscoliosis and a scar over the back. I thought that there might be arachnodactyly and an arthropathy of the fingers.

I was asked to give my findings and to suggest the most likely diagnosis. I answered that it was likely to be ankylosing spondylitis with pulmonary fibrosis and that the dyspnoea may be caused by a chest wall deformity and a restricted ventilatory defect. After the exam, I met the patient in the car park and she told me that she had Marfan's syndrome!*

Examine this patient's abdomen.

The patient was moderately jaundiced with a possible parotid swelling and numerous spider naevi. The jugular venous pressure (JVP) was not raised. There was 4 finger-breadth hepatomegaly which was firm and non-tender. However, there was no splenomegaly and no oedema.

I was asked for a differential diagnosis.

Station 2

This 36-year-old lady has had arthritis for 3 years. There is a history of bronchial asthma and she is on oral steroids, and ventolin and becotide inhalers. There has been an increase in the joint pains. Please ask her some questions.

I obtained a history of a progressive polyarthritis, mainly affecting the small joints of the hands, elbows and knees. There was significant early morning stiffness and Raynaud's phenomenon but there was no photosensitivity, fever or any other extra-articular features. There was ankle swelling but the asthma was stable. There had been no response to the steroids despite the side-effects of weight gain and hypertension. The chest X-ray showed possible fibrosis.

I was asked for the likely causes of both lung and joint disease. Finally, the examiner confirmed that it was rheumatoid arthritis with lung involvement and I was asked about the management in terms of drug treatment with disease-modifying agents such as azathioprine and

---

* For respiratory complications of Marfan's syndrome see p. 407, *An Aid to the MRCP PACES*, Volume 1.

methotrexate. I then had to enumerate the side-effects of methotrexate.

Station 3

The GP has referred this 72-year-old lady with a murmur. Please examine her.

Examination showed that the patient was in atrial fibrillation although the pulse was strong and the carotid pulse was visible. There was a systolic murmur at the mitral area with no radiation. The murmur was also heard at the left sternal edge but not at the carotid root. Both heart sounds were normal with no other murmurs.

I was asked for a diagnosis and I offered a differential of mitral regurgitation and hypertrophic obstructive cardiomyopathy (HOCM). The discussion then centred on mitral regurgitation. I was asked again for a differential diagnosis and what would I consider if the patient's condition deteriorated. I suggested infective endocarditis and, possibly, pulmonary oedema.

Look at this patient and examine neurologically.

There was frontal balding with a bilateral partial ptosis. I also found weakness of the facial muscles and wasting of the small muscles. There was no gynaecomastia or myotonia.

The examiner asked me what I thought the diagnosis was, so I suggested myotonic dystrophy or myasthenia gravis. He asked how I would differentiate between the two and which did I think was the most likely? I was then asked how to confirm the diagnosis and for the investigation and management of myotonic dystrophy. He asked me, 'What is myotonia?' and 'What is the prognosis?'

Station 4

You are the SHO in chest medicine. A 57-year-old lady was admitted about 5 weeks ago with pneumonia. She has small muscle wasting and diaphragmatic weakness. A neurologist has been consulted and thinks this is motor neurone disease. You plan to do an electromyographical (EMG) study but the patient wants to know what is wrong. Please tell the patient about her condition, the management plan and the prognosis.

I explained about motor neurone disease and that the diagnosis is by exclusion of other causes. I told her that the management is very multidisciplinary rather than with a specific drug treatment. She wanted a second opinion and to know the prognosis. She wanted to know about any feeding and respiratory difficulties. I explained that her pneumonia was probably a result of aspiration because of difficulty with swallowing and that

she might need a percutaneous endoscopic gastrostomy (PEG) in the future. I also told her of the poor prognosis but that we needed to exclude other possibilities.

The examiners asked about the fact that the patient lived alone. Would she need residential or nursing home care at some stage? 'Should the patient be allowed a second opinion?' 'Yes', I said, 'she has a right to that'. 'Are there any newer treatments?' 'Yes, there is riluzole which improves the quality of life but does not improve survival.'

Station 5

Look at this patient.

I noticed the obvious features of acromegaly and I was asked about the investigations and management.

This elderly man has had a sudden onset of blindness in his right eye. Please examine him and explain why.

There was right-sided optic atrophy with attenuation of the vessels in the right temporal region but there was no cherry-red spot.

I was asked for the diagnosis and suggested either central retinal artery occlusion or an ischaemic optic neuropathy.

This is a lady of about 80 years. Please look at her hands.

She had a bilateral symmetrical arthropathy with the distal interphalangeal joints involved as well. There were Heberden's nodes and gouty tophi and subluxation of the metacarpophalangeal joints.

I was asked for a differential diagnosis and then asked which features were in favour of rheumatoid arthritis and which were against this possibility. Also, which features were for and against osteoarthritis.

Look at this patient's face.

I saw lupus pernio and lots of telangiectasiae.

I was asked for the diagnosis so said, 'Lupus pernio, and possibly hereditary haemorrhagic telangiectasiae (HHT) as well'. I was then asked to outline how to investigate and confirm a diagnosis of sarcoid.

> **Comments**
>
> It was unusual to have a patient with Marfan's syndrome as the respiratory case. The patient did not exhibit typical Marfan's syndrome because the kyphoscoliosis made him look much shorter and the flexion deformity of the fingers obscured the arachnodactyly.

11 *I thought he was normal! But managed to persuade myself that he had short 4th and 5th metacarpals!*

Station 1

This lady is short of breath, please examine her respiratory system.

The patient was on oxygen, had central cyanosis and was clubbed. On auscultation, there were widespread crackles.

I was asked about long-term oxygen trials (LTOT),* steroid trials and pulmonary function tests. I was also asked for the causes of pulmonary fibrosis and which questions I would ask the patient.

I was given some haematology results which were suggestive that the patient might have splenomegaly.

I could not find a spleen and I was sent back to have another look! I think he also had cervical lymph nodes. I was asked how I could confirm a spleen if I was not sure clinically. Then I had to list the causes of splenomegaly.

Station 2

This 30-year-old lady has had fits and needs to be started on antiepileptics. However, she is thinking of starting a family—please advise.

She had had about four grand mal seizures in the last couple of months. Her mother had a brain tumour. She was on the oral contraceptive pill but wanted to stop it and start a family. She was not keen to have any tablets that could be harmful to a baby. We talked about doing a CT scan and an electroencephalogram (EEG) to investigate for possible causes, about not driving, and about taking the contraceptive pill until all the investigations were complete. I explained that antiepileptics are teratogenic but that the risks are less if one takes folate supplements. I explained that having a seizure could be more harmful.

The examiner kept dwelling on the blood tests that would be useful to investigate the cause—I think he was driving at systemic lupus erythematosus (she was Afro-Caribbean).

* Long-term oxygen trials (LTOT) were carried out to look at the effect of oxygen given for over 15 h/day on survival in patients with chronic obstructive pulmonary disease (COPD)—it did and in fact is the only pharmacological treatment for COPD that has shown a benefit on survival. Inhalers that we all spend millions on do not. Oxygen therapy has not been shown to improve longevity in pulmonary fibrosis but keeping saturations of oxygen above 92% obviously has other benefits, e.g. quality of life, prevention of polycythaemia and also mental/psychological parameters.

We suspect this case was a pulmonary fibrosis patient but LTOT trials questions would be more relevant in COPD patients as there are guidelines on when to prescribe these in COPD and the evidence is convincing.

Station 3

This patient had a myocardial infarct 1 year ago. Please examine the cardiovascular system.

There was an ejection systolic murmur at the aortic area with no radiation. The pulse and blood pressure were both normal. However, there was also a pansystolic murmur at the apex. There was no overt cardiac failure.

The examiner asked me: 'What is the most significant lesion and the probable cause for it?', 'How would you investigate?', 'What would be a significant gradient across the aortic valve?'

This patient has a 20-year history of weakness in the right arm and shoulder.

I found asymmetry, wasting and fasciculation over the right shoulder and some areas of the arm—I thought it could be a C5 radiculopathy.

'What are the causes?' I suggested motor neurone disease, polio and syringomyelia. 'Which is the most likely?' 'Which nerves/roots are involved and why?'

Station 4

A 55-year-old man has recently been admitted with an aspiration pneumonia. He is at the end-stage of motor neurone disease. His chest is now better and he is going home. You need to speak to his wife and discuss his resuscitation status, his suitability or not for ITU, withholding antibiotics and the use or not of non-invasive positive pressure ventilation (NIPPV) on future admissions.

I explained to the wife that he was at the end-stage of the disease and that it was probably unkind to prolong his suffering. We discussed whether he should stay at home when he gets the next chest infection and to arrange for different agencies to come in to help her, such as the GP, the district nurse and palliative care nurses. He could be given oxygen at home and be given a syringe driver to relieve unpleasant symptoms. By the end of the discussion she appeared quite happy with the above.

I was asked to explain how I could be sure that she had got the message and who was going to follow this up if he is going home today.

Station 5

Please examine this patient's hands. He is a 15-year-old boy who presented with carpopedal spasm as a child.

I thought he was normal but managed to persuade myself that he had short fourth and fifth metacarpals!

The examiner exclaimed, 'Isn't he a bit tall for pseudohypoparathyroidism?' He went on to ask, 'How is it inherited?' and 'Could it be anything else?'

Examine this patient's fundus.
There were bilateral cataracts and photocoagulation scars.

The examiner wanted to know how I would prevent further retinal damage and asked what the ideal cholesterol level was. 'What tablets should she be on if she has high blood pressure and proteinuria?'

Examine this patient's hands.
There were multiple neurofibromas over the hands and also over the trunk.

I had to discuss inheritance, complications and family screening.

Examine this patient's foot.
The patient had a diabetic foot ulcer. The feet were cold, with reduced sensation including vibration sense and also the arterial pulses were absent.

The examiner asked me, 'How can you best prevent these ulcers?', 'What is the best method of treatment and what further investigations would you do?' I talked about Doppler ultrasound and angiograms.

Comments

Everyone was nice. It was good to have a 5-min break between each station and to know that the next two examiners are totally objective and are not aware of how you did at the previous station.

---

12 *The examiner asked me why the patient was pale, what are the mechanisms of anaemia in renal failure and is there any condition in which the patients are not anaemic.*

Station 1
This man has a long history of breathlessness. Please examine his respiratory system.
On examination, there was no clubbing but he had fine, end-inspiratory crackles and so I diagnosed pulmonary fibrosis.

The examiner asked me for the causes of pulmonary fibrosis and what did I think was the significance of this patient having a parrot at home. He asked what tests I would perform and I had to explain what is meant by the transfer factor. He concluded by asking me what treatment I would give this patient.

This patient attends the renal clinic with hypertension. Please examine his abdominal system.
I found the patient to have an arteriovenous fistula with a scar in the lower abdomen. A transplanted kidney was palpable. However, I could not feel any polycystic kidneys.

The examiner asked me why the patient was pale, what are the mechanisms of anaemia in renal failure and is there any condition in which the patients are not anaemic. He then asked me why this patient was in end-stage renal failure and why had he had a transplant? He also wanted to know what medication he should be on post-transplant, why is he hypertensive and what would be the treatment for the hypertension?

Station 2
This 30-year-old lady has a previous history of back pain which was thought to be renal colic. She now presents with further back pain. Her past medical history also includes amenorrhoea for which she is on bromocriptine and a recent abdominal X-ray shows nephrocalcinosis. Please take a history.
During the history taking we discussed her back pain which was similar to her previous episodes. We discussed her amenorrhoea and associated galactorrhoea and the fact that she was now menstruating. Scans performed at the time had shown a pituitary 'problem' which I assumed was a prolactinoma.

The examiner wanted to know the overall diagnosis and I suggested multiple endocrine neoplasia (MEN) type 1 (see pp. 429 and 441, *An AID to the MRCP Paces*, Volume 1). He asked me what the components of this were, what investigations I would perform and then we had a discussion about pituitary function tests.

Station 3
This man has been complaining of chest pain and palpitations. Please examine the cardiovascular system.
I was not very sure about my findings but thought he had an ejection systolic murmur so I thought the diagnosis should be aortic stenosis.

At first I said he had mitral stenosis! We talked about an opening snap, the duration of the murmur and the loud first heart sound. The discussion then went on to the clinical indicators for the severity of aortic stenosis.

This patient has problems with his balance. Please examine his cerebellar system.
I found left-sided cerebellar signs with increased tone and hyperreflexia and a probable internuclear ophthalmoplegia.

The examiners wanted to know the causes of a cerebellar syndrome and what the likely cause was in this patient. I suggested multiple sclerosis and he asked me what investigations I would perform and what treatment I would give. He asked me who decides about who gets interferon.

Station 4

This is a young asthmatic who has had a recent severe exacerbation. He is due to go home but is worried about this happening again. Please discuss his concerns.

This patient's main questions were, 'Will this happen again?', 'How can I prevent it?', 'Can I exercise now?' 'This episode started while I was decorating my house, should I stop doing this?' He was also confused about his inhalers and thought that they were making his cough worse.

The examiner asked me to summarize the situation and then asked me how I felt the conversation went. He asked if I thought that the patient was satisfied and had he understood about peak flow monitoring and the use of inhalers.

Station 5

This lady has had recent headaches. Please examine the appropriate systems.

The patient was obviously acromegalic and the examiner asked me why she was acromegalic and what else would I like to examine. He asked what investigations would I perform and what treatment would I give. He asked me what I needed to be worried about postoperatively in such patients.

This patient is blind. Examine his fundi.

I found he had cataracts and also retinitis pigmentosa. The examiners did not ask me any additional questions.

Look at, and examine, this man's legs.

He had wasting of the quadriceps and a scar from a muscle biopsy.

I was asked for the causes of a proximal myopathy and why did he have a muscle biopsy scar. I was then asked for the associations of polymyositis, its treatment and prognosis.

Describe this lady's abnormalities.

She had sclerodactyly, telangiectasiae and microstomia so I suggested limited systemic sclerosis as the underlying diagnosis.

The examiners requested that I ask the patient some questions, then they asked me what functional disabilities might she have and what problems can one get in diffuse systemic sclerosis.

> **Comments**
>
> In general, this exam was very fair and the examiners were nice. Often, I was looking for a hidden agenda but it was really just straightforward.

13 *They asked 'What difference would it make in terms of the anatomical site of problem whether the hemianopia had macular sparing or not?'*

Station 1

This patient presented with worsening shortness of breath. Please examine his chest.

I found bibasal end-inspiratory fine crepitations. There was no clubbing and no signs of scleroderma.

I was asked about the possible causes of pulmonary fibrosis and how I would investigate this patient.

Please examine this gentleman's abdominal system and comment on the findings.

There were multiple spider naevi over the chest. There was ascites with dullness in the loins and a caput medusa. I was not asked any additional questions.

Station 2

A 26-year-old bartender presented with a history of two episodes of tingling over the right side of the body each lasting 10–15 min. She has one daughter. She is a smoker and takes the oral contraceptive pill. Please take a history and discuss with the examiners. You are not expected to examine the patient.

She was a 26-year-old lady who smoked 10–15 cigarettes/day and had been on the oral contraceptive pill for 2 years. She presented as above. Both of the episodes were associated with tingling over the right side of the face, upper and lower limbs. There was no motor weakness and no loss of consciousness. On both occasions she had taken one tablet of 'speed' (she did not tell the GP about that, so it was not mentioned in the GP letter). Otherwise she was fit and well. She was on no other medication and no over-the-counter tablets. There were no symptoms of worsening weakness or general tiredness. There was no history of previous spontaneous abortions, nor of photosensitivity nor deep vein thromboses. She had no mouth or genital ulcers and no gait abnormalities.

The examiners asked me for a differential as to the most likely possibility and then we went on to a discussion about other possible causes. They wanted to know what the appropriate investigations would include.

Station 3

This lady has a heart murmur. Please examine her cardiovascular system.

On inspection, there was a left valvotomy scar and all the signs of a left hemiplegia. There was a tapping apex beat, an opening snap and the classical diastolic murmur of mitral stenosis.

No questions were asked.

Examine this patient's cranial nerves.

I examined the cranial nerve and told them the patient had a right homonymous hemianopia with macular sparing.

They asked, 'What difference would it make in terms of the anatomical site of the problem whether the hemianopia had macular sparing or not?'

Station 4

This patient presents with chorea. His father died of Huntington's disease and his sister has the disease. He is in the neurology clinic to see the consultant who has had to leave early and you are left with him. Please counsel him about his chorea. You are almost certain that he has the disease. He is not at all happy that the consultant is not in the clinic.

I apologized for the situation. I then asked him if he had any idea as to what might be the cause of his symptoms. I asked him what he knew about the disease and I gave him time to express his worries. (His wife, who was not with him was very concerned and he did not want to cause stress to his family, particularly as his 12-year-old son was taking exams.) He has two sons aged 12 and 4, and a 9-year-old daughter. I asked him if he thought that he might be willing to speak to his children regarding genetic testing. At the end I offered for him to return to the clinic with his wife to meet both me and the consultant.

The examiner wanted to know if I thought that offering genetic testing on the children was possible without the consent of the children. He then went on, 'As antenatal testing for Huntington's disease is possible, do you think that it is fair to put the 50% of fetuses who do not have the disease under the risk of amniocentesis?' Then he said, 'At what age do the human rights of the individual start?'

Station 5

This patient has a goitre. Please examine her.

I found exophthalmos and a homogeneous, nonnodular goitre but the patient was clinically euthyroid.

There were no questions.

Examine the patient's fundi.

A 25-year-old man was sitting in a conservatory at 12

midday with the curtains open! However, I did manage to see background proliferative diabetic retinopathy with photocoagulation scars and flame-shaped haemorrhages.

I had to explain how I would differentiate between old and new photocoagulation scars on fundoscopy.

Examine this patient's spine (patient sitting on a chair reading a newspaper).

There was ankylosing spondylitis and I listened to his heart and found aortic regurgitation.

The examiners moved on without asking anything else.

What is the diagnosis?

I found a psoriatic erythema and no questions were asked.

14 *On this attempt (my fourth) I treated the exam as a ward round and did not feel the examiners could 'hurt' me any more. Perhaps in hindsight that is the reason I passed. With re-accreditation looming I think it would be worthwhile getting MRCP examiners to actually sit the MRCP PACES exam under exam conditions—that would be fun!*

Station 1

This gentleman has been getting more breathless in recent months. Please examine his chest.

The patient was tachypnoeic and tachycardic. The trachea was deviated to the left. There was reduced air entry* on the left side with reduced expansion on that side of the chest and there was also a left-sided thoracotomy scar.

The examiner asked me for my findings and then asked me to show him how I assessed the position of the trachea. 'What do you think is the reason for your findings and why do you think the patient is breathless?'

Examine this gentleman's abdomen.

This was a man with dark glasses and a walking stick. I found that he was jaundiced with spider naevi, hepatomegaly and ascites but he had no significant central or peripheral oedema.

The examiner asked me to give my findings and to tell him about the pathophysiology of ascites, what metabolic abnormalities might be present and to describe a management plan.

Station 2

Take a history from this business manager who is stressed at work and describes abdominal symptoms.

He described symptoms of difficulty with defaecation

---

* It is more accurate to say reduced breath sounds.

and passing pellet-like stools. He also described rectal bleeding and was concerned because his father had died in his fifties from colonic cancer. He was stressed at work but had no actual weight loss. He did not think he had haemorrhoids and had had no significant change in his bowel habit. He was very anxious about his condition as he had a wife and three children to support.

The examiner asked me what I thought this gentleman's main concerns were and what plan of management would I propose. He then asked me what did I know about heredity factors in colonic neoplasms.

Station 3

Examine this man's cardiovascular system.
The gentleman was elderly, fully dressed and sitting in a chair. I was required to get him onto the bed and into the correct position. I found that he had a slow-rising pulse with an ejection systolic murmur radiating to the carotids.

The examiner wanted me to give my findings and to demonstrate the position of the apex beat. I had to roll the patient over to do this. He asked me what features of the history might be of relevance, what investigations would I perform and, on a cardiac echogram, what gradient would concern me.

Examine the legs of this lady.
She was about 40 years of age and I found upper motor neurone signs with an element of a sensory deficit. I thought she had hereditary motor and sensory neuropathy (HMSN) and I was asked to demonstrate all the methods of eliciting a plantar response, i.e. Babinski, Oppenheim, Gordon, etc., and then to demonstrate the presence of clonus.

Station 4

This 88-year-old lady has had a dense, completed stroke. She is extremely unwell and is unable to take adequate nutrition. The team have decided that her outlook is poor. Please talk to her daughter about the issue of 'not for resuscitation'.
The patient has two daughters, one of whom is in Japan. The daughter I was speaking to was keen that her mother be kept comfortable and that she was 'not for resuscitation' (NFR). However, the daughter in Japan wanted everything to be done for her mother in terms of active management. I had to delve into the daughter's assessment of her mother's health and her premorbid state and discuss issues regarding a living will. At the end of the discussion an agreement was reached for her to be NFR.

I was asked about the scenario of the daughter leaving and the mother arresting, would we resuscitate? I was also asked about the issues of documenting the decision in the notes.

Station 5

Look at this patient's eyes.
The patient had bilateral exophthalmos and also had a frosted left lens in his glasses.

No additional questions were asked by the examiner.

Please examine this patient's fundi.
I found background diabetic retinopathy and I was not asked any further questions.

Look at this patient's hand and legs.
The patient had sclerodactyly and an ulcer on the leg.

The examiner asked me what type of ulcer was it and I suggested that it could be vasculitic.

Look at this patient's skin.
I found some weird-looking lesions that did not fit into any characteristic appearance of psoriasis but, because of the distribution, I plumped for that as a diagnosis.

I was then asked about the treatment, management and complications of psoriasis so perhaps I had been right with the diagnosis!

Comments

Having failed the short cases many times before I passed this time but, if truth be told, I was least prepared this time.

I do not believe that the exam has become more objective.

On this attempt (my fourth) I treated the exam as a ward round and I did not feel that the examiners could 'hurt' me any more. Perhaps with hindsight that is the reason I passed.

With re-accreditation looming I think it would be worthwhile getting MRCP examiners to actually sit the MRCP PACES exam under exam conditions — that would be fun!

---

15 *This man's skin was really red. There were no plaques or scales but I said he had psoriasis. The Examiners asked me how I would manage this man if it was a Friday at 5.30 p.m. and I was in the Accident and Emergency Department and I could not get in touch with a dermatologist.*

Station 1

This lady is breathless. Please examine her chest.

The patient had simple emphysema. It was a ward patient who had been brought along at the last minute as the expected patient had not arrived.

I was asked how to differentiate the different types of lung disease.

Examine this patient's abdominal system.

I found hepatosplenomegaly and the stigmata of chronic liver disease but the patient was not jaundiced.

The examiner asked me about the management of acute gastrointestinal bleeding in a patient with liver disease and the emphasis was on the 'ABC', etc.

Station 2

This 40-year-old lady has presented with a persistent cough and shortness of breath. Inhalers have not helped and a chest X-ray carried out by the GP has been reported as normal. Please take a history.

The patient was living in the East End of London surrounded by people with tuberculosis. She was a smoker and had a family history of thrombotic events.

The examiners asked me what investigations I would do and what I thought the likely outcomes of these investigations would be.

Station 3

This patient has had an acute episode of breathlessness. Please examine the cardiovascular system.

I found evidence of aortic stenosis. I thought it was clinically mild but I was subsequently told that the gradient was 70 mmHg.

The examiner asked me if I was surprised at the gradient. He told me that the patient was unfit for surgery and so how would I follow him up, and in which way might he deteriorate. The discussion covered ischaemic heart disease, left ventricular failure, Adams–Stokes attacks and subacute bacterial endocarditis.

This lady has difficulty doing the housework, especially with taking things out of cupboards. Look at her face and examine her hands.

She had the classic features of myotonic dystrophy.

The examiner said to me, 'She wants to have children, how would you advise her?' He then asked me how the condition might progress and what else might be affected.

Station 4

You see a heavy goods vehicle (HGV) driver in the casualty department who has had several funny turns in the past but today has had one that was definitely an epileptic seizure. Counsel him about the implications of this diagnosis.

I explained to him that he does have epilepsy. (He argued.) I explained to him that he must stop driving. (He protested.) I explained about the financial benefits that are available to compensate for the loss of earnings and that he could find other work. I explained that medication controls the epilepsy but that he still cannot drive. I emphasized that this was because of safety for himself and for other people on the road. I was unsure as to whether he would *ever* be able to drive HGV vehicles again but said that I would find out straight after the consultation and get back to him and that I would ring a social worker about any available financial benefits.

I thought the conversation went very well. The examiners asked me about any possible situations in which one can legally break confidentiality. We talked more about driving and epilepsy and I was asked how would I know whether he was continuing to drive or not.

Station 5

Examine this patient's neck.

The patient had a goitre but was euthyroid.

I had to list the possible complications of a goitre including dysphagia, stridor, etc., and what could be some causes of a sudden deterioration, e.g. bleeding into a nodule. They wanted to know how I would detect stridor.

Examine this patient's fundi.

I found dot haemorrhages on the right side, with silver wiring and arteriovenous nipping bilaterally.

The examiners wanted a classification of diabetic retinopathy but I cannot remember the rest of the questions!

Examine this patient's hands.

He had obvious psoriatic arthropathy although it looked somewhat like rheumatoid arthritis but there were psoriatic plaques.

I am sure that I was asked some questions at this point but I cannot remember what they were.

Look at this patient.

This man's skin was really red. There were no plaques or scales but I said that he had psoriasis.

The examiners asked me how I would manage this man if it was Friday evening at 5.30 p.m. and I was in the casualty department and I could not get in touch with a dermatologist. I said that I would rehydrate, that I would treat any infection aggressively and that I would use simple aqueous creams. I passed the exam but on reflection I realized that I should have said that he had a drug reaction because as I was walking away the examiner said, 'Did you really think it was psoriasis?' and I said, 'No!' They smiled.

> **Comments**
>
> I would definitely have benefited from more practice in history taking and in communication skills before the exam.

16 *I finished the history taking very quickly so had to sit in silence until time was up. That was awful!*

Station 1
This patient is complaining of shortness of breath. Please examine the chest.
I found a left-sided pleural effusion.

I was asked what the important points in the history-taking would be and for the further investigations and management. There was a discussion about pleural plaques.

This patient has been referred from the cardiology clinic with sweats and a mass in the abdomen. Please examine.
I found splenomegaly which was apparently secondary to infective endocarditis.

I was asked for the differential diagnosis of splenomegaly, the treatment of chronic lymphatic leukaemia and the diagnosis, and management, of endocarditis.

Station 2
This man has had palpitations and has been started on amiodarone. He is now hyperthyroid and has been started on carbimazole 5 mg b.d. The thyroid-stimulating hormone (TSH) is still very low.* Take a history.

* Amiodarone contains iodine and can cause disorders of thyroid function; both hypothyroidism and hyperthyroidism may occur. Clinical assessment alone is unreliable, and laboratory tests should be performed before treatment and every 6 months. Thyroxine (T4) may be raised in the absence of hyperthyroidism; therefore tri-iodothyronine (T3), T4, and thyroid-stimulating hormone (TSH) should all be measured. A raised T3 and T4 with a very low or undetectable TSH concentration suggests the development of thyrotoxicosis. The thyrotoxicosis may be very refractory, and amiodarone should usually be withdrawn at least temporarily to help achieve control; treatment with carbimazole may be required. Hypothyroidism can be treated with replacement therapy without withdrawing amiodarone if it is essential.

I took a cardiac history and asked about the palpitations for which he had been started on amiodarone. He was sweaty and agitated, and the thyroxine (T4) was still high with a low TSH. He had been started on carbimazole but was not really any better.

I was asked how I would alter his drug management and about his social history. The examiners also asked me about the mode of action of amiodarone.

Station 3
This patient is short of breath. Please examine the heart.
I found mixed aortic valve disease.

The examiners asked me to measure the blood pressure and to say which was the most serious lesion. I was then asked for the diagnostic tests and the management of aortic regurgitation and aortic stenosis.

This patient has had weakness of the legs for 3 years. Please examine the legs and find out why.
The patient had a spastic right leg but the left was normal.

I was asked to give the causes of a spastic paraparesis but then there was no time left for a discussion or any further questions.

Station 4
This man, with a long history of alcohol abuse, has had to wait 8 weeks for an outpatient appointment. The ultrasound scan of his abdomen has shown a 10 cm lesion in the liver. This has been biopsied and found to be a hepatocellular carcinoma. The patient is happy for you to speak to his wife. You have to break the bad news to the wife who does not want her husband to be told.
I explained the diagnosis and she definitely did not want her husband to be told. However, I explained the problems with this approach and she eventually relented. I explained about further treatment and management.

I was asked by the examiners how I thought the conversation had gone and did I think that I handled it as well as I thought I could?

Station 5
This woman has glycosuria. Look at her and examine anything that is relevant.
The patient was obviously acromegalic so I examined for, and demonstrated, xanthelasma and a bitemporal hemianopia.

I was asked how the xanthelasma could be associated with acromegaly and why should there be glycosuria.

This patient feels as if he is walking on cotton wool and has had recurrent Bell's palsies. Please examine his eyes.

There was a preproliferative diabetic retinopathy but no laser burns were visible.

The examiner asked if he had had any treatment to his eyes and why did he have altered sensation in his feet. He also asked me for a reason for the recurrent Bell's palsies and to explain what is meant by Bell's phenomenon.

This patient is tired all the time. Why is that?
There was koilonychia so the patient must have had an iron-deficiency anaemia but there was no time for any discussion.

Examine the patient's hands and any other relevant joints.
The patient had CRST and also there were nodules at the elbows.

I was asked how I would differentiate between CRST and rheumatoid arthritis, what is the treatment for CRST and what further questions would I ask the patient?

Comments

The exam felt very rushed. There was not enough time to examine patients fully and to discuss the findings with the examiners.

I finished the history taking at Station 2 very quickly and then had to sit in silence until time was up. That was awful!

---

17 *Despite being told how difficult it is to cope with the indifference with which some examiners treat you, when it actually happened it was far more devastating than I was prepared for.*

Station 1
Examine this man's respiratory system.
I cannot remember anything about the Station 1 respiratory case!

Examine this man's abdomen and tell me what you find.
I found most of the signs of chronic liver disease—liver palms, spider naevi and ascites, in a thin and wasted man.

The examiner asked for possible causes and the investigations that are needed to make a diagnosis of liver disease.

Station 2
Please see this middle-aged lady who is feeling lethargic. The GP has performed some blood tests and has discovered abnormal liver function tests with a hepatitic picture. She is being referred for further investigations.

The patient was a 46-year-old married lady who is a teacher. She had noticed progressively worsening lethargy but she had very little in the way of other symptoms. It was probably all a result of alcohol consumption.

The examiner wanted me to give some possible causes for her symptoms and the abnormal liver function tests. He asked if I thought that the alcohol was a probable cause but I had not taken a very good alcohol history! He asked me about primary biliary cirrhosis and I thought that her symptoms could be caused by that. He finally asked if there were any other things that I should have asked her and I had to admit that I had also forgotten to ask about any intravenous drug usage.

Station 3
The GP has noted a murmur—can you tell me what you think?
I found the murmurs of mixed aortic valve disease.

The examiner asked if I was sure and how would I judge the significance of the predominant murmur?

This man has had a collapse—please examine his limbs.
There was evidence of a facial weakness and a left hemiplegia.

I was asked for possible causes and I had noted that he was in atrial fibrillation. I had to list the investigations that I would do (routine blood tests, ECG, CT scan of the brain, etc.) and they wanted to know my treatment plans. I talked about physiotherapy and anticoagulation.

Station 4
This gentleman has recently had a cardiac arrest. He has been left with severe marked cerebral damage and is in need of huge amounts of inotropic support. Please discuss the resuscitation status with his son.
The conversation that I had with the son included having to tell him how sick his father was and that any attempt at resuscitation was unlikely to be successful. I had to explain about the severity of the brain impairment and that I did not think that cardiopulmonary resuscitation would be in his best interest as he was unlikely to recover from this acute episode.

The examiner asked me if I thought that the son understood what I was trying to explain and I replied that I thought he had understood. I was then asked to discuss the prognostic indicators for a patient after a cardiac arrest.

Station 5
What do you think of this lady?
She was a Cushingoid lady and I was asked for the pos-

sible causes and the complications of long-term steroid use.

Examine this person's eyes.
I found tunnel vision, and on fundoscopy there was retinitis pigmentosa although it was not very florid at all.

The examiner did not ask me any questions—he just grunted and walked off!

Examine this man's hands.
He had rheumatoid hands and scars from what I assumed were bilateral decompressions for carpal tunnel syndrome.

The examiner asked what I thought the scars were caused by and why was he on methotrexate.

Take a look at this lady's rash.
She had a widespread, macular, erythematous rash and the examiners told me that the dermatologists did not know the diagnosis! I described the rash and explained that I would take a full history including a drug history and if in doubt I would do some blood tests and biopsy the lesion.

They did not ask me any questions.

Comments

Despite being told how difficult it is to cope with the indifference with which some examiners treat you, when it actually happened it was far more devastating than I was prepared for. This occurred in the first station and I felt dreadful but I remembered having been told that the next case is a new case and treat it as such otherwise one can fall into a downward spiral. It worked for me and I got into the 'swing' of the exam. I think it was the most dreadful experience of my life and I felt emotionally drained after it. Thank God I passed! The very best reason to pass the exam first time is that you never have to take the bloody thing again!

---

18 *In the ensuing questions I was asked about what ethical issues this scenario raised and explain 'duty to act justly'.*

Station 1
This man has developed a productive cough. Please examine his chest and suggest a cause.

The patient had bilateral, upper lobe, fine crepitations and I suggested a diagnosis of pulmonary fibrosis.

The examiners showed me the chest X-ray and there was an opacity in both upper lobes. I suggested aspergillosis affecting old tuberculous cavities and they asked me what further investigations I would do. I suggested sputum for culture and sensitivity/cytology/acid-alcohol-fast bacilli.

This lady has been having abdominal pain. Please examine and suggest a cause.
I found evidence of polycystic kidneys and a polycystic liver. There were multiple scars from previous operations to drain the cysts. There were no arteriovenous fistulae. She had palmar erythema but was not jaundiced and the abdomen was generally tender.

The examiners asked me questions about polycystic kidney disease, i.e. chromosomal abnormalities and what possible complications could occur.

Station 2
The GP letter describes a history of funny turns and then subsequent development of a right hemiplegia. The letter asks for a review of the diagnosis of a stroke and then to suggest further appropriate management.
The patient was a 68-year-old lady who, 4 months previously, had noticed intermittent episodes of a dizzy feeling. She denied vertigo or any other associated neurological or cardiac symptoms. A month later, she developed a right-sided weakness which had been preceded by impaired coordination. There had been no headaches, no loss of consciousness and no visual disturbances. Now her function was improving although she still had difficulty with stairs, tired easily and was frustrated that she could no longer work in the family pet shop. Her risk factors included the fact that her father had ischaemic heart disease, there was no family history of stroke and she was found to have hypertension. She did not smoke and did not have diabetes mellitus. There was no other past medical history. Her drug history included antihypertensives and aspirin and she was unclear as to whether she had had her serum cholesterol level measured.

The examiners asked me what I thought about her presentation and the differential diagnosis of her funny turns. They asked if I thought she was depressed and what questions I would ask her to establish this.

Station 3
This patient presented with shortness of breath. Please examine the cardiovascular system.

The patient definitely had mixed mitral valve disease and was in atrial fibrillation. However, it was difficult to ascertain the predominant lesion. I thought there was also a murmur of aortic sclerosis.

There then followed a discussion about atrial fibrillation, its management and possible complications and the examiners wanted to know how I could clinically assess for the dominant valvular lesion.

This man has difficulty walking and has falls, especially at night. Examine his gait and then his legs.

His gait was very unsteady. It was broad-based and the Romberg's test was positive. There were definite cerebellar signs and I also thought there was a sensory neuropathy.

The examiners wanted me to suggest possible causes.

Station 4

You are the resident medical officer and a 37-week pregnant woman presents to the casualty department with symptoms suggestive of a pulmonary embolus. Please discuss the likely diagnosis and outline management plans.

I discussed with her the possible diagnosis and important investigations. I then explained the benefit vs. the risk to the baby of appropriate management and treatment and the reasons why pulmonary emboli occurred during pregnancy.

In the ensuing questions I was asked about what ethical issues this scenario raised and to explain 'duty to act justly'.

Station 5

This woman presents with painful eyes. Please examine her.

There was quite marked chemosis of the eyes and an obvious goitre. They also wanted me to examine her thyroid status.

This man had sudden onset of blindness. Please look at the fundi and suggest why.

He had glaucoma with marked cupping of the discs. I wondered if he had had a retinal artery occlusion as well and we discussed the possible causes of sudden blindness.

This man has a painful knee. Please examine his hands and suggest why.

He had an asymmetrical arthropathy with gouty tophi.

The following discussion was about gout, its management, investigations and complications.

This lady complains of some abnormalities in her gums. Please examine her.

She had the classic features of lichen planus and I also saw a lesion of lichen planus on her skin.

The examiners wanted to know if I knew any other causes of gum hyperplasia.

19 *I was asked about the mechanism of the reflex arc.*

Station 1

Examine this patient's chest.

I found a right-sided pleural effusion and was asked for the possible causes, the investigations that should be carried out in their order of priority and, finally, for the management of a pleural effusion.

This patient is complaining of tiredness. Examine his abdomen.

I found hepatosplenomegaly and clinical anaemia in a patient who also had rheumatoid hands.

I was asked for causes of hepatosplenomegaly and the most likely cause in this patient. I was then asked for further possible explanations for the anaemia.

Station 2

This lady with Crohn's disease has recently had an ileal resection for fistulating disease. She now has abdominal pain and has noticed some hair loss. She was discharged from hospital on 6-mercaptopurine.

The patient had a history of Crohn's disease which had not settled with 5-aminosalicylic acid (5-ASA) and prednisolone. She subsequently had surgery and had undergone multiple operations. The pain had now improved but not totally gone and her main concern currently was the hair loss. The patient and I discussed the options of changing the therapy and of further investigations for the hair loss.

The examiners asked me, 'What is the most likely cause for her hair loss?', 'Do you think that her Crohn's disease is active?', 'What alternative therapy could be used?' and 'What would be your further management?'

Station 3

Examine this gentleman's heart. He has been complaining of palpitations.

I found atrial fibrillation with a mitral stenotic murmur. There was no valvotomy scar and there was no evidence of cardiac failure.

I was asked about the likely cause for the mitral stenosis, the treatment of atrial fibrillation and what was the cause of the opening snap.

This gentleman has noticed a tendency to drop objects. Please examine his motor system.
I found the patient to have a right hemiparesis and I was asked about the mechanism of the reflex arc.

Station 4
A patient under your care has been diagnosed with Huntington's chorea. Her daughter would like to discuss her mother's condition.
We discussed the need for consent to discuss her mother's condition with her. I gave an explanation of the diagnosis of Huntington's chorea and how it had so far affected her mother. We talked about the process of genetic screening, whether this was indicated for her, and how this may affect her life. I outlined the further support and treatment that would be planned to help her mother in the future.

I was asked about the problems of consent to test for Huntington's chorea if the patient refused and whether it would be beneficial for the daughter to be tested. I was asked how I thought the interview went.

Station 5
Examine this gentleman. What do you notice?
The patient had marked Cushingoid features and I was asked the possible reasons for the patient being on steroid therapy.

Examine this patient's fundi.
The patient had unilateral optic atrophy and angioid streaks.
I was asked for the causes of optic atrophy.

Examine the patient's eyes.
The patient had a unilateral III, IV and VI nerve palsy which was caused by a cavernous sinus thrombosis (see pp. 204, 426, 437, 489, *An Aid to the MRCP PACES*, Volume 1).

Examine this patient's hands.
The patient had marked rheumatoid hands with nodules.

Examine this patient.
She had peripheral and central cyanosis with warm swollen hands and I was asked for the cause.

> **Comments**
>
> There is plenty of time to examine thoroughly and the questions are usually management based.
>
> On Station 5, I had two eye cases so I had a total of five patients at that station. This station seemed much more flexible than the others, with no written instructions.

20 *They asked for causes of dysarthria so I volunteered bulbar and pseudo bulbar and of course they wanted causes for both!*

Station 1
This man has noisy breathing. Please examine his chest to find out why.
The man had no signs in his chest at all but I did notice that on his skin he had a very large (10–20 cm) psoriatic plaque.

The examiners asked me where I thought the lesion was likely to be and I said in his upper airway. They asked how I would confirm this diagnosis and I said by performing a respiratory flow loop test. They asked me what it would look like but at that point the bell went.

Examine this patient's abdomen.
I found hepatosplenomegaly with minimal ascites but there was no evidence of chronic liver disease.

They asked me why I thought the swelling on the left side of his abdomen was a spleen and not a kidney and then they asked if I had checked for a notch, but of course I had not!

Station 2
This 40-year-old lady has suffered from chronic intermittent diarrhoea and back pain. She took a holiday to India last year with her family. Please take a history.
I asked her for further details about the diarrhoea and the back pain and most of her history pointed to a diagnosis of irritable bowel syndrome. However, I tried to exclude inflammatory bowel disease. It was all very straightforward but I made sure that I included questions about her menstrual history and her social history.

Station 3
Please examine this patient's cardiovascular system.
The patient had a midline sternotomy scar and there was a systolic murmur which I thought could be a flow murmur or could be a result of mitral valve disease.

They wanted to know what I thought the scar was for and I suggested that it was either for a valve replacement or a coronary artery bypass graft.

This patient has difficulty in walking. Please examine him.
There was subtle, left-sided dysdiadochokinesis and he could not do the tandem walking test so I concluded that he had cerebellar signs but I was not that convinced about any dysarthria. I was then asked to examine the facial nerve and found that he also had a left facial palsy which I thought was supranuclear.

I was asked to link all this together so I suggested cerebrovascular disease or multiple sclerosis. They asked for the causes of dysarthria so I volunteered bulbar and pseudobulbar and of course they then wanted causes for both! They asked for other causes of dysarthria and I suggested that a large tongue could be responsible for it.

Station 4

An elderly lady had a cerebrovascular accident (CVA) last year and is on aspirin medication. She lives alone and now presents with a gastrointestinal bleed. She is refusing to have an endoscopy (OGD) and is 'fed up'. The daughter still wants her to have the investigation against her wishes.
The discussion centred on the ethical implications of this.

The examiner asked if the patient was mentally competent or was she depressed or demented.

Station 5

This lady has had headaches. Please examine her.
She had very subtle facial changes of acromegaly and, in addition, I noticed bilateral scars at her wrists from treatment for carpal tunnel syndrome.

This patient has rheumatoid arthritis. Please check the functional status.
The patient was unable to pick up a coin or to do up buttons. There was no pincer grasp at all.

I had to discuss the treatment options for rheumatoid disease.

You must know the diagnosis of this patient.
I think the patient had the typical, multiple lesions of neurofibromatosis and as I gave this diagnosis they jumped straight into the questions.

They wanted to know the possible neurological complications and I gave them a satisfactory list. They asked, 'What can be the cardiovascular complications?' I did not know the answer to that one at all!

21 *'This took me by surprise as I was prepared to take a history rather than to be asked questions by the patient.'*

Station 1

Examine this gentleman's respiratory system.
The young man had a sternotomy scar. There was no clubbing, and auscultation was normal.

I was told that he had had a lung transplant and I was asked for the symptoms and signs of organ rejection. I was then 'grilled' on bronchiolitis obliterans!

Examine this lady's abdominal system.
She had hepatomegaly and inguinal lymphadenopathy and I was asked to offer a differential diagnosis.

Station 2

This gentleman attends the outpatient clinic referred by his GP with possible lung fibrosis secondary to methotrexate. Please proceed as necessary.
The patient immediately asked several questions including, 'Do I need home oxygen?', 'How long have I got to live?', and 'Is it secondary to the methotrexate?' I proceeded to take a history about the background of the problems, i.e. rheumatoid arthritis, and about the symptoms and signs of the breathlessness.

I failed this station outright and my impression was that the examiners wanted me to answer the patient's questions rather than take a history, although it *was* the history taking station. This took me by surprise as I was prepared to take a history rather than be asked questions by the patient!

Station 3

Examine this gentleman's cardiovascular system.
The patient was a young man who had clubbing, a sternotomy scar and a pansystolic murmur in the aortic region.

I was asked for a differential diagnosis and in retrospect I wonder if it was some form of cyanotic congenital heart disease and that perhaps he had a corrected Fallot's tetralogy.

Examine this lady's lower limbs.
I found pes cavus, ataxia and distal weakness.

I was asked for a differential diagnosis and I offered Charcot–Marie–Tooth disease which I was told was incorrect so I then suggested Friedreich's ataxia.

Station 4

A 40-year-old man who had some coryzal symptoms was admitted to hospital following a collapse and an epileptic fit at work. A lumbar puncture has shown meningococcal meningitis. His Glasgow Coma Scale (GCS) is now 8/15. Please explain the situation to his wife.

I explained the diagnosis and the surrounding details. She asked about their child who was also exhibiting similar coryzal symptoms. I explained about the infection control department and the need for prophylactic antibiotics.

The examiners then asked me to outline the poor prognostic indicators in meningococcal septicaemia.

Station 5

Look at this patient.

The patient had obvious acromegaly and I was not asked any additional questions.

Examine this patient's eyes.

This patient had a complete third nerve palsy and I was asked to list the possible causes.

Examine this patient's hands.

The only abnormality here was squaring of the hand with no other signs. The patient must have had osteoarthrosis.

The examiner asked me the name of the joint involved in 'squaring of the hand' and what was the differential diagnosis.

Examine this lady's face and hands.

The patient looked Cushingoid and there were multiple warts on her hands.

I was not asked any questions here but in retrospect I wonder whether she had human papillomavirus following a transplant.

Comments

I felt that the cases were comparatively hard and unusual. The instructions were not always made clear, especially in the history taking station. I had expected to examine some fundi but this was not requested at all in this exam.

---

22 *Lots of empathy was needed and I tried to structure the conversation into sections. I can't remember the details about the discussion with the examiners but I do know that whilst talking to the daughter I got some of the details about*

the inheritance/penetrance/blood testing wong but I came clean about this during the discussion. I still passed!

Station 1

Examine this patient's chest.

I found all the features of bronchiectasis and was asked to give the details and significance of any investigations and what possible treatments were there for this condition.

Examine this patient's abdomen.

This was a young man who also had some 'chest problems'. I found him to have hepatosplenomegaly and ascites and the examiners wanted a list of possible causes.

Station 2

This man has paroxysmal atrial fibrillation. Please take a history.

It was a very complicated history and I cannot remember all the details. Quite a few of his different conditions meant that certain agents would be contraindicated in his management.

However, the examiners asked me to outline a management plan for him and would I anticoagulate him with warfarin or not? They asked me about the use of amiodarone and beta-blockers, but the patient had asthma.

Station 3

Examine this man's cardiovascular system.

He had atrial fibrillation and a prosthetic mitral valve.

The examiners wanted to know about investigations and possible complications.

Examine this man's neurological system.

He had a proximal myopathy, foot drop, a peripheral neuropathy and ulcers on his toes. I thought he probably had diabetes mellitus and the examiners asked me for my views on his further management.

PS. Don't forget to examine the patient's gait!

Station 4

A lady has been diagnosed with Huntington's disease. Please discuss the implications with her daughter.

There was far too much information to fit into too short a time. However, we talked about the clinical features, the differential diagnosis, inheritance, support networks and discharge planning. The daughter was very concerned about whether her son—the patient's grandson—would get it. Lots of empathy was needed and I tried to structure the conversation into sections.

I cannot remember the details about the discussion with the examiners but I do know that while talking to the daughter I got some of the details about the inheritance/penetrance/blood testing wrong but I came clean about this during the discussion and I still passed!

Station 5
Look at this man and examine him as you feel appropriate.
He had all the features of acromegaly and I was asked what investigations I would do.

Examine this man's eyes.
He had Graves' eye disease. He was supposed to have diplopia at the extremes of vision but not even the examiner could demonstrate it!

Examine the patient's hands.
The patient had a deforming arthropathy and I was asked to give a differential diagnosis and to give the differing features between each possible cause.

Examine this lady's skin.
This lady had neurofibromas (but not many of them) together with axillary freckling and *café au lait* spots. I diagnosed von Recklinghausen's disease (neurofibromatosis type 1).

I was asked for the associations with this condition and the differing features from neurofibromatosis type 2.

Comments

Both the history section and the communication/ethics section are very rushed in the exam. It *will* feel very artificial because you will find there is too much to cover in 14 min (plus 1 min for reflection and then 5 min of questions) but persevere and be empathic.

If you do not know the answer to a question do not make it up but say, 'I will find out the answer and we will talk again soon'. It worked for me.

---

23 *The examiners asked me what I would say to the patient if he had asked me to help him end his life.*

Station 1
Examine this patient's chest.
There was a chest drain on the left side with an effusion still draining.

I was asked about the likely aetiologies of a pleural effusion.

This patient's abdomen has shown intermittent swelling— what could one cause be?
The patient had many of the signs of alcoholic liver disease with minimal ascites. He also had hereditary haemorrhagic telangiectasia.

I was asked for the cause of the abdominal swelling.

Station 2
This patient has had a cough for some time. The chest X-ray last year was normal. There was some initial improvement with inhalers. Now nothing seems to work. Please take a history.
There was no shortness of breath on exertion and the only problem seemed to be the cough. There was a history of excessive smoking and the patient had no previous industrial exposure nor had he kept any pets.

I was asked about the likely cause of the cough and what investigations were needed.

Station 3
This patient has been having palpitations— can you find a cause?
The patient was in atrial fibrillation but I could not hear a mitral stenotic murmur.

We had a discussion about whether or not mitral stenosis was present and then on how to manage the atrial fibrillation.

This patient has a worsening tremor of his upper limbs. Please give some reasons.
There was an intention tremor which was worse in the right arm. There were no other cerebellar signs but there was a patchy peripheral sensory neuropathy.

I was asked what the cause could be, given the above findings.

Station 4
This patient has been admitted with an aspiration pneumonia and it is now thought that he has motor neurone disease. He has seen a neurologist who is planning further investigations but he has already told the patient that this is the likely diagnosis. The patient has some questions to ask and you are the on-call doctor.
The patient was concerned about any cognitive decline and about any possible cardiovascular complications. The patient did not want to be a burden on his family and wanted to know if there were any treatments and

whether there were any better treatment options in the USA where his daughter lived.

The examiners asked me what I would say to the patient if he had asked me to help him end his life.

Station 5

This patient has noticed a swelling in his neck — please examine.
There was a large goitre and the right lobe, in particular, was very swollen.

I was asked what investigations were needed and whether the patient was euthyroid.

Examine the eyes of this diabetic patient.
There was evidence of panretinal photocoagulation with hard exudates near the macula.

Look at this patient.
She had scleroderma and I was asked about the CRST syndrome.

Look at this patient's hands.
There was rheumatoid arthritis but without any significant deformity.

I was asked what treatments were available.

24 *This is a discussion about living wills, euthanasia, options for pain control and her anger at the 'delayed/missed' diagnosis.*

Station 1

Examine this man.
There was a collecting bag on the right posterior chest wall containing fluid. Presumably a chest drain had fallen out. There was lymphoedema of the left arm.

I was asked for the likely causes.

This man has pain on walking. Please examine him.
He had a ruddy complexion and hepatosplenomegaly.

I was asked for the diagnosis which was probably polycythaemia rubra vera. I was then asked to describe the position and the anatomy of the spleen and the treatment for polycythaemia for which I volunteered venesection.

Station 2

Take a history.
The patient had peripheral vascular disease, hypertension, diabetes mellitus, renal artery stenosis and impaired left ventricular function.

There was a discussion with the examiners about renal failure and the role of ACE inhibitors in this patient.

Station 3

Examine the patient's heart.
There were the features of mitral stenosis.

I was asked about the methods of treatment and I offered valvotomy, valve replacement, rate control of the atrial fibrillation and thromboprophylaxis.

Examine the patient's legs but omit looking at the gait.
I found a sensory neuropathy in a stocking distribution, upper motor neurone signs including brisk knee jerks, absent ankle jerks and upgoing plantars.

I was asked for the causes and I suggested probable subacute combined degeneration of the cord.

Station 4

The lady has metastatic carcinoma of the breast. Discuss the diagnosis and management with her.
This included a discussion about living wills, euthanasia, options for pain control and her anger at the 'delayed/missed' diagnosis.

Station 5

Look at this patient.
The patient had acromegaly with a bitemporal hemianopia, an old transfrontal scar at the right inner canthus and a carpal tunnel scar.

We discussed replacement therapy and the different zones of the adrenal gland.

Look at the patient's fundi.
I found proliferative diabetic retinopathy with new vessels and photocoagulation scars.

I was asked about the cofactors for eye disease (hypertension, lipids, etc.). The eyes were not dilated, the room was not darkened and the signs were very subtle!

Examine the patient's hands.
I found the signs of chronic tophaceous gout.

I was then asked about the management and treatment of chronic gout.

Look at the patient's face.
The patient had obvious hereditary haemorrhagic telangiectasia.

I was asked about iron-deficiency anaemia in this condition and about the need to investigate with endoscopy to exclude any other coexistent bowel pathology.

25 *I found very little and the whole case was just a nightmare!!*

Station 1

Examine this lady's chest.
I found that she had had a bilateral lower lobectomy and there was fibrosis in the left lung.

I was asked for a cause.

Examine this gentleman's abdomen.
The patient had alcoholic liver disease with many of the signs of chronic liver disease, encephalopathy and tender hepatomegaly.

I was asked for all the other possible causes apart from alcohol.

Station 2

Take a history.
The patient had atypical chest pain which was probably pericarditis.

I can remember talking about a rash and arthralgia and I was asked about the risks of systemic lupus erythematosus.

Station 3

Examine the cardiovascular system.
I found a jerky pulse, cardiomegaly and quiet heart sounds. I diagnosed hypertrophic obstructive cardiomyopathy.*

I was asked about the causes, risks and treatment.

Examine the gait and anything else which is relevant.
I found very little and the whole case was just a nightmare!

Station 4

This patient possibly has hyperthyroidism. She is in atrial fibrillation.

* These days the condition is referred to as hypertrophic cardiomyopathy.

Please discuss the diagnosis, the causes of atrial fibrillation, the risks and the management.

Station 5

Examine the patient's eyes and anything else appropriate.
The patient had Graves' eye disease and all the other features of Graves'.

Examine the patient's fundi. The patient has a central scotoma.
I diagnosed retinitis pigmentosa and diabetic maculopathy.

The examiner wanted to know what questions I would ask the patient. I said family history, whether he was diabetic, smoked and had good or poor night vision.

Examine the patient's hands.
The patient had the signs of rheumatoid disease and was wearing a cervical collar.

The examiner asked me about treatment including the new advances, tumour necrosis factor α (TNFα) and the risks.

Examine this patient's skin.
The patient had psoriasis and I was asked about treatment.

26 *The examiners wanted to know which anti-epileptic is the safest in pregnancy.*

Station 1

Examine this lady's respiratory system from the front.
About half a minute later I was asked to examine her chest from the back. I found that the patient had had a previous right pneumonectomy.

The examiners wanted to know how common lung cancer was in women.

This 62-year-old man has a lymphocytosis. Please examine his abdomen.
I found him to have splenomegaly.

The examiners wanted to know what further investigations were required and what would one see on a peripheral blood smear.

Station 2

Miss Green is a 30-year-old flower shop assistant with a history of two fits, one of which was associated with incontinence and was witnessed by her fiancé. She had been started on antiepileptic pills by her GP but she stopped taking them after 2 weeks as she wanted to conceive and she had heard that antiepileptic medications could have side-effects on the baby. Please take a detailed history and address the patient's concerns.

The history-taking went quite well and the examiners wanted to know which antiepileptic is the safest in pregnancy.

Station 3

Examine the patient's cardiovascular system.

The patient was in her late seventies. There was a midline sternotomy scar and there was evidence of a prosthetic valve.

The examiners wanted to know which valve had been replaced.

Examine this patient's upper limbs. There has been a weakness for about the last 5 years.

I found proximal weakness in the left upper limb with fasciculation over both arms and I suggested a diagnosis of motor neurone disease.

Station 4

This young lady with meningitis has three children at home. She wants to discharge herself. Please convince the patient that hospital treatment is essential.

We discussed why the treatment was important but I also empathized with the fact that she had three children and was relying on neighbours, friends and relatives to look after them. We eventually compromised on her staying in to complete intravenous antibiotics and that she could go home as soon as she could go on oral medication.

Station 5

Please examine this patient's eyes.

I found the patient to have exophthalmos and there was a discussion regarding the eye signs.

Please have a look at this patient's eyes.

I found a third nerve palsy and was asked for the causes.

Please look at this patient's ankles and feet.

There was an ulcer on one heel with a Charcot joint at that ankle. I was asked for possible causes.

Examine this patient's shin.

There was obvious neurofibromatosis and I was then asked for the possible associations.

27 *There was diabetic maculopathy and I was asked to draw my findings!*

Station 1

This young man is breathless. Please examine his chest.

I found evidence of chronic obstructive pulmonary disease. The examiners asked me about the likely forced expiratory volume (*FEV*) and what was a possible aetiology—in fact he had alpha 1 antitrypsin deficiency. He also had a subcutaneous infusion running but I was not sure what it was although the examiners did try to get me to give an answer.

Please examine the abdomen of this man who is complaining of pruritus.

The patient looked unwell. He had a continuous ambulatory peritoneal dialysis catheter *in situ* and I could feel a right polycystic kidney.

The examiners wanted to know what his glomerular filtration rate would be.

Station 2

Take a history from this young professional woman who is diabetic and who is having recurrent hypoglycaemic episodes.

She also had an infected foot ulcer and was driving a car on a regular basis.

Station 3

Please examine the cardiovascular system.

I found mixed aortic valve disease.

Examine this patient's legs.

There were all the features of a mixed upper and lower motor neurone disorder and they questioned me about the possible aetiology.

Station 4

I had to interview a patient with possible Huntington's disease and I had to discuss the implications for the family and for family screening.

Station 5

Please look at this patient.

He had definite acromegaly.

This patient has visual loss. Please examine the fundi.
There was diabetic maculopathy and I was asked to draw
my findings!

Look at this patient's hands.
The only abnormality that I could find was a single, swan
neck deformity. It was very difficult!

This patient is diabetic. Please look at the feet.
There was a unilateral sensory loss and absent dorsalis
pedis pulses. There was a Charcot joint at the ankle.
    I was asked for a diagnosis.

Additional Station 2 experiences

28 *You are the SHO in the department and you are told
that you should present this patient at a regional haematology meeting. Take his history and summarize.*
The patient was a young man with multiple myeloma
who had been treated with C-VAMP (cyclosphos-
phamine, vincristine, adriamycin, methyl prednisolone), the treatment being complicated by
infections. He was awaiting an autologous bone marrow
transplant with high-dose melphalan. He was very
anxious.
    The examiners asked about the social aspects of the
diagnosis. Would haematologists at a regional meeting
really be interested and what was the evidence for an
autologous bone marrow transplant in multiple
myeloma?

29 *I was given a GP letter regarding a lady with worsening shortness of breath, who had a past cardiac, respiratory
and thyroid history.*
She described increasing shortness of breath and fatigue.
She had started smoking again and had had significant
life events. I thought she could be depressed as well as
having cardiac problems with being on amiodarone and
the previous hypothyroidism.
    I was asked about further management and for a dif-
ferential diagnosis.

30 *I was given quite a long letter regarding a lady on
digoxin and carbimazole who had presented with episodes
of fainting and nausea.*
It was a difficult case as the patient did not appear to have
been primed that it was a role play and answered most of
the questions about her fainting episodes by saying that

they were months ago and now resolved. The essentials
were that she had amiodarone-induced thyrotoxicosis
(she was in atrial fibrillation) and so she had been
switched to digoxin and was probably now experiencing
bradyarrhythmias. She had therefore had her dosage reduced. Now her main complaint was of tiredness.
    I was not helped by the examiners getting the timing
wrong and stopping me after 10 min! The questioning
centred on the differential diagnosis of faints and
tiredness.

31 *I had to see a middle-aged gentleman with recurrent
abdominal pains. He had had a recent admission for surgery when normal bloods and normal findings on OGD
were obtained. The GP had referred him to the medical
clinic.*
I obtained a history of recurrent abdominal pains over
the last 20 years. There were lots of stress factors in his life,
especially relating to his work. There was hardly any
weight loss, no blood passed per rectum and only occasional mucus. There was no history of diabetes mellitus,
heavy metal poisoning or of porphyria. The patient had
obvious concerns regarding a possible malignancy as he
had a positive family history for colonic carcinoma.
    The examiner asked me how I would write back to the
GP, what invasive investigations would I do and what did
I think was the most likely cause? I said, 'Irritable bowel
syndrome'.

32 *I was given a detailed GP letter. It was regarding a lady
in her seventies with congestive cardiac failure. She was
known to have ischaemic heart disease with a previous myocardial infarction. She had hypertension and chronic*

renal impairment. The GP requested advice on further investigations and management. She was taking atenolol, bendrofluazide (bendroflumethiazide), frusemide (furosemide) 40 mg and aspirin 75 mg. Her blood pressure was 160/90 mmHg and relevant blood investigations showed a urea of 20 mmol/L, creatinine 250 µmol/L and cholesterol 8 mmol/L.

The history was quite straightforward. A 70-year-old lady with hypertension, hypercholesterolaemia and chronic renal failure who had had a small myocardial infarction several years ago presenting now with shortness of breath on exertion and orthopnoea. She had been started on diuretics by the GP. She lived with her husband and had no social problems.

I was asked to give a problem list and to dictate the letter to the GP as if I had just seen the patient in clinic but, with the examiners and the patient watching this, it was not easy! I was asked what investigations I would do and what changes to her treatment I would arrange in the clinic. They really wanted to see what I would actually do if I had this patient in front of me in outpatients.

33 *I was asked to see a 50-year-old lady who presents to the clinic with diarrhoea which has lasted for more than a few weeks.*

The history evolved like a case of thyrotoxicosis with a past history of increasing appetite and loss of weight with a goitre. She even mentioned her staring appearance. I remembered to sum up my plan for investigations to the patient before time was up.

I was then asked about the investigations that I would do, the treatment that I would start her on and the management of thyroid eye disease.

34 *The GP requests a further assessment of a 63-year-old known diabetic who has had a coronary artery bypass graft in the past. He is now complaining of increasing frequency of angina. He has had a left, below knee amputation and has methicillin-resistant* Staphylococcus aureus *(MRSA) in an ulcer on his right foot.*

There were many, many problems! I ran out of time on the social history. He had angina and reduced mobility as a result of this and his limb prosthesis. He was blind in the right eye and was still smoking and had numerous social problems!

The examiners asked me how I would investigate the angina and what was the feasibility of nuclear scanning. They asked me how I would treat his MRSA ulcer and, finally, they wanted to know what I thought his prognosis was.

35 *I was given a GP referral letter for a patient who had developed a 1-month history of chest pain and had a past history of multiple joint pains and backache.*

The 43-year-old lady had a 1-month history of tight, retrosternal chest pain which was worse on exertion and on lying flat and which was associated with shortness of breath on exertion. She had a past history of pericarditis diagnosed by the GP 9 years previously but this had required no treatment. She had a family history of ischaemic heart disease with both her mother and brother dying in their fifties. The pain was not like the pain of her pericarditis, there was no history of diabetes mellitus or of hypertension. She was a non-smoker and had minimal alcohol intake. She also had a flitting arthralgia which was not a true arthritis as there was no swelling. I finished the history taking by outlining to the patient the physical examination I would perform and the investigations I would request which would be looking into the possibility of ischaemic heart disease, peptic ulcer disease, systemic lupus erythematosus (SLE) and musculoskeletal pain.

I was then asked to outline my differential diagnosis and was asked what investigations I would perform, so I suggested an ECG, an exercise ECG and an echocardiogram. They asked me what would be the diagnosis if the ECG showed ST elevation in all leads. They briefly asked me about SLE but then the bell went.

36 *I had to take a history from a lady who presented with a 6-month history of a cough. She had been on ACE inhibitors for the last 18 months.*

She had a dry cough which was associated with panicking. There were no features of asthma or of left ventricular failure and the most likely diagnosis was a cough resulting from ACE inhibition.

They asked me what I would put in the GP letter so I said I would stop the ACE inhibitors and change her to AT II RA (angiotersin II receptor antagonists) and that I would do a peak flow rate and arrange for pulmonary function tests.

37 *There was a very long GP letter giving the patient's past history of ulcerative colitis. The main concerns of the GP were about recent per rectum (PR) bleeding and about the use of steroids.*

The history I obtained consisted of a recent onset of PR bleeding which was dark in colour. There was no weight loss or loss of appetite. She had long-standing ulcerative colitis but was stable with no increased frequency of bowel movements or diarrhoea. She was taking nonsteroidals and steroids. She also had psoriasis but it was well controlled. The patient's concern was whether this was colonic carcinoma.

The examiners asked me what investigations I would do and how would I deal with the side-effects of steroids.

38 *I had to see a 36-year-old lady with insulin-dependent diabetes mellitus who had had a recent admission for a foot ulcer. All peripheral pulses were intact. The GP had referred her to the clinic because of the ulcer and was requesting measures to encourage the ulcer to heal. I was given the blood pressure of 130/80 mmHg.*

She had previous poor diabetic control and was unaware of any hypoglycaemic episodes. She was a non-smoker. She had two children and as her family was now complete her husband had had a vasectomy. She drank three glasses of wine every day. She had a low BM in the mornings and was on Insulatard and Actrapid t.d.s. She had a painless ulcer and had not seen the chiropodist recently.

I was asked about the role of the diabetic nurse and the chiropodist. The patient did not drive but the examiners asked me anyway whether she should have been advised against driving and I said, 'Yes, the patient should not really drive'.

39 *There was a GP letter asking whether this 72-year-old lady with weakness of her right arm and leg had had a stroke and what should be the management.*

The patient was a real inpatient and was a *very* bad historian! She had a 6-month history of falls and now had weakness of the right arm and leg. She was virtually unable to stand unaided and was not able to give a clear history of the duration or the onset or of any progression of her symptoms. She also complained of *incontinence, unsteadiness* and *confusion*—the triad of normal pressure hydrocephalus (NPH). She had no headaches and had had no social input as she 'hated' the social services, etc.

The examiners asked me the following questions: 'What differential diagnosis would you give in a letter to the GP?' and 'What action would you take?' I said I would admit the patient but that made it a very confusing scenario. 'What investigations would you do?' and 'What differential diagnosis would you write on the CT scan request?' We then had a long discussion as I had not mentioned a space-occupying lesion which the examiner clearly had as the top priority in his own mind. I thought he was wanting NPH. This was a very frustrating station as the patient was not a good history giver.

40 *The patient was an elderly man with chronic obstructive pulmonary disease (COPD) and social problems.*

There was also a previous history of an operation for small bowel obstruction.

I was asked for my management plans and the likely underlying causes of the small bowel obstruction.

41 *Speak to this 36-year-old diabetic lady who is on insulin and who has recently been treated for a diabetic foot ulcer. Take a history from her and explain to her the important problems that she now has.*

She was a 36-year-old lady who looked healthy. She was on regular insulin but her home BM readings varied quite considerably. She had one daughter aged 3 years and she had no other past medical illnesses. She had had a recent foot ulcer which had now healed well. She complained of a tingling sensation over both feet. She had already been seen in the ophthalmology clinic for an eye check. She had had no hypoglycaemic episodes but was adjusting the insulin dosage herself according to her BM results. The GP had planned to check her HbA1c. She was not on any drugs for pain relief and the GP notes said that both her dorsalis pedis pulses were palpable.

I was asked several questions by the examiners. 'What is the cause of her leg pain?' I said it would be either neuropathic or ischaemic and as her dorsalis pedis pulses were palpable then it was more likely to be neuropathic. 'What is the treatment if it is indeed neuropathic pain?' I said I would try carbamazepine but the examiners asked if that really was the first line of treatment. 'Is there any history of claudication?', 'What about her eye signs?' I explained to the examiner that the patient had told me that she had seen the ophthalmologist and had been told that her vision was normal. 'Is she driving now?' 'Yes', I said, 'but she does have to inform the DVLA and she cannot drive heavy goods vehicles'. The examiner asked me, 'What is the main problem that you have identified?' I replied, 'Neuropathic leg pain'. 'So how will you manage that?' I replied, 'With strict BM control, and carbamazepine or gabapentin'. 'What will you advise in the letter to the GP about this patient and her diabetes?'

42 *I missed this station because I arrived late! It is not a good idea to miss one complete station! It is still possible to pass the exam but one would need to get 100% on the other four stations and also if you are late for the first station you are likely to be flustered for the remainder of the exam. It is best to travel to the exam the night before and to be relaxed when you arrive.*

43 *The patient is a 60-year-old man with Parkinson's disease and on long-term medication. Recently, he has de-*

veloped worsening of the tremor. He has a history of a myocardial infarction with a coronary artery bypass graft and also he has prostatism. Explore his Parkinson's disease and suggest any further intervention and medication.

I took a history regarding the Parkinson's disease and the drugs that he had been on. He had recently been affected by worsening symptoms and I had to delve into the other features of his disease. I asked him how his symptoms affected him in different ways, such as physical/social. I also enquired about his myocardial infarction and took a history about chest pain/angina. I asked him about his prostatism and in fact he was due to have a repeat prostate operation. I included the other routine sections of the history taking including family history, allergies, social history, etc.

The examiners asked me how I could improve his symptoms. I was not asked about any specialized drugs as the scenario was not centred on a specialist neurological clinic. They asked me how I would seek out further information if I was unsure as to what to give. I said I would refer to a specialist clinic or look up the literature. The examiner asked me about the risks of having a repeat operation for his prostate and, finally, how were his symptoms related to micturition.

44 Take a history from this patient and think of how to reply to the GP.

The patient was a 65-year-old with symptoms of a transient ischaemic attack with slurred speech and weakness. The patient also had Hodgkin's disease. The GP was worried about disease recurrence.

I was asked about the psychosocial factors and whether the patient could have a superior vena caval obstruction.

45 I was given a GP letter regarding a patient with arthritis who had had recurrent falls and was not coping at home. The patient herself was not concerned but her family had gone to see the GP with their concerns for their mother. She had had recurrent falls and had burnt-out rheumatoid arthritis. There was no active disease and she was on no treatment. She had a regular home help.

I was asked whether I should be talking to the relatives without the patient's knowledge.

46 A 57-year-old Chinese gentleman is referred by his GP, diagnosed to have hypertension about 18 months ago. He has been treated with beta-blockers and hydrochlorothiazide but the BP has remained uncontrolled. He was subsequently changed to an ACE inhibitor but the patient has defaulted with his medication. His blood pressure is now 185/105 mmHg and investigations have revealed urinary glycosuria, blood sugar 8 mmol/L, blood urea 7 mMol/L and serum creatinine 145 µMol/L.

I introduced myself and asked him how the hypertension was diagnosed. Apparently he had had a headache and saw his GP who noted the high blood pressure. He was not aware of any sweating or palpitations. I explored any possible complications of hypertension such as chest pain and he did describe atypical chest pain on effort but the ECG had been normal. There was no paroxysmal nocturnal dyspnoea or orthopnoea, he had no intermittent claudication but did have transient weakness of his limbs. There was no focal neurological deficit and he had no symptoms of diabetes with no polyuria, polydipsia or excessive nocturia. He understood his diagnosis so I then went on to assess his cardiovascular risk. He was a chronic smoker, previously smoking 2 packets/day for 18 years, but had now reduced to 10 cigarettes/day. He consumed 3 units of alcohol/day. He played golf twice a week and I suggested a brisk walk in addition. He was overweight with hyperlipidaemia and had an excessive salt intake. I asked why he was not compliant to the medication and he explained that he was experiencing side-effects with erectile dysfunction from the beta-blockers and a dry, irritating cough from the ACE inhibitors. I asked about any family history of hypertension, diabetes or ischaemic heart disease and I enquired about his psychosocial history with regards to occupation, stress, family, etc.

His problem list was that he had hypertension which was not controlled because of poor compliance as experiencing side-effects from the medication. I also said that I would have to rule out a secondary cause for the hypertension. He had atypical chest pain which needed to be followed up by an exercise stress test. He had glycosuria which needed to be further investigated with a fasting blood sugar. I listed his risk factors for ischaemic heart disease in terms of age, sex, hypertension, smoking, alcohol, weight and hyperlipidaemia. I told him that he needed some lifestyle modification.

47 You are asked to see a 20-year-old with a headache. The GP wonders if he has had a subarachnoid haemorrhage. He was seen by the neurosurgeons as a child.

He had had a ventriculoperitoneal (VP) shunt inserted in infancy for hydrocephalus and this had been revised at the age of 10. The history was clearly not of a subarachnoid haemorrhage and there was a positive family history for migraine. He had no aura before the headaches, which were focal on the right side, although he was under considerable stress as he was studying and also working part time. I felt the differential diagnosis here was of migraine.

The examiners asked me for a differential diagnosis for the headache and what were the complications of a VP shunt and expected me to include a subependymal abscess! I was asked how to investigate headaches and how to treat migraine. They asked me what percentage of patients get an aura.

48 *Please see this 50-year-old lady with type 2 diabetes diagnosed 1 year ago. She takes gliclazide. She developed watery diarrhoea while on holiday in Greece and this has persisted for 4 weeks after her return. She has had one negative stool sample. Please advise.*

She had had weight loss, polyuria and polydipsia, all of which had begun before her holiday and had continued subsequently. There were no symptoms suggestive of in-flammatory bowel disease. Her home BM checks had been acceptable and no other family members who were on holiday with her had been affected.

I was asked about the causes for the symptoms and the signs of poorly controlled diabetes such as infection. 'What investigations would you like to do?' We returned to the possible causes and eventually I mentioned hyper-thyroidism which appeared to be what they were looking for!

49 *Please could you advise on this 60-year-old man with chronic respiratory problems.*

He had had bronchial asthma for 50 years. For the previous year he had had recurrent chest infections, which had improved with steroids given by his GP. However, his chest X-ray now showed a lesion. I thought the diagnosis could be bronchopulmonary aspergillosis.

Additional Station 4 experiences

50 *A retired nurse, who had worked in Hong Kong, had an elective hip operation cancelled because she was hepatitis C antibody-positive. She was told this without any explanation and just sent home. She found out more about hepatitis C herself and was concerned about the possibility of either a hepatoma or cirrhosis developing. She comes to casualty very upset.*

The discussion centred on her concerns regarding, 'Have I got HIV?', 'Have I got cirrhosis/hepatoma?', 'Will I ever have my hip operation?', 'Why did they do the test without telling me and why did they not explain anything?' It was probably because they were surgeons!

The questions were, 'Was their attitude ethical in doing the hepatitis screen without informing her', and how would I have investigated her.

51 *A lady has come back to clinic and you are the only doctor there. All the others are away. She has recently been investigated for multiple sclerosis and you have to give her the diagnosis.*

The conversation centred on the above and she wanted to know about the diagnosis and whether she could work. She asked if she could still drive, if she could have children and were there any treatment options.

I was asked what I would do if her boyfriend tele-phoned me and asked me to tell him about the consulta-tion because she would not discuss it with him.

52 *Breaking bad news—multiple sclerosis. You have come to clinic early today and you are the only person available.*

The patient did not know much about multiple sclerosis and so I had to go back to basics. The patient asked me very limited questions and I finished by asking her to come to an appointment the following day with her part-ner. The examiner said to me that her partner telephones you at 5 p.m. demanding to know what she has been told. What would you do? The examiner also says that the pa-tient has asked about interferon. How would I manage that?

53 *I was given a clinical scenario of a man with recently diagnosed carcinoma of the lung. I was asked to tell the patient his diagnosis and to ask for his consent for a bronchoscopy.*

I went over with the patient the symptoms he had pre-sented with and then broke the bad news. I paused fre-quently, which I felt was very important, and I listened to his concerns. He did not want his wife to know so I ex-plored why and managed to convince him that I should see them together. He was happy about that. We dis-cussed the prognosis and he thought he was going to die in the next few weeks. He was concerned about having the bronchoscopy as a friend of his had had a bad experi-ence with a rigid bronchoscope. I explained to him that the modern procedure uses a thin, flexible tube and that sedation is given. However, I did not have enough time to tell him about the dangers of bronchoscopy.

The examiners asked me about these dangers and about what I would do if his wife wanted to know the diagnosis and the patient was not there, which raised the issues of confidentiality, etc.

54 *A 55-year-old lady who had had previous radical radiotherapy for carcinoma of the lung had recently been for her 6-month check up which was OK. She now presents with back pain, and both a bone scan and a CT scan have shown bony metastases in her spine, pelvis and ribs with an unstable L2 vertebra. Explain the results of her tests.*
She was a nurse but played a good patient. She was 'in denial'. The family did not know anything and she did not want them to until they had been on their holiday to France. I explained the situation and offered support and suggested that I could talk to her husband with her. I said that she was free to go on holiday but that she should really see the orthopaedic surgeon and the radiotherapist to get an opinion on the stability of her spine before she went.

I was asked about her rights.

55 *You are about to see a 24-weeks pregnant lady who has swelling of her leg. She has taken antibiotics which did not help. Discuss with her the methods of investigating for a deep vein thrombosis.*
The patient was worried about the risks from any radiological investigation and we then discussed methods for anticoagulation.

I was asked about the dilemmas of investigation and treatment with low molecular weight heparin.

56 *Explain to this lady that her mother probably has Huntington's chorea with a recent relapse.*
The 'relative' appeared well-educated and was asking many questions. She wanted to know about investigations, prognosis, any possible cure and future implications.

It all went very well and the examiners looked pleased.

57 *You are the SHO on call and you have been asked to talk to the daughter of a patient who is being tested for Huntington's disease. The genetic tests are not back yet but the daughter is very concerned.*
I asked her how much she knew already and what provisional diagnosis she had been given. I explained about Huntington's disease in relation to the patient having choreiform movements. She wanted to know all the implications for the family and I explained these. She was concerned about if her mother did not want the family to

know then could we tell her the diagnosis as it may affect her and her children. Confidentiality was discussed at length and we also briefly touched on genetic counselling.

The examiner asked me if we could break confidentiality here and could I outline any diseases where confidentiality could and should be broken. I needed to be prompted with a scenario of a teacher being diagnosed with tuberculosis before I mentioned that notifiable diseases was an area where confidentiality had to be broken. I was then asked to define a notifiable disease.

58 *You have to see a heavy goods vehicle driver who was diagnosed 3 months ago with insulin-dependent diabetes mellitus and you have to advise him that he cannot drive HGVs any more.*
We discussed the history of his diabetes and his recent review at which he had been started on insulin. He had not been told that he must stop driving at that review although I explained to him that he was legally required to renounce his HGV licence. He was unwilling to consider this as he was the only wage earner in the family and it would affect his livelihood and that of his family. We discussed the legal position and whether the police would need to be informed.

I was asked who I would discuss this with and I suggested that his GP should be informed as well as the DVLA and my senior colleague.

59 *A young woman is admitted to the casualty department with a hypoglycaemic episode. She has type 1 diabetes mellitus and is a heavy goods vehicle driver. You have to ensure that she informs the DVLA and stops driving HGV vehicles.*
The whole conversation was very difficult! The actor performed as a stubborn patient. She was not listening to any of my arguments. We tried to establish the cause for the hypoglycaemic episodes and I tried to suggest that we get the GP and the diabetic nurse involved/informed.

The examiner asked me what I would have done next if the patient persisted in driving.

60 *You occasionally attend the neurology clinics and are called to outpatients as a lady has arrived without a clinic appointment wanting to know the results of her investigations. She has had internuclear ophthalmoplegia and investigations have shown an oligoclonal band in the cerebrospinal fluid and an MRI scan is suggestive of multiple sclerosis. Please tell her that she has multiple sclerosis and that the consultant neurologist is busy elsewhere.*
It was awful! There was a large table between us so I moved my chair closer to the patient and then had the ex-

aminers right in front of me and I also had difficulty in seeing the clock. The 'patient' was obviously neither a patient nor a good actress and showed very little emotion. I did not want to get into the finer details of multiple sclerosis so I established early on that the patient ought to return with her fiancé and she had no further questions. We finished early and then had 2 min of complete silence!

The examiner asked me how I thought the patient would feel when she got home and should she have been given some warning before the investigations were carried out that she might have multiple sclerosis. One examiner gave me a clear pass on all aspects and the other just on the conduct of the interview.

61 *This lady's father has recently been diagnosed with Huntington's disease. She has some information about the condition from the Internet but wants to discuss the inheritance risks and her concerns about starting a family.*

I started off by ascertaining her understanding of her father's condition and what her main concerns were. I explained that the inheritance was autosomal dominant, i.e. 50% risk of passing the condition on to any child. I asked her if she had discussed this with her husband and suggested that she bring her husband in to discuss these issues. We also discussed what support had already been given to her father. The 'relative'/actress appeared well informed and was, I think, an SpR in medicine who appeared to be totally unemotional.

The examiner asked me what her husband's views were likely to be. Would I have informed her of the 50% inheritance risk if the husband had been present? We then went on to talk about the ethics of advanced directives and how often advanced directives needed to be updated.

62 *You see an 18-year-old girl who is a newly diagnosed insulin-dependent diabetic. She had presented with ketonuria and hyperglycaemia. Explain the diagnosis and its implications to her.*

She was a typical teenage girl with diabetes who refused to know about her diagnosis and kept changing the subject. She asked about driving but then moved to the next question before I was able to say anything about notifying the DVLA. I was able to bring it up again later and I then noticed the examiners were changing their marksheets!

The examiner asked me what I would do if the patient decided to leave without accepting insulin therapy.

63 *You must speak to the son of a 76-year-old man who has bronchogenic carcinoma and who is refusing to under-*

go treatment. You must discuss with the son your management strategy and his father's resuscitation status.

The son was keen for no further treatment as his father was suffering quite a lot. I told the examiner that if the patient is mentally fit and not depressed then we cannot force treatment. If he is not mentally fit then the consultant has to decide the management after consulting with the relatives. Regarding resuscitation status I needed to talk to the patient in order to make a decision.

64 *You are about to see a young lady with lymphoma and you have to break the bad news to her.*

The patient was very emotional and I was unable to control the situation. I felt that I did really badly here and in fact I had a clear fail.

65 *I had to see a 30-year-old lady with probable multiple sclerosis. She was working full-time and this was her first consultation after having been referred from the GP after an episode of loss of vision in one eye which had now resolved. She had problems with shaking/tremor in her hands and diplopia. She had been advised to come in for further investigations. A previous CT brain scan was normal.*

I was asked to speak to the patient about the possibility of multiple sclerosis but to explain that we needed to confirm the diagnosis by doing further investigations in hospital and this would require admission. I was asked to explain about an MRI scan and a lumbar puncture. The patient had some social concerns about going to work, the probable chance of having multiple sclerosis and the implications for her teenage daughter.

66 *You have to see the daughter of a lady who is very unwell and likely to succumb to a severe pneumonia. Please counsel the daughter regarding resuscitation status.*

The whole counselling, with a very agreeable and cooperative 'relative', lasted a mere 7 min!

The examiners asked me about the principles of ethics in terms of autonomy and paternalism.

67 *You are about to see a patient with atrial fibrillation who is taking amiodarone. Talk to the patient about starting warfarin.*

We discussed the pros and cons of warfarin therapy and discussed risk vs. benefit.

68 *This 27-year-old lady was diagnosed as having migraine. She has a strong family history of migraine including her sister and mother. She has expressed her concern regarding worsening headaches and requests a CT scan. She* is also concerned about the renal complications following prolonged analgesic ingestion. One of her friends has just died of a brain haemorrhage. On a previous occasion you have examined her and found no serious pathology.

I explained to the patient that I had been asked to explain to her the plan of management. I asked her to tell me more about her concerns and then tried to address these. I attempted to evaluate the headache, enquiring about the site, nature, frequency and duration of the pain and about whether there were any sinister symptoms and signs. I asked about recent changes in lifestyle and in particular about any recent precipitating foods, stress, poor sleep, etc. I enquired about the medication she was on in terms of type and frequency of medication. I explored any occupational stress, interpersonal relationships with staff at work and regarding her family support. I explained to her that both the history and physical examination had not revealed any serious pathology in her brain. I tried to reassure her and provide support. I explained about avoiding precipitating factors, e.g. tyramine-containing foods and to take her migraine prophylactic drugs and then we discussed any possible side-effects. I touched on stress management with breathing exercises, yoga and medication and arranged a follow-up appointment for 1 month's time. I explained that if she had improved by then that all would be well, but that if no improvement was obvious then one would have to consider a CT scan. Meanwhile I explained to her that a CT brain scan was not required as it was costly and may pick up minor abnormalities which would further worry the patient. I addressed her concerns regarding kidney function and reassured her that the frequency and dosage of tablets would be minimal and that one can assess renal function by investigations. I said that if she had any serious symptoms she was to return to clinic sooner than the given appointment.

69 *A young female patient who had had her first fit returns to clinic. You must discuss the implications of this with her. She is a keen sportswoman and drives a car having just passed her test. Her occupation is in computing.*
The patient asked me lots of questions including, 'Is this epilepsy?', 'Will I fit again?', 'Why can I not drive?' The patient was upset at having had this fit and was very concerned about the stigma of epilepsy.

70 *A 55-year-old lady, who had had a mastectomy 10 years ago for carcinoma, now presents with hypercalcaemia and back pain and is found to have metastatic recurrence. You are the SHO on the ward and must tell the patient the*

diagnosis, the need to refer her to the oncologist and the likely treatment options.
I broke the news early on. The patient was very shocked and then became angry, particularly stating that she was not told 10 years ago that the disease could return. She asked me if I thought it was wrong not to have told her. I did not agree or disagree with her but merely expressed my regret and sorrow. We discussed chemotherapy and radiotherapy and I tried to emphasize the seriousness of the condition and the fact that this was unlikely to be curable. I asked her about her other concerns. Her mother had recently died an 'undignified' death and the patient asked me about the possibility of euthanasia. I explained that this is illegal in this country and then went into the specifics of palliative care in an attempt to address her particular concerns of pain, etc.

The examiner asked me what should one do when a patient criticizes another doctor and then about whether the decision to resuscitate should always be discussed with the patient.

Invigilators diaries—Station 2 and 4

Poor start
On starting the consultation, the candidate's first sentence was, 'Sorry, but I have forgotten your name.' Another first sentence was, 'Right then, how can I help?'

First impressions
On approaching the patient, the candidate sneezed into his hands, and then shook the patient's hand.

Keeping eye contact
The candidate was so involved in taking notes during the history taking, that he missed how the patient described her chest pain, a sweep of the hand from the epigastric area to the throat mimicking her heartburn.

In a rush
A candidate mistimed the whole station; he raced through the history of the presenting complaint in about 1 min, proceeded to briefly take the rest of the history, and then realized he had 9 min left. The silence was broken by, 'OK then, tell me about these palpitations again.'

Interruptions
A patient with a previous history of ischaemic cardiac pain, angioplasty and coronary artery stenting was describing her present chest pain (resulting from oesophageal reflux) and just about to say that this present pain is different from her previous chest pain, when the

candidate interrupted and said, 'So, tell me more about your angioplasty.'

Specific questioning

When asking about smoking history, the candidate could not keep the questioning as open as possible and asked, 'how many cigarettes do you smoke a day, 10, 20, 30 or 40?'

Ignoring the past medical history

A patient presents with breathlessness and is on amiodarone for atrial fibrillation. She has had a coronary artery bypass graft in the past. The candidate asks the patient, 'Have you had any operations in the past?' 'Yes, a heart operation,' was the reply. The candidate followed this by saying, 'Oh, that's interesting. Moving on, tell me, do you smoke?'

Inability to pick up hints of emotions and lacking tact

The consultation revolved around a patient with blurred vision. The young patient was worried she may have multiple sclerosis. The patient says to the candidate, 'I'm worried this may be something serious.' The candidate replied 'That doesn't surprise me.'

Any questions?

After a consultation with a patient presenting with haemoptysis, the candidate asked the patient, 'Any questions?' The reply from the patient was, 'So, what is the problem.' The candidate then said, 'I don't know but I will refer you on to a respiratory specialist.'

End of station 2

A candidate, after seeing a patient with funny turns, gave no indication of any tests to be performed, any follow-up or any thoughts about the possible causes for the funny turns, ended the consultation by saying, 'Thanks, we've finished now.'

Experiences

These accounts from the pre MRCP PACES short cases start with four detailed experiences followed by a medley of short scenarios of individual cases. These are relevant to the current PACES format; because the same short cases are presented, albeit in different stations, a competent performance is expected, and the examiners ask the same sort of questions. Important learning points emerge from each experience, which should be incorporated in your examination technique. We have highlighted some key points in the footnotes.

'The examiners let him realize that he had missed coarctation of the aorta.'
1 In his first case (first attempt) a candidate was asked to: 'Examine this man's heart'. He found a short systolic murmur in a hypertensive patient and diagnosed aortic sclerosis. He did not look for radiofemoral delay because he had been asked to examine the heart and not the cardiovascular system.

The examiners let him realize that he had missed coarctation of the aorta. Filled with anger and dismay at this injustice he was taken to the next case where he was asked to listen to the *back* of a woman's chest. He had a quick look at the *front* (was not asked to) and spotted the radiation marks (he felt that the examiners were trying to hide this clue from him). He looked purposefully at the back and noted pleural aspiration marks. He therefore suspected a pleural effusion and performed the relevant clinical steps to confirm this impression. He was asked the probable cause and without hesitation gave the diagnosis of bronchial carcinoma along with the supportive evidence.

He was then asked to examine a man's cranial nerves. He performed a rapid, efficient screen and reported left VIth, VIIth, XIIth nerve palsies and left lateral nystagmus but he was not asked for a diagnosis. For his fourth case he was asked to look at a man and he gave the spot diagnosis of acromegaly. When asked how to diagnose the condition he suggested imaging of the pituitary fossa, glucose tolerance test (GTT) with growth hormone levels, etc. Next, he was asked to look at a patient's arm and he instantly recognized the 'plucked chicken skin' appearance of pseudoxanthoma elasticum in the antecubital fossa. Finally, he was asked to look at a woman's face where he saw nothing obvious until he spotted a small left pupil and slight ptosis. He immediately diagnosed a left Horner's syndrome and was asked for, and gave, the possible causes.

Although his performance in all but the first case had been impeccable he was convinced, until the result arrived, that he had failed because of that first case. In retrospect, his reaction to the first case may have had a positive effect on the subsequent performance. Instead of going to pieces (e.g. experience 2 below, and quotations 46 and 49, p. 366) he felt angry at being asked to examine the heart when the key finding was at the femoral pulse. He conducted the rest of the exam with ruthless efficiency and avenged himself by looking for more than he was asked to. The parting words of the examiner were: 'You'll never miss radiofemoral delay again, will you?' (Pass)

'He looked down on two thin legs, imagined two inverted champagne bottles, and before he could stop himself, heard himself saying "Charcot–Marie–Tooth disease".'
2 On his second attempt another candidate was asked first to, 'Examine the abdomen'. Without looking anywhere else he coned down on the abdomen and felt the liver edge. After a long time, and some persuasion, he noticed the palmar erythema, anaemia, gynaecomastia and decreased body hair. These signs, in particular the gynaecomastia, together with the diagnosis of cirrhosis had to be dragged out of him by the examiners. The candidate had been nervous before the start and now, realizing that he had performed badly on the first case through lack of proper inspection, was already becoming engulfed in the 'downward spiral syndrome'.

At the second case the examiner said, 'We haven't much time so just quickly feel the pulse and listen over the apex and base'. He was confused as he did not know where the base was so he listened at the lower left sternal edge and the apex. He did not look at the neck or at the praecordium. He felt a collapsing pulse, heard a systolic murmur and diagnosed mitral incompetence. In retrospect, he thought that he must have missed mixed aortic valve disease.

On the next case he was asked to examine the patient's legs. He realized that things were going very badly and that he had to score highly from then on. He looked down on two thin legs, imagined two inverted champagne bottles and, before he could stop himself, heard himself saying 'Charcot–Marie–Tooth disease'. The examiner, who was apparently becoming increasingly doubtful about the candidate's capability of performing a competent clinical examination, had to drag a hesitant, unstructured examination out of him which revealed spastic paraparesis. A discussion followed on the possible causes.

In the next case the candidate looked at a fundus with whiteness around the disc and diagnosed myelinated nerve fibres. In his last case he examined a patient's hands with swollen metacarpophalangeal and proximal interphalangeal joints, tapered fingers, wasted intrinsic muscles and papery, thin skin. With his morale gone, it took a long time before he saw any of the abnormalities and longer still to suggest rheumatoid arthritis (?on steroids). (Fail)

'He was side-tracked into saying that she could have hereditary haemorrhagic telangiectasia.'
3 After an indifferent start in the short cases, a candidate was asked to examine a man's pulse. He found it regular and the rate was 40 beats/min. He was then asked to listen to the precordium but he failed to comment on the variable intensity of the first heart sound which could have led him to the diagnosis of complete heart block.

He was next asked to look at a woman's face. There was perioral tethering and telangiectasis, but as he had not performed a *visual survey* and his presentation was loose, he was side-tracked into saying that she could have hereditary haemorrhagic telangiectasia. It eventually became obvious to him (he was asked to look at the hands — sclerodactyly) that the patient had scleroderma. The examiner then asked him: 'On which part of the tongue would you say the telangiectasiae would most likely be found in hereditary haemorrhagic telangiectasia, if you were teaching a class of medical students?'

Having been unable to impress the examiners so far, he was asked to look at a man's neck. (The bell went almost immediately signalling the end of the exam.) The patient was lying down and his neck movements were completely restricted. The candidate diagnosed cervical spondylosis. The typical 'question mark' posture of ankylosing spondylitis only became recognizable when the patient sat up!

In his second attempt, this candidate was asked to examine a middle-aged woman with a goitre — he felt it was really quite straightforward. The goitre was asymmetrical but he annoyed one examiner by using the term 'slightly asymmetrical'. He also let out the word 'tumour' in front of the patient when asked to discuss management. (Fail)

'During the examination he was interrupted at various times.'
4 A candidate on his first attempt was asked to look at a man's legs (the examiner pulled the pyjamas to the lower end of the patella, leaving a lateral scar covered — which the candidate did not see until the end). He found a swollen, warm left leg and diagnosed a deep venous thrombosis. He was asked for other possibilities and said ruptured Baker's cyst. The examiner said he would not

ask who Baker was but wanted an explanation of the term. The examiners probed for further possibilities such as cellulitis, muscle rupture and also asked about ruptured plantaris muscle.

On his next case he was asked to look at the patient's hands and describe them. He diagnosed rheumatoid arthritis and was asked to explain the reasons for ulnar deviation, subluxation and boutonnière deformity. The examiner asked: 'Why is it called boutonnière? Have you ever seen a button hook? Why is the wrist like that? What are the important functions of the hand?' He was then asked to look at the knees of the same patient. He found a swollen, painful right knee which he thought resulted from synovial swelling. He said he had been about to say: 'Charcot's joint' but realized it was painful. He diagnosed rheumatoid arthritis of the knee and was then asked how he knew it was synovial swelling.

At the next patient the examiners said: 'I think we would be interested in this lady's precordium'. During the examination he was interrupted at various times: 'What do you think of the pulse?'; 'What do you think of the jugular venous pressure?'; and they stopped him before he had finished and asked for the findings. He diagnosed mixed mitral valve disease but had missed the mitral valvotomy scar.

The examiner then handed him an ophthalmoscope and said: 'We would like you to use this on the next patient'. The candidate noticed that this patient showed some incoordination and a spastic leg so he expected to find optic atrophy. When he mentioned this diagnosis the examiner asked him if he knew what sort of visual field defect he would expect and then asked him to test the visual fields.

On the last case he was asked to feel the patient's abdomen. He found an inguinal hernia, a palpable aorta and a palpable liver edge at about 2 cm below the right costal margin. He said he did not think it was hepatomegaly. The examiners asked what signs he would look for if the patient did have hepatomegaly! (Pass)

In the following examples the examiner seems to be probing the power and range of the candidate's observations

5 A candidate was asked to examine the motor system of a man's legs. She found global weakness, wasting and loss of reflexes. She gave a differential diagnosis of lower motor neurone paralysis that included a disc lesion, spinal canal problems, degenerative disorders and motor neurone disease. The examiners asked her to look at the patient's tongue—it was fasciculating. She was then able

to narrow the differential diagnosis to the last-mentioned possibility. (Pass)

6 A candidate was asked: 'Look at this man's chest and then examine his respiratory system'. The patient had a right mastectomy scar and the skin changes of previous radiotherapy. There was dullness to percussion and reduced breath sounds at the right base. The candidate diagnosed carcinoma of the breast with a right pleural effusion. (Pass)

7 A candidate was asked to listen only to a patient's heart. No other cardiovascular examination was expected. She found the features of mitral stenosis but did not notice the valvotomy scar. The examiner pointed this out to her. (Pass)

8a A candidate was asked to look at a woman's hands. He found the changes of rheumatoid arthritis. A description was not wanted, only the diagnosis. The examiner then asked him: 'Why is she wearing a cervical collar?' The candidate, who had noticed it but not mentioned it, said that it could be because of atlantoaxial subluxation. (Pass)

8b After mistaking a malar flush for SLE in a patient who had mitral stenosis, a candidate was asked to examine a woman's hands. She diagnosed acromegaly. Although the patient had wasting of the thenar eminence she missed this, and the diagnosis of carpal tunnel syndrome, until the examiner told her about the patient's symptoms. The candidate diagnosed optic atrophy, splenomegaly and hepatosplenomegaly successively in three other short cases and was then shown a patient and asked: 'On general appearance what is wrong with this man?' She thought that he had a myopathic facies and diagnosed dystrophia myotonica. The examiner asked why she thought he had a hearing aid. She looked at the head again and realized that the patient had an enlarged cranium, rather than wasted facial muscles, and diagnosed Paget's disease. (Fail)

9 A candidate was shown a patient and asked: 'On general appearance what is wrong with this man?' She thought that he had a myopathic facies and diagnosed myotonic dystrophy. The examiner asked why she thought he had a hearing aid. She looked at the head again and realized that the patient had an enlarged cranium, rather than wasted facial muscles, and diagnosed Paget's disease.* (Fail)

10 A candidate was asked to examine a man's abdomen. She found an enlarged, knobbly liver and diagnosed hepatic secondaries but forgot to test for ascites. She was asked if there was any free peritoneal fluid. The examiners watched intently as she demonstrated the presence of ascites. (Pass)

* It may be that in PACES such a case would be less likely to occur.

11 A candidate was asked to examine the patient's abdomen. He found bilateral masses in the loins and diagnosed polycystic kidneys. The patient also had a craniotomy scar from a repair of a ruptured berry aneurysm. On another case, he was able to diagnose hypothyroidism by looking at a woman's face. The examiner asked why she was in a surgical ward and he suggested severe constipation as a reason. (Pass)

12 A candidate was asked to, 'Examine this lady's cardiovascular system, commenting as you go'. He diagnosed mixed mitral valve disease but missed the cardiac cachexia and the left mastectomy scar. The examiners wanted him to comment that she was very ill and to suggest why. They also asked for comments as to whether the mitral stenosis or mitral incompetence was dominant. (Fail)

13 A candidate was asked to, 'Comment on this patient's appearance. Pretend he is sitting opposite you on the underground train and perform one clinical test.' The candidate noted frontal bossing, bilateral ptosis, deafness, missing fingers on the right hand and a saddle-shaped nose. Initially, the candidate thought he had congenital syphilis and wanted to do a Romberg's test. The examiner manipulated the discussion and got him round to thinking about myotonic dystrophy. After this, the candidate suggested a handshake as the one clinical test.

He was then asked to examine the abdomen of the next patient. He found bilateral, enlarged, 'lumpy' kidneys which were easily palpable and he diagnosed polycystic kidneys. The candidate was shown the patient's left forearm and, having worked on a renal unit, he immediately recognized the presence of an arteriovenous fistula for haemodialysis. The examiners seemed quite impressed with this. (Pass)

14 Another candidate was shown the same patient with myotonic dystrophy and asked: 'What observations do you make?' He commented on the bilateral ptosis, wasted sternomastoid and temporalis muscles and, after demonstrating myotonia in the hands, was able to make the diagnosis. There then followed a brief viva on cardiomyopathy in this condition. (Pass)

15 A candidate was asked to listen to a patient's heart. He found mitral incompetence and noted that the patient's face looked acromegalic. However, he did not mention the acromegaly until he was directly asked about it. (Fail)

16 A candidate was taken to a patient with a recent laparotomy scar and asked to examine his neck. He noticed a biopsy scar and, on palpation, found matted glands. He diagnosed Hodgkin's disease and the examiner just asked him for a differential diagnosis. (Pass)

17 'Look at this patient from here. What would you like to do now?' The candidate noticed a man with long extremities, muscle wasting, a pustular rash, paronychia, nicotine-stained fingers and pectus excavatum. He had to be prompted to the diagnosis of Marfan's syndrome. He was then asked to look into the patient's mouth (high-arched palate) and to listen to his heart (aortic incompetence). He found both of these but did not mention the hyperextensible joints. (Pass)

18a For the cardiovascular case, a candidate's instruction was: 'This lady is breathless—listen to her heart'. He diagnosed mitral stenosis but the examiners pointed out that he had not noticed that the lady had rheumatoid arthritis as well.

Later on, for his respiratory case, he was told: 'This patient is breathless—examine the respiratory system'. He found crepitations and basal dullness so he diagnosed pulmonary fibrosis with a pleural effusion. Having learned from the earlier case, he was able to relate both to the rheumatoid arthritis which he had already observed in this patient. (Pass)

18b After having difficulty deciding whether a patient had diabetic or hypertensive retinopathy, a candidate was asked to examine another patient's neck. He diagnosed a small multinodular goitre but the examiners remained dissatisfied. They asked if the patient was thyrotoxic or not. While he examined for a tremor he noticed the gross rheumatoid arthritis in the hands. He reported that the examiners were looking for the diagnosis of autoimmune thyroid disease. (Fail)

19 A candidate was invited to look at a patient's face. The face was normal when looking straight ahead but on further examination he discovered weakness of the lower part of the right side of the face and he diagnosed a right upper motor neurone VIIth nerve palsy.* He missed the surgical scar just below the jaw on the right side and, in retrospect, felt it was a partial right lower motor neurone VIIth nerve palsy. (Fail)

20 A candidate was asked to look at a patient's face. He said: 'Acromegaly'. The examiner asked if he was happy with that in such a way that he implied to the candidate that he should look for more physical signs. At once the candidate said that he would like to look for complications such as a bitemporal hemianopia, hypertension, cardiomegaly or evidence of treatment already given. The patient did, in fact, have a hemianopia. (Pass)

* The correct expression would be 'upper motor neurone *facial muscular*' palsy, because the lesion has to be above the nucleus of the VIIth cranial nerve.

In the experiences that follow the spotlight seems to be on the candidate's examination technique

21 A candidate was asked to make a neurological examination of a patient's legs. He found bilateral upper motor neurone signs and was then asked the level of the lesion. The candidate proceeded to examine the arms and found upper motor neurone signs in one arm. He then tested the jaw jerk, which was normal. No further questions were asked. (Pass)

22 A candidate was asked to examine a patient's abdomen. He found an enlarged organ in the left hypochondrium and thought that it was a polycystic kidney but he admits that his examination was 'cack-handed'. In retrospect, he thinks it was a spleen. For his eye case he was asked to look at a patient's fundi. He diagnosed choroiditis but, in retrospect, he feels that it was probably a diabetic retinopathy with laser burns. (Fail)

23 A candidate was asked to examine a woman's fundi, to look for pyramidal signs in her hands and to elicit her plantar responses. He found early papilloedema on the left, an increased finger jerk and supernator jerk on the right and a right extensor plantar. He admitted that he had made a mess of doing the finger jerks and did not know the two ways of eliciting these; the examiner had to demonstrate the tests. He was about to test the plantar response with the end of the patella hammer when he was stopped by the examiner who gave him a thin wooden orange stick! (Pass)

24 A candidate was asked to look at, and then examine, the legs of a man who complained of unsteadiness. He found ataxia, pyramidal weakness with clonus in both legs and bilateral extensor plantar responses and he diagnosed multiple sclerosis. However, the examiner was not at all happy with his neurological examination technique and, in fact, showed him how to do it! (Fail)

25 A candidate was asked to watch a patient walk and to examine his lower limbs. He could see bilateral foot-drop with wasted anterior compartments but did not make the diagnosis of Charcot–Marie–Tooth disease. The examiners criticized the way in which he examined the reflexes. (Fail)

26 A candidate was told: 'This man has gone off his feet. Examine the legs and say why.' He found gross wasting, fasciculation, absent ankle jerks and flexor plantar responses and he diagnosed progressive muscular atrophy (motor neurone disease). He commented to us that he had to wait for what seemed to be 3–4 min before any fasciculation was seen, although when it did come it was very obvious. (Pass)

27 A candidate was asked to examine a patient's eyes. He

was almost blind in the left eye with a left VIth nerve palsy. He commented that he might well have failed the examination had he not tested visual acuity and thus found the explanation for the absence of diplopia. (Pass)

28 A candidate was asked to examine neurologically a man's hand. The patient had gross wasting and weakness of the small muscles of the hand. Although the candidate diagnosed a T1 lesion he admitted that he looked very confused examining the hands.

A little unsettled by this experience, he was later asked to examine another patient's abdomen and jugular venous pressure. He found a pulsatile liver and giant *v* waves. He diagnosed tricuspid incompetence but admitted that he lacked confidence and this showed in the way he carried out the examination.

For the respiratory case, he was asked to examine the chest of a patient who had a thoracotomy scar, stridor and clubbing. He did not notice the stridor and also missed the pleural effusion. (Fail)

29 On being asked to examine the abdomen of a patient, a candidate found bilateral subcostal masses. He gave the findings and said the diagnosis was probably polycystic kidneys. The left-sided mass could have been a small spleen moving diagonally across the abdomen from under the rib cage on inspiration but it was bimanually ballottable. He gave the findings and persevered with the diagnosis of polycystic kidneys. The examiners persisted in discussing the possibility that the mass was a spleen but the candidate stuck to his diagnosis which he thinks was right. (Pass)

30 A candidate was asked: 'Examine this man's chest. Is there anything else you would look for?' He found ankylosing spondylitis with poor expansion of the chest, but commented that he had to get the patient out of bed before he appreciated the typical 'question mark' posture of ankylosing spondylitis. There was no evidence of aortic regurgitation or upper lobe fibrosis. (Pass)

31 A candidate examined the abdomen of a 35-year-old Afro-Caribbean woman and found a 6-cm spherical mass in the left upper quadrant. He commented that he was allowed to 'go through the routine'—nodes, mouth, hands, etc. He said it was not a spleen or a kidney and he explained why. He gave a brief differential diagnosis. 'Expressionless and without comment they led me away.' (Pass)

32 A candidate was asked to: 'Show me how you examine the reflexes in the legs'. He found absent knee and ankle jerks and extensor plantar responses. He offered the differential diagnosis of tabes dorsalis, subacute combined degeneration of the cord and a hereditary neuropathy such as Friedreich's ataxia. He was asked what else he would like to examine and he suggested the pupillary reflexes. He found small, irregular pupils which reacted to light and accommodation, but more to accommodation. He was asked if these were Argyll Robertson pupils and he answered: 'No'. The other examiner said: 'You said that this picture in the legs may be caused by tabes dorsalis. How do you explain the extensor plantars?' He answered that this indicates pyramidal tract involvement. The examiner pointed out that this is called taboparesis, not tabes dorsalis. The candidate felt that his unfamiliarity with the different manifestations of neurosyphilis let him down, and he had failed to recognize Argyll Robertson pupils. (Fail)

33 A candidate was asked to: 'Examine the abdomen'. He found an enlarged liver of 3 finger-breadths and a spleen of 4 finger-breadths and diagnosed hepatosplenomegaly. The examiner's parting comment was: 'It is no good only making a diagnosis;* there is a proper method to examine the patient!' (Fail)

34 A candidate was asked to examine the back of a young man's chest. He diagnosed* bilateral pleural effusions and he felt that these probably resulted from nephrotic syndrome. He believes the examiners agreed. However, he had forgotten to test for vocal resonance or tactile vocal fremitus. (Fail)

35 A candidate was asked to examine a patient's heart. He went through all the correct examination steps except that he forgot to lift up the arm and feel for a collapsing pulse. He diagnosed mixed mitral valve disease. One examiner proceeded to listen to the heart while the other examiner asked if the candidate had felt for a collapsing pulse. The candidate now wonders if he missed aortic valve disease. (Fail)

36 A candidate was asked to examine the eyes of a young woman aged about 20–30 years. He went comprehensively through the routine, checking visual acuity and visual fields before testing eye movements. He felt that the examiners were impatient at the delay in finding the nystagmus that was present. The examiners asked what he wanted to examine next. The candidate, thinking that the diagnosis was likely to be multiple sclerosis, and assuming the presence of cerebellar signs, said he wanted to look at the fundi (for optic atrophy). He could not understand why the examiners seemed so irritated by this. They wanted him to demonstrate the cerebellar signs that were present. The candidate felt that this was an easy case on which he had made no great errors and yet the

examiners seemed to have been unimpressed by his performance.† (Fail)

37 A candidate was asked to examine a patient's legs neurologically and then to ask him some questions. He found global aphasia and a profound right-sided spastic hemiparesis. He diagnosed a dominant hemisphere vascular lesion. He was asked: 'What might be the cause? The patient is 40', (pause), 'Feel the pulse'. He was in atrial fibrillation. 'What do you think the cause is now?' (Pass)

38 A candidate was shown a woman with a spastic paraparesis which she correctly diagnosed. After she had been taken to the next case, the examiners said: 'By the way, which side of the fire does that previous lady usually sit by?' Luckily, she had noticed the erythema ab igne on the legs. (Pass)

A lack of polish and fluidity may make the examiners reflect on the clinical competence of a candidate. In the following examples, the examiners seem to be endeavouring to find the real clinical depth

39 The instruction in a patient with typical rheumatoid hands was: 'This lady had a fit 6 months ago, examine her hands'. During his examination the candidate found no skin rash or nodules. He diagnosed systemic lupus erythematosus in view of the fit. However, in retrospect, he still wonders if the diagnosis was just rheumatoid arthritis. (Pass)

40 A candidate was asked to examine a patient's cardiovascular system. He found a slow rising pulse, an ejection systolic murmur and an early diastolic murmur. He diagnosed mixed aortic valve disease with predominant aortic stenosis. The examiners asked him to guess the patient's blood pressure. (Pass)

41 In the neurological case, after correctly diagnosing a spastic paraparesis, a candidate was asked to give the differences between upper and lower motor neurone lesions. In the cardiovascular case he was asked to feel a man's pulse. He suggested slow atrial fibrillation but, in retrospect, he thinks it may have been complete heart block as there then followed a discussion about the differential diagnosis and the management of complete heart block including a discussion about the different types of pacemakers. (Fail)

42 A candidate who was taking the examination for the fourth time was taken to his cardiovascular case and asked: 'Feel this patient's pulse and apex beat, and listen

---

* The purpose of the examination is to demonstrate the difference between a guess and the diagnosis.

† Having noticed the nystagmus, the examiners probably wanted him to move on to demonstrate cerebellar signs with little or no prompting.

to the base of the heart'. He was required to give a full description of the findings and the probable diagnosis at each stage. He found pulsus bisferiens, a displaced apex, an ejection systolic and an early diastolic murmur. (Pass)

43 A candidate, who was unhappy with his examination technique and the mistakes he had made in an easy first case, was asked to examine the right arm of a 40-year-old man. He reports finding a 'flail' arm with increased reflexes. He thought his method of examination was poor and he was unsure of the diagnosis. He was then asked to examine the same man's abdomen and reports finding bilateral, large, smooth, more or less symmetrical masses in the lumbar regions which he diagnosed as bilateral hydronephrotic kidneys.* (Fail)

44 A candidate was asked to: 'Examine the eyes from a neurological point of view'. He found bilateral ptosis and a homonymous hemianopia and he said to the examiner that he could not explain the findings by one lesion. The examiner said: 'Examine the hands'. The candidate became preoccupied with the obvious rheumatoid arthritis and came up with the suggestion of rheumatoid arthritis associated with myasthenia gravis, which would explain the ptosis but not the hemianopia. The examiner said: 'Feel the pulse'. The candidate found an irregular pulse and diagnosed atrial fibrillation causing a cerebral embolus. (Pass)

45 A candidate examined the back of a patient's chest and found a pleural effusion. He had to go through the full examination and was asked what he was doing at every move, what each finding was caused by and how he interpreted it, e.g. breath sounds, crepitations, etc. (Pass)

Common errors

46 A candidate was asked to give a running commentary as he examined a patient's cardiovascular system. He commented on a collapsing pulse and on a mitral valvotomy scar but found no murmurs. He diagnosed mitral stenosis and became involved in a long discussion on the causes of a collapsing pulse. (Fail)

47 A candidate was asked to listen to a woman's heart. He found systolic and diastolic murmurs maximal at the base of the heart, to the left of the sternum. He diagnosed mixed aortic valve disease. In retrospect, he is sure that he missed the typical machinery murmur of a patent ductus arteriosus.† (Fail)

48 A candidate was asked to examine a man's chest, commenting as he went along. Although he thought the patient had chronic obstructive airways disease he was not actually asked for a diagnosis, but instead became caught up in a discussion on the distinction between a wheeze and stridor. (Pass)

49 A candidate examined the fundus of a patient whose pupil had been dilated. He could not find much wrong and wondered if there was some vascular abnormality. He made a wild guess at diabetic retinopathy and wonders, in retrospect, if this was a branch retinal vein or artery occlusion. His comment was: 'I was totally lost by this time!' (Fail)

50 A candidate examined the fundi of a patient and diagnosed bilateral optic atrophy and background diabetic retinopathy. He told us he had blurted out his impressions before stopping and thinking. Even in retrospect he does not know what the diagnosis was. (Fail)

51 A candidate was asked to examine the fundi of a patient (dilated pupils, dark room). He saw haemorrhages, exudates and some whiteness around the disc. He was put off by the examiners talking in the background and by his paranoia that the examiners were thinking that he was taking too long so he stopped before he had finished. He offered the diagnosis of diabetic retinopathy and myelinated nerve fibres. One examiner looked in the fundi while the other enquired if any microaneurysms had been seen. The candidate was not sure. There was then a discussion about the treatment of diabetic retinopathy and when photocoagulation was mentioned the examiner asked if there was any evidence of this. In retrospect, the candidate felt diabetic retinopathy was probably right but wonders about the possibility of having missed hypertensive retinopathy and papilloedema. He felt that if only he had continued examining longer to elicit the exact findings present he would have saved himself the cost of another attempt at the exam. (Fail)

52 A candidate was asked to feel the pulse of a patient. She was unable to feel it and guessed that atrial fibrillation must be present. (She failed.) Another candidate was taken to the same patient and admitted that she could feel neither the radials, brachials nor carotids (the patient was in low output cardiac failure). Afterwards she was told by the examiners that they had re-examined the patient and agreed with her. (Pass)

53 A candidate was asked to examine the back of the chest of a patient with bronchiectasis. During ausculta-

---

* We wonder if this patient had polycystic kidneys and an old cerebrovascular accident (ruptured berry aneurysm/hypertension).

† Confusing a continuous murmur of a patent ductus arteriosus for systolic and diastolic murmurs of aortic valve disease is a sin not easily forgiven. Paul Wood, a famous British cardiologist, is re-

ported to have remarked that the two sets of murmurs are so distinct from each other there should be no confusion in recognizing them (see p. 161, *An Aid to the MRCP PACES*, Volume 1).

tion the patient, in her enthusiasm to cooperate, breathed deeply and expired forcibly, generating upper airways wheeze.* The candidate, who already had his stethoscope in his ears, was unaware of the racket the patient was making. He reported the finding of widespread wheeze (the basal crepitations were completely drowned) although there was no wheezing at all when the patient was asked to breath deeply in and out in a relaxed fashion.

Look first

54 A candidate was asked to listen to the back of a lady's chest. Although only asked to listen, she examined expansion, percussion, palpation and finally auscultation, thinking that they would stop her if all they wanted her to do was to listen. They did not interrupt. She presented her findings of bilateral mid to late inspiratory crackles up to the mid zone and her diagnosis of fibrosing alveolitis. The examiners asked: 'Look at the patient and tell us what you think is the cause in her case'. At first the candidate could see no obvious cause from the face and therefore looked at her hands and immediately *spotted the changes of systemic sclerosis*. She then looked at the face again and the telangiectasia and tight skin were evident. (Pass)

55 A candidate was asked to examine a lady's neck. The candidate started off looking at the patient generally. No jugular venous pressure was obvious. She started feeling for lymph nodes. The examiners said: 'What are you doing?' so she explained that she was looking for lymph nodes—they asked why. She explained that she could not see anything else abnormal and then *spotted the glass of water* on the window sill and 'twigged'. She then started a thyroid examination and found a left thyroid nodule which was both visible and palpable on swallowing. A discussion followed about the possible causes. (Pass)

56 A candidate was asked to examine a patient's legs. He initially noticed gross ataxia, nystagmus and dysarthria when he introduced himself and shook the patient's hand. However, he still managed to fail to make a diagnosis of Friedreich's ataxia ('youthful ignorance' was his own comment about this!) and also ignored the examin-

er's prompt when he offered him a tuning fork and a patella hammer! (Fail)

Double pathology

57 A candidate was asked to examine neurologically a woman's legs. She found absent ankle jerks, increased knee reflexes and equivocal plantars. She was told that the patient was a diabetic and she noticed that she was wearing a cervical collar. Her mind was alerted to the possibility that there was a combination of a peripheral neuropathy and cervical spondylosis. (Pass)

58 A candidate was asked to look at the face of a woman who had presented with melaena. In retrospect, he felt the patient had acromegaly and Peutz–Jeghers syndrome (!) but he had not spotted the latter condition quickly enough. He was asked to examine the visual fields and, having mentioned the presence of greasy skin, was drawn into a discussion on skin function. (Fail)

59 A candidate was asked to comment on the appearance of a patient. She had proptosis and a prosthetic eye. In addition, there was a thyroidectomy scar, evidence of thyroid acropachy and pretibial myxoedema. She had also had a recent amputation. He was asked to examine the fundi and it was obvious that she was also a diabetic. (Pass)

60 A candidate was asked to examine the legs of a man whom he was told had diabetes mellitus. He found a peripheral neuropathy and peripheral vascular disease. He also spotted that the patient had coexistent facioscapular dystrophy. (Pass)

61 A candidate was asked to examine just the heart of a patient. He found mixed aortic valve disease. He also suspected mitral stenosis but did not mention it as he had 'not expected to find double valve pathology'. (Fail)

Tell them of the expert that told you

62 A candidate was examined on a patient with acromegaly and feels that he performed reasonably well. In the discussion as to why he had used a red pin to test visual fields, he told them that a neurologist whom he had worked for had recommended it for the peripheral fields. The examiners seemed happy with that explanation. (Pass)

Apologies accepted

63 A candidate was asked to look in the eyes of a patient. He thought the disc margins were blurred and said so. The examiners asked him if he could see venous pulsation. The candidate pointed out that he would not recognize it if he saw it! He said that the examiners appeared to

---

* You can generate upper airways wheeze yourself by expiring hard at the same time as voluntarily narrowing your upper airways. If in doubt in the hysterical asthmatic, ask the patient to purse his or her lips as he or she breathes. This manoeuvre will abolish factitious wheeze. Although the wheeze of such a patient may be heard down the corridor, the pulse is not significantly elevated in the absence of true severe asthma (unless the acute asthma is caused by the inappropriate prescription of a beta-blocker!).

like this response and went on to grill him on the different causes of blurred disc margins. The diagnosis was apparently hypermetropia. (Pass)

64 A candidate was asked to examine the fundi of a patient who was diabetic. She explained that she could not see with her left eye and could only undertake ophthalmoscopy with her right eye. The examiners responded: 'As long as you are competent, we do not care how you do it'. (Pass)

65 A candidate was asked to examine the precordium of a 55-year-old female patient. He found atrial fibrillation and mitral stenosis and a long discussion followed about 'How do you know it's atrial fibrillation?' He forgot to mention the variable first heart sound. He reports that he made a big blunder when he said that the tapping apex was caused by a big left atrium. Thirty seconds later, he said: 'Sir, I was wrong earlier. The tapping apex is not caused by a big left atrium.' The examiner looked relieved and went on to ask where the candidate would feel for a big left atrium.* Luckily, the bell went at that moment and the candidate was not required to answer. (Pass)

'Even though I didn't mean to say it—I did; I opened my mouth and all this rubbish came out

66 A candidate, nervous on his first attempt, was asked to palpate the abdomen. He found bilateral masses in the upper quadrants but states that he was interrupted before he could examine them properly. He thought they were polycystic kidneys but in the stress of the moment he found himself saying hepatosplenomegaly before he could stop himself! (Fail)

67 A candidate was asked to examine a woman's abdomen. She found a deeply jaundiced woman with cachexia and a hard, craggy liver. She did not detect ascites nor, convincingly, a spleen. However, when asked to give her findings, she found herself saying 'and she has a 2-cm spleen'. She reports that she heard herself lying but was unable to stop herself. The examiner was not convinced either and the candidate then started talking about 'a difficult to define mass in the left hypochondrium which could be splenic'. She said the examiner seemed happier with this but did not ask how to differentiate left hypochondrial masses. (Fail)

68 A candidate was asked to examine the cardiovascular system. He reports that he was stopped after examining the precordium before feeling the carotids and that although the signs had fitted with aortic stenosis, he was unsure whether the murmur was classically

---

* First heart sound is palpable; left atrium is not palpable.

crescendo–decrescendo and he found himself giving the diagnosis of ventricular septal defect. The examiners made it obvious that they disagreed with this diagnosis. (Pass)

69 A candidate was asked to examine the fundi of a 19-year-old asymptomatic girl. On looking at the right fundus, she could not see the disc but the vessels and background were normal. She assumes now that there must have been papilloedema but it was the first case, she was in a complete panic and found herself saying that she did not know the diagnosis. She was told that she must know the diagnosis and then said: 'Hypertension'. The examiners walked out without comment. (Pass)

70 A candidate was told that a female patient was breathless and he was asked to examine her abdomen and to explain her breathlessness. He found massive hepatosplenomegaly plus anaemia but instead of coming out with myelosclerosis as the diagnosis, he said sarcoidosis! At this stage the examiners, who had been very pleasant until then, began to look impatient! (Fail)

71 'Examine the heart.' Having done so, it would have been easy to start by saying, 'This chap, who is comfortable at rest with a midline sternotomy scar, has mitral regurgitation'. However, my mouth went into action before my brain and a load of verbal diarrhoea came out. The diagnosis was correct but the delivery was awful. (Fail)

Invigilators' diaries

72 A candidate was asked to examine the legs of a patient. He was allowed to carry out a large proportion of a full neurological examination before he became aware, with prodding from the examiner, of the large skull, hearing aid and the bowed tibiae of Paget's disease. The examiner commented that if he had *looked* at the patient first he might have saved himself the time wasted on the unnecessary neurological examination. (This would not happen now as this patient would be in Station 5 for a spot diagnosis.)

73 A candidate was asked to examine the eyes of a patient. He had examined the eye movements before he noticed the obvious blue sclerae of osteogenesis imperfecta. The examiner was irritated by this and commented that the candidate had wasted several minutes of the examiner's time by not looking at the eyes properly and noticing an obvious physical sign.

74 A candidate was asked to examine the fundi of a patient with diabetic retinopathy and laser photocoagulation scars. It was the end of the afternoon and the tropicamide drops, which had been put in that morning to dilate the pupil, had worn off. The candidate said she could see nothing and asked to take the patient into a darkened room. A side room was found but it was only semidark. She still said she could see nothing. The examiner was very unimpressed that she had missed what he considered to be a very easy case of diabetic retinopathy. When the invigilator tried to help save the candidate by apologizing that the drops had worn off, the examiner retorted that 'the pupils would not be dilated in the casualty department'.

75 A patient in the examination had a 'full house' of mixed mitral and aortic valve disease. The examiner commented that candidates kept failing to hear all the murmurs. He suspected that having heard one or two loud ones, candidates stopped listening for the others which were less obvious.

76 A candidate was asked to look at a lady's hands. He described Heberden's nodes, spindling of the fingers and proximal joint swelling, all of which the patient had. He suggested combined osteoarthrosis and rheumatoid arthritis. When the examiner asked about conditions associated with rheumatoid arthritis, the candidate looked beyond the hands and noticed the generalized pigmentation and then the palmar crease pigmentation of Addison's disease. The latter condition was the reason for the patient's inclusion in the examination—the joint changes had not been noted before!

77 A patient known to have Behçet's disease was included as a fundus case with optic atrophy. On fundoscopy, he had optic atrophy, choroidoretinitis and also sheathing of the vessel walls. All the examiners agreed that they had not seen a fundus like it before and that it was a 'museum' case. The underlying cause was not discussed with any of the candidates who were only expected to see what was there and describe it accurately. Calling the vessel sheathing 'silver wiring', as one candidate did, was considered unacceptable.

78 A candidate was asked to examine the heart of a patient with mitral valve prolapse. Unfortunately, the backrest collapsed while he was examining and could not be repaired so the patient could only be examined lying flat or sitting upright. Although the examiners accepted that this was off-putting, they did not feel that it justified missing all the signs and getting systole and diastole the wrong way round!

79 An MRCP examiner was heard telling a group of students that many candidates fail to recognize atrial fibrillation. Furthermore, in his experience, about 20% of candidates cannot accurately demonstrate the second left intercostal space. He had also noticed that candidates were often poor in their technique of examining ankle jerks.

80 A candidate was asked to examine the fundi of a patient with diabetic retinopathy and obvious laser scars. She diagnosed diabetic retinopathy but when asked if she had seen any microaneurysms or photocoagulation scars she was not sure.

81 A candidate was shown a euthyroid diabetic patient with necrobiosis lipoidica diabeticorum and he had been given some of the patient's symptoms which were vaguely suggestive of hyperthyroidism. He was then asked to assess the girl's thyroid status. Despite the normal pulse rate and lack of other supportive signs the candidate apparently managed to diagnose hyperthyroidism!

82 An examiner was watching a candidate feeling for the apex beat of a female patient. The rough handling of the patient's breast irritated the examiner who later commented: 'That sort of behaviour brings a candidate immediately to the pass/fail borderline'.

83 After observing some candidates examining a patient with rheumatoid hands, a 'fly on the wall' advised: 'Don't give too much prominence to the possibility of psoriatic arthropathy in an obvious case of rheumatoid. If you are considering psoriatic arthropathy then look particularly for nail changes. If there are boutonnière and swan neck deformities, say so rather than spending ages describing what's happening at each metacarpophalangeal and interphalangeal joint.'

84 A flustered and overanxious candidate marked himself out by spending an inordinate amount of time fixing the patient's blanket and putting the patient's pyjamas back on rather than following the examiners to the next case—they had to come back for him twice. 'Oh heck!', he remarked at their second return for him. On another occasion he was still shaking hands with the last patient when the examiners were trying to get him to start on the next! After forgetting to listen to the neck in a patient with a systolic murmur in the aortic area, he elected to draw the examiner's attention to this without prompting: 'I'm sorry, I didn't listen to the neck!' He was generally slow and took ages describing, hesitantly, peripheral and unimportant things, digging holes when it would have been better to come out immediately and say confidently: 'I think this patient has aortic stenosis'. On the rheumatoid hands case he spent ages trying to describe what was happening at each metacarpophalangeal and interphalangeal joint, struggling in his panic to find the right words when it would have been better to get straight to the diagnosis with just a few key extras such as 'boutonnière', 'swan neck', 'ulnar deviation', etc. The examiner commented: 'He looked as though he was going to fall apart at any moment; he didn't seem to be used to examining people; I wonder if he is in public health!' It was estimated that during the 30 min he had said 'Sir' about 84 times!

85 A candidate was taken to see a patient with one leg that was slightly shorter and wasted compared to the other. The candidate did not think of polio and the examiner had to admit that: 'A lot of young people won't have seen it'.

86 A candidate was asked to examine the hands of a patient with gross, generalized wasting and frontal baldness. The candidate carried out a long, detailed examination of the hands before reaching the diagnosis (myotonic dystrophy) after finally being prompted to shake hands with the patient.

87a A candidate on her first case had a patient with lymphoma presenting with a right iliac fossa mass, splenomegaly and generalized lymphadenopathy. The candidate missed the spleen, got bogged down in standard lists of causes of a right iliac fossa mass including irrelevant ones such as an appendix abscess!

87b Before one examination session all the examiners gathered around a patient to be shown his signs, which were said to include splenomegaly. Two or three of the examiners felt the abdomen and agreed that they could not feel the spleen. After these had moved on, another of the examiners examined the abdomen and called the invigilator over, saying: 'Put your hand here, like this—the spleen is palpable—can you feel it?'

Fly on the wall—complete accounts

In the same way that later in this section we have some complete first-hand accounts of candidates' experiences during the short cases, the following are two fuller accounts from one sitting, followed by two more detailed accounts from the same morning of another sitting— these are the notes of a 'fly on the wall'.

The second examiner chipped in: 'Can you have an opening snap in the presence of atrial fibrillation?'—the candidate looked nonplussed, hesitated and could not come up with an answer.

88 The first patient had hepatosplenomegaly and polycythaemia. He had a red face that was not noticed, or mentioned, by the candidate. Asked to look at the abdomen from the end of the bed while the patient breathed, the candidate did not notice the liver moving up and down. The fact that the liver was palpable was dragged out of her slowly. The examiner asked the candidate to mark the position of the spleen on the skin with a finger so that the size of the spleen could be verified.

For the next case, the examiner said: 'Check the pulse, jugular venous pressure and precordium'. The candidate proceeded to irritate him by examining the fingernails. The patient had loud mitral stenosis. The examiner

instructed: 'Give me your diagnosis or findings— whichever you choose'. The candidate said mitral stenosis. Examiner: 'Why mitral stenosis, was there an opening snap?' The candidate was unsure, asked to listen again and then said that there was an opening snap. The examiner asked: 'What is an opening snap, what causes it?' As they were leaving the patient the second examiner chipped in: 'Can you have an opening snap in the presence of atrial fibrillation?' The candidate looked nonplussed, hesitated and did not come up with an answer. The examiner said afterwards he thought this was a very relevant question which the candidate ought to have been able to answer.

The next patient had hereditary haemorrhagic telangiectasia and congenital nystagmus. The candidate moved hesitantly to the first diagnosis. She was asked why there was a scar on the left side of the chest. The candidate suggested an arteriovenous fistula. The examiner asked if there was a better, more commonly used term. The candidate was very slow to answer 'Arteriovenous shunt and arteriovenous malformations'. She was slow to get congenital nystagmus as the cause of the nystagmus and was asked how she could tell it was congenital and not brought about by any other cause. She did not really know, but the fact that it was present in all directions was dragged out of her. The examiner (a neurologist) explained that the nystagmus was coarse, in the same plane as the eye movement, of variable frequency, with the fast phase sometimes in one direction and sometimes in another! She was asked if she knew of another condition that went with congenital nystagmus and she did not. The examiner explained that there were little nodding movements of the head that the patient sometimes exhibited which are called 'spasmus nutans'!

The next patient had psoriasis of the soles of the feet which the candidate got and also gave the differential diagnosis, when asked, of keratoderma blenorrhagica in association with Reiter's syndrome.

The next patient had rheumatoid hands with swan neck and boutonnière deformities. The candidate was asked about the cause of the swan neck deformity and he started talking about the small muscles of the hand. The examiner said: 'I wouldn't have said that but as you mention it, what small muscles of the hand?' The candidate was very hesitant and eventually said: 'flexor digito . . .' 'You are talking rubbish', said the examiner, 'it is the interossei and lumbricals'. As the examiner moved on to the next case, the candidate said that there were also boutonnière deformities.

The examiner was about to ask the candidate to look into the eyes of the next patient when he stopped, reached in his pocket and pulled out an instrument and asked the candidate what the instrument was. She did not know it was a two-point sensation discriminator. 'Can be very useful in testing sensation', said the examiner. The candidate's next case was diabetic retinopathy which she got right, including the fact that there were hard exudates near the macula.

In view of the previous, fairly disastrous, abdomen, the candidate was taken to look at the abdomen of another patient, who had hepatosplenomegaly; she got it this time and when asked the cause suggested 'a myeloproliferative disease' which was correct. She was asked to draw the edge of the spleen again. (Bare fail)

Other candidates in the same sitting had diagnosed the old choroiditis and not called it papilloedema; had diagnosed the retinopathy and not called it optic atrophy; had identified the palpable kidney and marked the correct size of the spleen, etc.

89 The first case was hepatosplenomegaly with the right kidney easily palpable. The candidate started off with: 'I would like to examine the patient from nipples to knees'. He was asked to concentrate on the abdomen. He said that he had found hepatosplenomegaly. He was asked to show the edge of the spleen and said it was 6 cm and marked it as such, when in fact it was just a palpable spleen tip. It was interesting to note that when he had actually been examining the spleen one could see where he was feeling and he must have felt just the spleen tip with the patient turned on the right side; yet he went on to describe it as 6 cm enlarged. He did not mention the bimanually ballottable right kidney which presumably he thought was the liver.

After this bad start he did reasonably well on the patient with mitral stenosis. He was asked to examine the pulse, the jugular venous pressure (JVP) and the precordium. After feeling the pulse, looking at the JVP and palpating the precordium, the examiner stopped him and asked his findings. He gave them as those of mitral stenosis and said he expected to hear the auscultatory findings which he subsequently did. However, he got into a mess when asked to describe the venous pressure and said that it was a single wave and when asked about the relevance of this started talking about atrial fibrillation and mitral stenosis. He said: '*cv* waves'. The examiner raised his eyebrows at this. The candidate did not mention tricuspid incompetence which was the cause of the pulsations in the neck. The examiner then asked if there was anything else he had noticed about the patient (this was not on the official documentation about the patient but the examiner was an endocrinologist) and after a

struggle the candidate said that there was a chest deformity and after a further struggle he mentioned kyphosis. There was more delay and struggling and then the examiner showed him the patient's axillae which had no hair. The candidate suggested that maybe the patient shaved and she said that she had not had hair for many years. The examiner asked if the candidate could tie up the absent axillary hair with the chest and spinal deformities and the candidate was unable to do so. It turned out that the patient had had an early menopause and had been oestrogen-deficient for many years.

The next case was a patient with a fundus with a patch of old choroiditis superior and just temporal to the macula. The candidate diagnosed papilloedema.

The next patient had polyarteritis and bilateral carpal tunnel syndrome. The candidate diagnosed rheumatoid arthritis and bilateral carpal tunnel syndrome. The examiner said: 'If she had a patch of numbness on her right leg here (pointing below the knee), what would you say?' The candidate answered: 'Mononeuritis multiplex'. This was accepted by the examiner.

The next case involved examining the visual fields in a patient with widespread cerebrovascular disease who presumably had a right homonymous hemianopia. The candidate found a defective temporal field in the right eye but also a defective nasal field and said that both nasal and temporal fields were diminished. The candidate was asked, without comment, to go on and examine the legs and he said that he had found 'pyramidal weakness of the right leg'. He was asked what this meant and responded 'weakness of flexion at the hip, the knee and dorsiflexion at the foot'. This was accepted. He also said that he felt the reflexes were brisk bilaterally. The examiner (?a neurologist) asked what other reflexes could be tested—in cases of doubt about the briskness of reflexes ('How can you tell if reflexes are brisk if they are bilaterally brisk?'). The candidate said, and tested, the adductor reflexes.* The examiner asked what it is that causes the brisk reflex. The candidate struggled and was unable to describe the reflex arc. He was then asked what causes increased tone and started talking about muscles being perpetually in contraction; and was then asked if he meant that the muscles are contracting all the time, to which he replied: 'No'. He was asked why there could be discordance between tone and jerks.

The last patient had grade III hypertensive retinopathy. The candidate said there was no retinopathy but that the discs were pale. (Fail)

---

* Probably the examiners were expecting him to say abdominal reflexes and clonus.

The candidate was asked to demonstrate with his finger exactly where the spleen and liver edges were.

90 His cardiology case was a youngish woman with mixed aortic valve disease and mixed mitral valve disease, although the mitral incompetence was debatable. He diagnosed mixed aortic valve disease but did not notice the mid-diastolic murmur, although the examiner did not seem perturbed by this. The candidate, when asked about whether the pulse was collapsing or not, said that it was not. The examiner then asked him for the peripheral signs of aortic incompetence and the discussion moved to the nail-fold sign. The candidate was asked what this was called and he said: 'Quincke's sign' and he was asked to see if the patient had this. The candidate thought he had and the examiner answered: 'I thought so too'.

The respiratory case was a patient with bronchiectasis and the candidate was asked to examine the chest. He examined first from the front and he was about to move to the back when the examiner said: 'Time is at a premium, could you discuss your findings so far?' During the examination the patient had given a rattly cough on several occasions. The candidate thought that the diagnosis was bronchiectasis but then went on to say that he thought the patient looked Cushingoid and wondered if he was on steroids for obstructive airways disease (he was not on steroids). The causes of bronchiectasis were asked for.

The candidate was then requested to look at a patient with Parkinson's disease and he spotted the diagnosis correctly and said he would like to examine the gait; he was allowed to do this. The only Parkinsonian feature in the gait was that one arm swung less than the other and he exhibited a slight tremor. When the candidate said this, the examiner asked what features he might have had. In the ensuing discussion the candidate was asked what 'festinant'* meant. He said he did not know. The examiner told him that it meant 'dancing' and asked him why he thought this word should be used to describe the Parkinsonian gait.

The next case was a patient with diabetic fundi, multiple laser burns and debatable new vessels on the disc. The candidate, during the discussions, said that the discs were normal and when pressed on this stuck to his decision that they were normal.

The next case was a patient with CRST syndrome and he was asked: 'What is your spot diagnosis?' The candidate immediately answered: 'Tophaceous gout'. When the examiner was obviously unhappy about this, the candidate explained that he was sorry that he had rushed to

---

* Festinant comes from the Latin verb festinare meaning 'to hurry'.

that diagnosis. The examiner told him that he should *never* rush to a diagnosis. The candidate then discussed systemic sclerosis and CRST syndrome and a discussion took place about difficulties with swallowing.

The next patient had neurofibromatosis and the candidate was asked to: 'Look at the hands and tell me what you see—spot diagnosis'. The candidate got the diagnosis at once.

The next patient had hereditary haemorrhagic telangiectasia and the candidate got this diagnosis at once. He was then asked if the patient had anything else and he answered to the effect that the patient had gross nystagmus. On being pressed on this, he said that there was also a squint and when being pressed further for a diagnosis, he suggested that the patient had congenital nystagmus (which was correct).

The next patient had had a cerebrovascular accident, with cerebellar signs and a carotid bruit. The examiner told the candidate that the patient had difficulty with walking and asked him to perform a neurological examination of the legs. The candidate started off with observation and after a brief pause the examiner asked him to 'move on if you want to finish on time'. He examined power and reflexes and found the reflexes diminished at the right knee compared to the left, so he started discussing an L3/4 root lesion as the cause. The examiner told him to leave sensation and what else would he like to examine. The candidate did not come up with a suggestion. Eventually, the examiner suggested that he should check coordination in the legs and the candidate was then led to examine for cerebellar signs in the arms. Cerebellar signs were found on the right. When asked about the possible diagnosis, the candidate suggested cerebellar syndrome and a lower motor neurone lesion at L3/4. The examiner suggested that this was a bizarre collection of physical signs and asked the candidate to listen to his neck. A right carotid bruit was found. The candidate then offered 'cerebellar infarction' as the cause, to which the examiner said: 'What about a middle cerebral artery stroke?' In the ensuing discussion the examiner said: 'Do you disagree with me? You can, if you want to, you know.'

The next patient had hepatosplenomegaly and the candidate started his presentation by saying that the patient was pigmented. The examiner said: 'Do you really think he is pigmented? Actually, he's tanned; he's just been to Cyprus for his holiday.' The candidate was asked to demonstrate with his finger where the spleen and liver edges exactly were. In the discussion about the cause, myeloproliferative disease was first suggested to which the examiner responded by saying that the patient had had the spleen for 30 years. The candidate then suggested an 'ethnic anaemia' and a discussion took place about why it was not thalassaemia minor or thalassaemia major, and when the candidate suggested sickle cell disease the examiner said to him: 'You didn't mean that, did you?' After the bell went he told the candidate that it was haemoglobin H disease but that the candidate need not worry because he was on the right lines. (Pass)

She got the patient to open his mouth and put his tongue out. The inside and outside of his mouth were covered with telangiectasiae—how did she not see them?
91 The first short case had systemic sclerosis which at first (on examining the hands) she called psoriasis, and then dermatomyositis, before coming to the right diagnosis.

The next patient had hepatosplenomegaly and she got it right without problems.

The next case was hereditary haemorrhagic telangiectasia and she was asked to examine the back. She found a thoracotomy scar and evidence of a lobectomy (presumably from removal of an arteriovenous shunt). Then, in a discussion which led to the fact that 'some lung had been removed', she was asked to discuss the possible reasons. (She was told the operation had been many years previously.) She suggested tuberculosis and this possible cause was accepted. 'Anything else?' She suggested there might be rheumatoid changes in the hands and this was accepted. 'Why would this lead to a thoracotomy?' The candidate started discussing pulmonary fibrosis before she realized that this would not lead to a thoracotomy. The examiner asked if she thought the patient was cyanosed. She got the patient to open his mouth and put his tongue out. The inside and outside of his mouth was covered with telangiectasiae—how did she not see them? She said she did not think there was cyanosis. Did she know why the patient might have had a thoracotomy?—'No'.

The next patient, she was told, was unsteady on the feet and she was asked to examine the arms. The patient had cerebellar signs following a cerebrovascular accident. She initially started discussing Parkinson's disease and cogwheeling and then retracted this. She was asked to examine the eyes for nystagmus and soon after she began she was asked: 'Has she got it?', to which the candidate immediately answered: 'Yes'. 'Tell us about the nystagmus.' She was asked to examine speech and eventually got the patient to have difficulty saying, 'West Register Street'.

She was asked for a spot diagnosis on a patient with neurofibromatosis and she got this. She was asked for a spot diagnosis on a patient with exophthalmos and got this too. When asked where else to look, she eventually said the shins for pretibial myxoedema which the patient had (debatably).

The next patient had a small to moderate multinodular goitre which the candidate said was a big goitre; initially that it was diffuse, although she later said it was nodular.

The next patient had mixed aortic valve disease and mixed mitral valve disease. The candidate confidently diagnosed aortic stenosis but nothing else.

The next patient had diabetic retinopathy with laser burns and the candidate got this.

The next patient had Parkinson's disease which she got. A discussion then took place on the causes of Parkinson's disease and when she ground to a halt after giving several possibilities, she was asked for any others. 'Have you heard of the expression "mad as a hatter"?'*

The next case was coarctation of the aorta. The examiner said that he wanted to put her in the area of the circulatory system but not to do a full examination of the heart because she had already done this. He led her to listen to the precordium and she heard something of a systolic murmur but the bell went before discussion could take place. She mentioned 'patent ductus' as she left the room. (Fail)

Ungentlemanly clinical methods
92 A candidate was asked to examine a patient's respiratory system. He found clubbing and basal crackles and diagnosed bronchiectasis. He confessed that he was helped along with this diagnosis as he could see it on the examiner's clipboard!
93 A candidate was asked to examine the fundi. The examiners were several yards away so as he was examining he quietly asked the patient if he was a diabetic, to which the patient answered, 'Yes'. The candidate diagnosed proliferative diabetic retinopathy with photocoagulation scars in one eye and a vitreous haemorrhage in the other. He was asked why it was difficult to see one of the fundi well and replied that it was because of the vitreous haemorrhage. (Pass)
94 A candidate reports: 'I was asked to "look at this lady's right eye". I saw a cataract, retinopathy and laser scars. I said 'diabetic retinopathy'—which was what I saw printed on the examiner's sheet!' (Pass)
95 A candidate reports: 'My last short case really made

* Chronic mercury poisoning (persistent involuntary movements, fatigue, insomnia, neuropathy, etc.) was probably the examiner's bee under the bonnet! Mercury was used by hat makers and chronic exposure caused poisoning with widespread manifestation in some of them. Although mercury is mentioned among the toxic causes of Parkinsonism, most neurologists admit that they have never seen a *bona fide* case of Parkinsonism attributable to mercury.

my day. Having arrived at the examination ward with little time to spare, I happened to meet an elderly woman going in the same direction who obviously was not a candidate and too polite to be an examiner! She asked if we were going to the same place and volunteered that she always came up for the examinations. She told me that they always looked at her eyes and shins, and then at her neck, volunteering that she had no scar but had "drunk iodine"! Sure enough, I was led to this same woman who smiled when I was told to examine her legs which showed pretibial myxoedema. I went on to demonstrate the exophthalmos with lid-lag, a multinodular goitre and no scar!' (Pass)

Miscellaneous 'pass' experiences

'The examiner said: "First class". This was the nicest remark made to me in the last 2 years!'

1 'Would you examine these hands? This chap has a weakness in his hands.' He had obvious bilateral *ulnar nerve palsy* and I was asked for the causes.

'Examine this patient's abdomen. He came in with anaemia.' There was obvious hepatosplenomegaly and I was asked for a differential diagnosis. I included *myelofibrosis* and was asked why it could be this condition. I said because of the large size of the spleen.

'Examine this patient's fundus.' There were haemorrhages and exudates with arteriovenous nipping. I suggested diabetic eye disease but the examiner then said: 'What if I tell you that the other eye is normal?' I then suggested a *retinal branch vein occlusion* to which the examiner said: 'First class'. This was the nicest remark made to me in the last 2 years!

'Listen to this lady's heart.' Before I went any further I checked to see if I was allowed to palpate, etc. 'No', said the examiner, 'auscultate only'. I found a *mitral diastolic murmur* with an opening snap and ?presystolic accentuation. The examiner asked if the patient was in sinus rhythm.* I said I could not tell just by auscultating, but he went on: 'What do you think?'

'This lady has a rash on her thighs'. It looked like purpura but then they showed me her shins. There was no lesion visible here. 'Does this put you off a diagnosis of purpura?' 'Yes', I said. 'Quite right', said the examiner. 'What if I told you she had pains in her joints and trouble with her kidneys?' I suggested polyarteritis nodosa. 'No',

---

* The question was prompted by the candidate's mention of presystolic accentuation, which would not occur if the rhythm had been atrial fibrillation. The examiner was exploring whether the candidate threw in 'presystolic accentuation' without realizing its significance.

said the examiner, 'but don't worry. I have only seen it once before!' (Apparently it was *Fabry's disease.*)

The next patient was in a side room which gave me a clue. I was told, 'This young man has lost weight and noticed these lesions on his chest. What are they?' They were definitely *Kaposi's sarcomas*. I was then asked the mechanism of diarrhoea in *AIDS*. (Pass—sixth and final attempt)

'On leaving the room the patient commented loudly on what a nice young man I was and how I had said it all so nicely!'

2 I was asked to look at the fundi of an elderly lady with widely dilated pupils. I tested her pupil reactions to light but not to accommodation and elicited a light reflex. I then examined the right fundus. It was obviously *background diabetic retinopathy* and after approximately 20 seconds I looked up and asked if they wanted me to specifically look into the left fundus. He said: 'Not if you are ready to present your findings'. I did present the findings, gave the diagnosis and emphasized that there were no proliferative or hypertensive changes or laser burns.

I was taken to a young woman with a mitral valvotomy scar, atrial fibrillation and the murmurs of *mixed mitral valve disease*. She was not short of breath or cyanosed. I presented the findings and continued to give my reasons why I believed the stenotic component was predominant. I was asked if the murmurs were haemodynamically significant. I replied that they were not and again gave my reasons.† The examiners and the patient all appeared pleased. In fact, on leaving the room the patient commented loudly on what a nice young man I was and how I had said it all so nicely!

I next saw a patient with obvious *severe rheumatoid arthritis* and evidence of previous joint replacements. I was asked to describe what I saw and then to look for additional evidence of rheumatoid arthritis, i.e. nodules. There were none present so they asked me where else they might be found. I replied: 'I would look on a chest X-ray'.

The next patient had pronounced *exophthalmos* and the examiner began by asking me to describe what I could see, saying: 'You can be as rude as you like about Mr L'. to which the patient laughed. I demonstrated the examination of exophthalmos and lid-lag and said that I could feel a goitre (which I think was present although not large). The examiner did not appear completely convinced but acceded to my observation. I was asked to

---

† The question of predominance of either lesion should not arise if the murmurs are not haemodynamically significant.

assess the thyroid state clinically. He was *euthyroid* and I gave my reasons for this.

I was then taken to a patient who was in bed with a cervical collar on. I was asked to examine his legs neurologically because 'he has difficulty in walking'. He had a smaller, wasted, areflexic left leg suggestive of *old polio* and a very brisk set of reflexes in the right leg. I suggested that he had old polio of the left leg with superimposed *cervical myelopathy* affecting the right leg.

I was then asked to examine the back of a man's chest. There was dullness to percussion and reduced chest wall movement on the right side, but the air entry* was not diminished greatly in comparison to the left side. I gave a tentative diagnosis of a right *pleural effusion* but added why I was uncertain. I was then asked to examine his abdomen 'because my houseman informs me that he has *hepatomegaly*'. The liver margin was in fact easily palpable. However, on percussion it appeared low lying and I therefore suggested this and the examiner appeared to agree.

For my last case I was asked to palpate the precordium only. There was a systolic apical thrill. I was asked to give a differential diagnosis but at this point my concentration was somewhat flagging and I could only mention mitral regurgitation and forgot *ventricular septal defect*. He asked again if there was anything else of note on palpation! I had nearly missed his bilateral *gynaecomastia*. I was asked what drugs might be the cause in this particular case. I gave a reasonable list but could not think of spironolactone. He repeated the question but somehow mixed up his words and actually said: 'What are the spiros . . .' I began to laugh as did both the patient and the other examiner who had been observing at this point. As the bell had now sounded they said that they would let me go. I thanked them and shook hands — phew! (Pass)

'I was then taken to see a gentleman who had a white stick and the examiner said: "This man is almost blind, please examine his eyes."'

3 'This lady came in to have her varicose veins done and something else was noted incidentally. Please examine her abdomen and tell us what you find that is abnormal.' On examination, there was gross, visible splenomegaly with mild anaemia. I was asked the causes of massive splenomegaly and the definition of splenomegaly. She had *myelofibrosis*.

---

* 'Air entry' is not a good expression. It is better to use the terms breath sounds present/absent/diminished. Breath sounds are *not* caused by the air entering into that part of the lung where they are heard, but rather generated in the major bronchi and *conducted* to the periphery.

'This man has a cough and fever. Examine the respiratory system.' He was an Asian gentleman who was dyspnoeic at rest and had clubbing of the fingers. He had superb signs. There was dullness to percussion with increased breath sounds (bronchial breathing) and there was increased vocal resonance at the left apex. I was asked for a differential diagnosis and, because he was Asian, I said tuberculosis and, because he was a smoker as detected by the discoloration of his nails, I also suggested carcinoma of the lung. The examiner told me that he did not like my technique for testing for tracheal deviation (thumb to each side separately) and he showed me his way of doing it and asked me to try it. I had to admit that the trachea probably was deviated to the left. There was then a long dissertation from the examiner regarding the physical findings in the left upper lobe, i.e. collapse vs. consolidation, and I was not really asked to contribute at all to this conversation!

I was then taken to see a gentleman who had a white stick and the examiner said: 'This man is almost blind, please examine his eyes'. I found no cataracts or corneal problems but there was gross *choroidoretinitis*. I desperately tried to find evidence of diabetic retinopathy to make this into laser therapy but I could not. Therefore, I thought it could be retinitis pigmentosa although I had never seen it before. I said this honestly to the examiners who agreed that the treatment of diabetic eye disease would be the most common cause of this type of thing but that: (a) it was a bit different; and (b) this is the MRCP exam! It was in fact *retinitis pigmentosa*. I wondered if it could have been *Refsum's syndrome* as the Whittington Hospital does have a patient with this.

My last patient was a lady and the examiner said: 'Tell me about her hands'. I had to be very quick as the bell had gone but she had gross *nodular rheumatoid*. I described the features as I was examining and I was also expected to perform a functional assessment. The examiners at the end said: 'Very good', and let me go. (Pass)

'I know this patient well, sir, this is Mrs L. and I biopsied her liver last year!'

4 I was asked to examine the precordium. She had *mitral stenosis* and atrial fibrillation. I was criticized for not actually counting the apical rate and only giving a 'guesstimate' of 130/min. I was then asked about the complications of mitral stenosis.

'This girl was admitted with an acute asthmatic attack. Can you find a cause for it?' After some prompting, I noticed a slight excoriation on the flexor creases and this was the only physical sign. I thought it was probably *atopic eczema.* The examiners then asked me what I would tell the girl's mother about her prognosis.

'Look at this patient's skin'. There were *café au lait* spots on the forearms and *neurofibromas* on the abdomen.

'Examine this patient's legs'. I recognized this patient—so I said: 'This is Mrs G. and she has *Charcot–Marie–Tooth disease*!' 'Examine this patient's abdomen'. 'I know this lady as well, sir. This is Mrs L. and *I biopsied her liver* last year!' The examiner said: 'Have you worked in this hospital before?' and I replied: 'Well, er, yes!' 'Palpate this patient's chest. No, feel again, there!' There was *aortic stenosis* with a systolic thrill which I missed initially. I was asked for further investigations so I mentioned echo and Doppler followed by cardiac catheterization.

'Look at this man's face.' He had definite facial flushing and we then discussed the features of the *carcinoid syndrome* and its treatment. The patient had had hepatic artery embolization.

I had been allocated to a hospital in which I had worked the previous year. My consultants advised me not to change as the examiners would not be prejudiced and I would not be at any disadvantage. However, I recognized two of the patients and I admitted to this. Although I was given credit for honesty it meant I missed out on the examination of two very good cases. The examiners told me afterwards that they had sat on the fence for the clinical but that I had passed comfortably in the other sections. I would advise any candidates finding themselves in a similar position to inform the College and to ask for a reallocation. Events such as this might easily upset one's whole performance. (Pass)

'Just because you are cool, it doesn't mean that you know the answers. But perhaps it helps convince the examiners that you do!'

5 *Gross acromegaly.* 'Examine this lady's hands. What do you notice?' The diagnosis was easy. He asked me to enumerate the features found in the hand in an acromegalic patient. 'And what else do you notice?' I listed all the facial features. 'What would you find in the other systems?' Again I gave a nice list. 'What are the treatments for this condition?' This was the perfect start to the short cases. I felt the examiners had warmed to me and it was all quite easy from here on.

Ventricular septal defect. 'Listen to this boy's heart.' He looked like a healthy teenager. Inspection of the apex was normal and his pulses were normal; however, palpation revealed a systolic thrill and on auscultation he had a systolic murmur only. I listened to his back. 'Why did you do that?' 'Because if he has a patent ductus the murmur

would be loudest at the back.' (The real reason was that I am terrible at interpreting murmurs and it gave me an extra few seconds to think.) Afterwards the examiner went back to listen.

Choroiditis. 'Look in this woman's eye. What do you see?' As I started to inspect her eye he said, 'No, just look at the fundus'. To begin with I could see nothing wrong but just as I turned to look away she changed her direction of gaze and I saw the grossly abnormal lesion. The moral must be to look everywhere in the retina.

Clubbing of the fingers. This was easy. I was allowed to ask some questions so I enquired how long the lady had had fingers like this. She was healthy and the answer was familial clubbing. I was then asked to recite the causes of clubbing.

Classical dermatomyositis. I had never seen this except in photographs and I almost missed it. She looked 'autoimmune' with white hair, pale skin and purplish eyelids and knuckles. I pointed this out but could not give a diagnosis. I was then asked to examine her arms where she had a small, healing, surgical scar over the triceps. Once I had 'clicked' that this was a muscle biopsy the diagnosis was easy. By now I was thoroughly enjoying myself and I turned to one of the examiners and said, 'I almost missed that'. 'Yes', he said, 'but you didn't!'

Paget's disease. This was bizarre. It was a lady of about 70 years whose radius and ulna of the right forearm were bent at 90°. I asked her if she had broken the arm and had a poor result from healing but the answer was no. I knew that there is a congenital cause of forearm deformity (Madelung's deformity?*) but this was not it so that left Paget's which I was told was the correct diagnosis.

IIIrd nerve palsy. It was a complete IIIrd nerve palsy. The examiner asked me to give the likely cause and the visible craniotomy scar gave me the answer.

Malignant melanoma with metastases. I was asked to examine this man's abdomen. He was deeply jaundiced and had a big, knobbly liver. I was then asked to describe the surface anatomy of the normal liver because his extended across to the left subcostal area and at first I thought he also had splenomegaly. However, the examiner demonstrated to our mutual satisfaction that he had hepatomegaly only. 'Now look in his eyes.' One was in the light and one was in shade so I looked at the one in the light. 'He is deeply jaundiced', I said. I was then asked why and instructed to look in both eyes. One had a white sclera! On asking the patient how long he had had his glass eye he said about 10 years and that he had had a

---

* In *Madelung's deformity* the arm is bent over the radial side as a result of the developmental overgrowth of the ulna.

tumour at the back of the eye! At this point the examiners did not ask me the diagnosis but simply thanked me and wished me good luck in the rest of the test. (Pass)

Afterwards the attending registrar said to me that I looked remarkably relaxed and cool under fire. I replied: 'Just because you're cool it doesn't mean that you know the answers'. But perhaps it helps convince the examiners that you do!

'The first thing I noticed was a puncture mark over the right lower chest suggesting a recent pleural aspiration.'
6 My first patient was introduced to me as a lady who was short of breath and would I do a cardiovascular examination to find out why. Just as I was about to listen to the lung fields at the end of my cardiovascular 'routine' I was stopped. My examiner asked if I had finished. I said: 'Yes'. And then I realized that I had not listened for an aortic diastolic murmur, but the examiner kindly allowed me to go back to do this. I was then asked for the diagnosis and I offered *mixed mitral valve disease* with a previous valvotomy. I was then asked which valve lesion was dominant. I plumped for stenosis by virtue of the loud first heart sound and was then pushed as to whether I wanted to change my mind. I did not so we passed on to the next case.

This was a lady whose neck I was asked to examine. It was obvious that she had a *goitre* but I tried to stop myself saying this before checking for other abnormalities. I showed them that I was examining for retrosternal extension and for bruits and then I was about to look for signs of hypo- or hyperthyroidism when they stopped me and asked me to describe my findings. As with the other cases, they let me start to show that I would extend my examination further and this seemed to impress but they always then stopped me in mid flow. I told them I had found a smoothly enlarged thyroid goitre and they then questioned me as to whether I was sure it was smooth. I was about to go back and re-examine but then realized that this would not look impressive. I did think it was smooth and so stuck to my original findings. I later discovered another candidate had been pushed on the same point and had also stuck firm.

I was then taken to a gentleman with frontal balding, mild ptosis and some facial muscle wasting and I was asked to hazard a diagnosis. I suggested *myotonic dystrophy* and was asked why. I explained my findings and made the mistake of saying 'myopathic facies'. My examiner looked puzzled and asked me what I meant. I explained about the muscle wasting that I could see although retracted my description of 'myopathic facies' as an unhelpful statement so he did not push me further.

I was then taken to a young lady with a large intravenous cannula in her right antecubital fossa and was asked to examine the back of her chest. The first thing I noticed was a puncture mark over the right lower chest suggesting a recent pleural aspiration. I quickly found a right *pleural effusion* and was asked to explain what brought me to that diagnosis and what was the most likely cause. In view of her age and the intravenous cannula I suggested pneumonia and was then asked the most likely microbiological cause for this lady and the most suitable antibiotic treatment.

I was then taken to another lady and was asked to examine her fundi and to describe my findings. I found early cataract formation, indistinct disc margins, arterial narrowing and patchy black *pigmentation* particularly in the *macular* region. I was asked where in the left eye was there a particularly dense black deposit. Unlike my first attempt, I did not try to pull the wool over their eyes with bluffing my way out. I was honest in saying I did not know where the densest deposit was and they allowed me a second look. I was then asked to hazard an attempt at putting all these features together and I was utterly stumped. However, my examiner just asked the cause of black pigmentation and we passed on to the next case.

I was asked to look at, and examine, a lady's hands. There was obvious *osteoarthrosis* but I did not want to be put off by this so I quickly checked for muscle wasting, clubbing and for a sensory loss. I was about to examine the elbows for gouty tophi and rheumatoid nodules, when I was stopped and directed to discuss my findings. I was asked what were the eponymous names for the swellings of the proximal and terminal interphalangeal joints.

I was finally taken to a middle-aged lady with a complete left *ptosis*. I was asked what I saw from the end of the bed and for the possible causes. I was then asked to examine further. I made a bit of a mess of this case. I examined the pupils and then proceeded to examine for diplopia which I was very ham-fisted about. I was desperately trying to keep the left eyelid open and examine visual movements by asking her to follow my finger and I got my arms all in a muddle! The examiner quickly intervened and asked me what I had found. I mentioned the pupillary reactions and the down and out position of the left eye and so he asked me for a diagnosis. I told him it was a *complete IIIrd nerve palsy* and he then requested me to ask the lady some questions to elucidate the cause. I asked about headache, thinking of a posterior communicating artery aneurysm, and that seemed to cause some surprise in the examiner. I then asked about diabetes. The lady was diabetic but I was told that in her case this was irrelevant and asked to hazard one more question. Fortunately, I was inspired to ask how long she had had the ptosis and discovered it was congenital. I was pushed on the difference between a complete and partial IIIrd nerve palsy and after describing the probable findings was asked the anatomical difference in the lesions. I thought I was being asked something esoteric and was somewhat annoyed when it transpired that all he wanted me to say was that in a partial nerve palsy only some of the IIIrd nerve fibres are affected!

My advice is to keep your head even when you have made a mistake. If you know you have made a mistake be quick to say so before your examiner has a chance to capitalize on it. If your examiner challenges, do not assume it means you have said something wrong. He may just be testing to see if you will stick firm to your diagnosis because you are absolutely certain of it. Practise, practise and practise, particularly in front of people who make you nervous. I also found it helpful to regard some of my outpatients as potential short cases. I think some of them had never been so thoroughly examined! Make every effort to show the examiner you can put the patient at ease. Introduce yourself and ask their permission to examine them and tell them exactly what you are going to do. Do not forget to thank them afterwards. It gives you time to calm down and think—and also it impresses the examiners. (Pass)

'The patient sounded most alarmed and said she hoped her daughter wouldn't get it.'

7 The first patient was an elderly, rather slow lady— 'Examine this lady's heart and chest'. (It'll take hours I thought!) I was almost panicked into combining my examination but then started doing the cardiovascular system alone. She was deaf and I felt I was not being very slick. I distinctly remember a wave of panic/fear that this was it! Anyhow, I found *mixed mitral valve disease* (MR > MS) and *aortic regurgitation*. I stood back and said this. The examiner nodded and said we would not bother with the chest. (My hands were cold when I started and the patient jumped which did not help my composure!)

The next patient was a young man with widespread *psoriasis* and a moon face. 'What do you think of this man?' I asked him if he had had any treatment, then stood back and said he had widespread psoriasis and could have been on systemic steroids. The examiner nodded, pointed out his palms and soles and asked what I would call this type of psoriasis. I answered: 'Pustular'. They agreed and moved on.

There was an ill-looking, jaundiced, old lady in a rather dimly lit bay. 'Examine this abdomen.' The examiners listened intently to my percussion but otherwise did not hassle me. I said I should like to go on to test for shifting dullness and to do a rectal exam, but did not attempt to move her for the former because she looked so ill. They accepted this and moved away from the bedside. I said I had found *hepatosplenomegaly* in a jaundiced patient and that I had noticed inguinal and supraclavicular nodes and a node biopsy scar in her groin. I suggested chronic myelocytic or lymphocytic leukaemia/non-Hodgkin's lymphoma, or metastatic carcinoma as the differential diagnosis. They asked how I would tell a student to examine the spleen and what its characteristic features were. (I wondered had I done it all wrong or felt a kidney instead!)

A lady with dilated pupils. 'Examine this fundus', they said and then wandered away a little. I looked in one eye and then asked if I could look in the other and got a rather non-committal 'if you must' expression. But I did anyway. I said I'd found *grade II hypertensive retinopathy* with silver wiring and arteriovenous nipping but no sign of haemorrhages, exudates or papilloedema. The examiner just said: 'Yes' and moved on.

A lady with florid *hereditary haemorrhagic telangiectasia* (HHT). 'What's the diagnosis?' When I got my tongue round it, I said the diagnosis in full! They said: 'What question would you like to ask?' I asked if anyone in the family had it. She said: 'No', and the examiners asked if I was surprised. I said it was an autosomal dominant trait and tended to run through the generations, to which the patient sounded most alarmed and said she hoped her daughter would not get it. The examiners placated her saying there was a 50% chance. I felt annoyed that it reflected badly on me upsetting her but surely the patient must have heard of it running in families before!

A lady with *neurofibromatosis*. They asked for a diagnosis and then for any neurological complications. I replied: 'Epilepsy, cord compression, carpal tunnel syndrome, tumours'.

A grossly *acromegalic* man. 'What's the diagnosis and what features would you like to demonstrate?' I described his facies, jaw and hands. They led me on to *carpal tunnel syndrome* and got me to demonstrate wasting and to try to show any sensory loss (intact!) and to talk about testing for median nerve motor function.

An old lady with denuded blisters and mouth lesions. The diagnosis was *pemphigus*. He asked me: 'Where's the split in the skin?' I said it was at the intraepidermal level.

Overall, my short cases went quite fluently. My worse moments were when I surprised a patient with my ice cold, stress-induced hands, and when I apparently upset the lady with HHT for mentioning that it ran in families.

One examiner questioned my use of 'He/she probably has . . .' when the diagnosis was obvious from just looking. By the end I was being more dogmatic which seemed to go down better. Even with no disasters it was hard to treat each case afresh but I am sure that is the knack of scoring highly. (Pass)

'Yes', said the examiner, 'tell me about the precursors of bilirubin.'
8 'Examine this man and shake hands with him.' The diagnosis was obviously *myotonic dystrophy*. The examiner asked me what else I would like to ask the patient. I suggested asking about family history and the examiner said: 'Good'.

'Look at this man, what is the diagnosis?' He had *pseudoxanthoma elasticum* and the examiner again said: 'Good'. He asked me what the description of the skin was and I replied: 'Plucked chicken skin' and again he said: 'Good! What would you expect to hear listening to his heart? That is what he is really here for.' I replied mitral valve prolapse. 'That's right', said the examiner.

'Look at this girl, what do you think? She is 25 years old.' I said: 'If she will forgive me, she is rather short'. 'That's right', said the examiner, 'what would you like to ask her?' I asked her how tall her parents were. 'Anything else?' said the examiner. I asked her when her periods started, if at all. The examiner said: 'That's a good question, what do you think of her face? She has *Crohn's disease.*' I replied that she had a Cushingoid moon face, and that steroids had probably been the cause of her short stature. 'Yes', said the examiner, 'in association with the malabsorption'.

'Look at this man.' He had obvious *acromegaly*. I was asked to examine his fundi and I found a pale left disc. 'Yes', said the examiner, 'I thought he had. Would you like to examine for a scotoma?' I produced a red hat pin and the patient volunteered that it changed colour. The examiners seemed satisfied.

'What is the diagnosis?' The patient had obvious *hereditary haemorrhagic telangiectasia* so I looked in the patient's mouth, which pleased the examiner. The examiner asked me what the other name of the condition was and I replied: 'Osler–Weber–Rendu syndrome'.

'What do you think about this man's feet?' He had definite *pustular psoriasis*. 'That's right', said the examiner, 'look at his hands'. He had the worst onycholysis that I have ever seen. 'Yes', said the examiner, 'that's the third time this has happened to this poor chap'.

'Look at this woman. What strikes you about her?' I replied that she appeared green in colour. 'That's right', said the examiner, 'why do you think that she is this colour?' I replied that I did not know but that perhaps it was very severe *jaundice*. 'Yes', said the examiner, 'tell me about the precursors of bilirubin?' I replied that it was biliverdin.

'Look at this woman's rash—this part in particular'. Some parts of the rash looked bullous and others appeared to have target lesions. I looked in her mouth. My first thought was that it was pemphigoid but eventually I came out with the right diagnosis of *erythema multiforme*.

'Look at this patient's hands.' I rolled up her sleeves that had been left down to her elbows and this revealed many *neurofibromas*. There was also partial amputation of several of her fingers. (Pass)

'The other examiner, who seemed annoyed at his colleague, took over and took the bull by the horns!'
9 The first examiner dithered and was an irritatingly slow 'dove'. He asked me to examine the respiratory system. I introduced myself, stood at the end of the bed and thought of the Newport course! He allowed me to examine fully both the anterior and posterior chest. I found an area of posterior consolidation on the right, with what I felt to be an area of anterior effusion. He mumbled something about 'overdiagnosing' but agreed with the *consolidation*.

The next case was a nightmare. I was asked to examine a man's legs neurologically. Again, I introduced myself and observed. I examined extensively and only found loss of proprioception. The examiner agreed and told me that was correct and other sensations were normal. He asked me to look at the man's face. He had a left-sided eye patch and underneath was a partial ptosis. No further examination was allowed and I was asked for my thoughts on a possible diagnosis. This really stumped me and there was an embarrassing pause of several seconds. My only thought was of luetic disease but he was not satisfied. Again, a number of long pauses. In the end he just wanted polyneuropathy! I was told subsequently by the registrar running the exam that this was the *Guillain–Barré Miller–Fisher variant*. Most neurologists I have talked to since have disagreed with this!*

The other examiner, who seemed annoyed at his colleague, took over and took the bull by the horns! At the next cubicle I was asked to look at a man and to say immediately if I had a diagnosis. It was clear from the

* This patient probably had external ophthalmoplegia (part of Miller–Fisher variant; p. 247, *An Aid to the MRCP PACES*, Volume 1) and the eye patch was used to obviate his diplopia. It would seem that the patient was in the recovery phase and some of the signs (areflexia, ataxia, etc.) had improved.

patient's expression (or lack of it) that he had *Parkinson's disease*. We quickly left the room.

The fourth case was again a spot diagnosis. The lady had glasses, a *Marfanoid appearance* and a high-arched palate. I gave the diagnosis and he agreed.

I was then asked to: 'Listen only', to a man's heart. I palpated the carotid but that was not much help. There was a very, very soft ejection systolic murmur at the left sternal edge with no radiation to the neck. I got up and he asked specifically for a diagnosis. I told him (quickly) my findings and plumped for early *aortic stenosis*. He said nothing but hurried me to the next case.

I was asked to look at the fundus of a lady doing some knitting close to her face. She had no cataracts and on inspection of the fundus she had what I am sure was *retinitis pigmentosa*, albeit not as typical as I had seen before.

With glee he then gave me the same instruction for the lady sitting next to her, also knitting but showing no family resemblance. She too had a very pigmented retina but this time it was *panretinal photocoagulation scars*.

For the next case I was asked to examine a lady's conjugate eye movements. She had a *bilateral VIth nerve palsy*. He agreed and asked me for the possible causes. I said the causes of mononeuritis multiplex and he seemed happy.

My next case was an elderly man with striking jaundice and firm irregular *hepatomegaly* with no spleen. He asked the most likely cause and I said malignancy. He agreed.

I cannot believe anybody comes out of the short cases thinking they have passed. My second case, in my own mind, was a disaster. I think it all comes down to how you look and the air of confidence you give. I heard them commenting on my good examination technique (learnt in Gwent) and I am sure this was the overriding factor that passed me. Finally, if disasters occur early, it is *not* all over. I survived and now have 'MRCP' to tell the tale! (Pass)

' "What else would you like to examine?" The patient started winking at me. "I'd like to examine his eyes, please." He had small, irregular pupils which did not react to light.'

10 The first patient was an elderly lady who was sitting upright. She was breathless at rest and quite cachectic. The examiner said to me: 'This lady is not very well so could you examine her chest from the back only?' I looked quickly at her hands and she had gross clubbing. The left side of her chest did not move on inspiration and it was dull to percussion. The examiner stopped me at this point and asked for a diagnosis so I said there was a large left *pleural effusion* but it could be consolidation. He

agreed and asked the most likely cause. I replied: '*NG*', as the patient was listening, and he agreed with me.

The next patient was a woman who was lying flat and I was asked to examine her abdomen. I looked at her hands, eyes, mouth, neck and axillae quite quickly and then moved on to the abdomen. She had *hepatosplenomegaly* but there was no ascites on testing for shifting dullness. The second examiner said that I should not bother to do shifting dullness if she was not stony dull in the flanks to percussion. I nodded. 'What do you think the diagnosis is?' I said that it was probably a lymphoreticular problem such as chronic lymphatic leukaemia or chronic myeloid leukaemia in view of the patient's age (she was about 60–70). 'What else could it be?' I suggested lymphoma but there were no nodes or it could be cirrhosis, malaria or another infection. The examiner said: 'No', to all of these suggestions so I have no idea what they were really after!

The third patient was another elderly woman sitting upright. The examiner asked me to feel her pulse. It was about 100 beats/min in atrial fibrillation. 'Is there anything else?' asked the examiner. 'No', I replied. 'OK', he said, 'then feel her apex beat'. Again, it was about 100 beats/min in atrial fibrillation and forceful. 'Forceful?'* asked the examiner. 'Yes', I said. 'OK, carry on and listen to her heart'. I started to position the patient correctly at 45°, etc. but the other examiner said to me: 'Don't bother with that, it wastes time'. So I just listened. My findings were that she had *isolated mitral stenosis*. I told them this and they nodded.

The next patient was a young boy about 20 years old who was grossly overweight. I was asked to look at his abdomen and to say what I thought the scar was caused by. It was a horizontal scar midway between the umbilicus and the groin. If he had been older I would have said it was for an aortic aneurysm but it was a bit too low so I eventually told them that I had never seen a scar like that before. The examiner said that it was for an *apronectomy* and he asked me why I thought he had had it performed. The patient did not look Cushingoid so I said it was probably for obesity as I did not think a surgeon would perform such an operation for a reversible metabolic cause. He laughed and said that was one way of looking at it! He asked if I thought he had *gynaecomastia*. I felt for breast tissue and said that there was. He then asked me to examine his testes which were very small. They took me outside and asked what I thought the diagnosis was. I said: 'Was it caused by alcoholism?' They said: 'No'. I explained

---

* The examiner must have been surprised to be told that the apex beat was forceful in a patient with lone mitral stenosis.

why I thought it was not Cushing's. They nodded: 'What else?' I suggested *Klinefelter's syndrome* because he was very tall. 'Yes', they said.

The next patient was sitting in a darkened room. 'Look at his fundi', they said. I thought he had proliferative diabetic retinopathy with extensive laser burns. However, there was no reply from the examiner. 'What else could it be?' I said it could be retinitis pigmentosa but explained how it looked different as the vessels were not usually traversed. 'Yes, but what else?' '*Choroidoretinitis* is another possibility but it isn't usually circumferential.' 'OK', they said.

For the sixth patient I had to 'Examine his visual fields'. I pulled up a chair and sat opposite to the patient at arm's length. I started to examine his visual fields but the examiners were walking about and talking and generally distracting the patient. I kept asking him to ignore them and to look at my nose! He had a *left homonymous hemianopia*. They asked me for the site of the lesion. He had no other gross signs of facial weakness or hemiplegia so I said it was probably a right middle cerebral artery cerebrovascular accident but that the lesion could be anywhere along the optic radiation and they agreed with this.

The next patient was a man about 50 years old who was lying in bed. 'Examine this man's legs', they said. He had a grossly deformed right ankle joint. I asked him if it was painful. He replied that it was not and never had been. I then said that it was a *Charcot's joint*. 'Caused by what?' they asked. 'Probably caused by *luetic disease*.' 'Yes, OK, what else would you like to examine?' I started to test the legs for sensation which was normal and for joint position sense which he did not allow me to do. 'What else?' The patient started to lift one of his feet and wiggle it about. 'Coordination', I suggested. 'Yes, OK.' I found that he was ataxic. 'What else would you like to examine?' The patient started winking at me. 'I'd like to examine his eyes, please.' He had small, irregular pupils which did not react to light. 'Does that confirm your suspicions?' I replied that it did and that was the end of the exam. (Pass)

'I would advise candidates that, whenever they are on call, to practise examining patients. I had the clinical on a Monday and was on call all weekend. As it turned out, this was very good practice.'

11 My first patient was a cyanosed, elderly man with clubbing and basal crackles. I said that *fibrosing alveolitis* was the most likely diagnosis. The examiner said: 'What else could it be?', so I suggested *occupational lung disease* and this seemed to suffice. The examiner then showed me the chest X-ray and expected me to describe the reticular pattern. He asked me for the Latin name for lacy! I did not know the word so the examiner moved on quickly.

The next patient was a young Asian man with an old ulcer on his shin. I was asked to say what had caused this so I suggested *sickle cell disease* and this was correct.

The next patient was an old, pale man with *hepatosplenomegaly*. The examiner asked how I knew that it was not polycystic kidney disease. I initially bluntly replied that I had not formally examined for the kidneys (which I had in fact forgotten to do) and the examiner looked a bit taken aback. However, I went on to say that he had no evidence of dialysis (shunts or peritoneal) and I could not get above the masses, etc. I feel that although I had forgotten to formally examine the kidneys he had obviously not noticed and my straightforward admission got me off the hook.

The next patient was a young lady and I was asked to examine her right hand. I noticed that both forearms seemed wasted distally. The right hand had both hypothenar and thenar wasting with clawing. I was asked first to describe this and then for what I thought it could be caused by (having briefly gone through a neurological motor and sensory examination and had demonstrated the most likely nerve lesions). I felt that it could be a *hereditary motor* and *sensory neuropathy* extending to the arms and said that I would want to see the legs. In retrospect, I think that this must have been correct. The examiner did not seem displeased but then asked for other possibilities. We got on to peripheral nerve lesions, brachial plexus lesions and syringomyelia, each of which I had to justify.

The next patient had *proliferative diabetic retinopathy*. The examiner asked me where the microaneurysms were so I said between the vessels. He then asked me why they were not right by the vessels. Seeing me struggle, he asked about Harvey's theories at which I realized that they must be aneurysms of the capillaries!

The next patient had complicated heart murmurs including *aortic regurgitation* and *mitral stenosis/ Austin Flint murmur* plus *mitral regurgitation*. She had had previous surgery and we got into a discussion about the indications for warfarinization with artificial pig valves.

The last patient had a straightforward *psoriatic arthropathy*.

I would advise candidates that, whenever they are on call, to practise examining patients. I had the clinical on a Monday and was on call all weekend. As it turned out this was very good practice as when seeing patients I would just concentrate on one particular system. (Pass)

'There was a loud stenotic murmur so I didn't mention that I had heard the regurgitant jet.'

12 'Examine this man's abdomen.' I started with the hands and was told (not unkindly) to move on. As soon as I had demonstrated the *spleen* they stopped me. 'What is your finding?' I said a large spleen. 'What is the cause in this man?' He was about 70–80 years and I had to modify my list accordingly, which I did rather poorly.

The second patient had a *diabetic retinopathy* with laser scars. The examiner asked me about his visual fields and whether the scars involved the macula. 'Yes', I said, 'so I expect a scotoma and a constrictive field defect'. 'Examine for this.' Of course, I found the patient had a completely normal blind spot and full fields!

The next patient had *optic atrophy*. It was an old man with hydrocephalus. I was asked what had caused his underlying optic atrophy and I replied that it was probably caused by chronic raised intracranial pressure. I had the impression that this was a case that they were not sure about including as they seemed pleased that I had made something of it.

For the next patient I was asked to feel the pulse. It was a collapsing pulse and I then had to examine the precordium. I heard the regurgitant murmur in the aortic area only. There was a loud stenotic murmur so I did not mention that I had heard the regurgitant jet. (I do not know why!) I said he had *aortic stenosis* but why the pulse? 'I would like to see the blood pressure', I said. This was 190/40. 'He must have *aortic regurgitation*.' The examiner said: 'Uuuh. Listen again', which I did and heard it again. (This time it was very loud!) However, I had been allowed to relisten to this patient. I felt that I could have done much better here in summing up the signs more sensibly.

The next patient was an elderly lady with a resting tremor, an intention tremor, titubation, a mini tracheostomy and clasp-knife tone. The examiner said: 'What do you notice?' I said: 'She has a mini tracheostomy'. 'Yes', said the examiner, 'the last candidate missed that'. My brief examination demonstrated all the above findings. The examiner said: 'What nerve supplies the larynx?' There was then a brief discussion on brainstem syndromes and I discovered afterwards that the eventual diagnosis here had been the *olivopontocerebellar degeneration syndrome*! (Pass)

'I said "Infectious mononucleosis" before I could stop myself.'

13 I was asked to examine the language function of a patient. This went well as she had an *expressive dysphasia*. I was then asked to examine her visual fields and she had a *homonymous hemianopia*. I was asked about the general management of stroke patients and the factors involved in their prognosis. They seemed happy with my answers.

I was then asked to examine the next patient's heart. I therefore listened and felt the carotid pulse at the same time. There was a plateau pulse plus aortic stenosis. I gave my findings and asked for the blood pressure. I was told it was 120/80. I made a diagnosis of *aortic stenosis* and had to explain why it was not aortic sclerosis. I was told that the patient had presented as a collapse so we talked about syncope secondary to aortic stenosis. I then got on to arrhythmias and Adams–Stokes attacks. I know that they were trying to change my mind about the diagnosis but I said clinically my diagnosis was of aortic stenosis and that an ECG and an echo and possibly catheter studies would help confirm this. I am sure I would have failed if I had changed my mind.

We went on to the next patient and I was asked to examine the abdomen, to explain what I was doing and to give my findings as I went along. They stopped me after I had found *hepatosplenomegaly* and then asked me for a differential diagnosis. I gave alcoholic liver disease with portal hypertension as the most likely cause and infection. 'What sort of infection?', they asked. I said 'Infectious mononucleosis' before I could stop myself and the examiner laughed and said: 'Is it likely?' I said: 'No, because the patient is in the wrong age group', and they seemed satisfied. I mentioned chronic myeloid leukaemia and they asked me about enzyme markers and that went OK.

For the next patient I had to examine the neck. There were large pulsating masses on both sides which were possibly *carotid aneurysms*. I examined the neck and then the examiner handed me my stethoscope! I presented my findings but was not asked for a diagnosis.

We moved on to the next patient: 'Examine these fundi'. The right fundus was normal but the left fundus had optic atrophy plus a small area of choroidoretinitis. They seemed surprised when they heard me describe what I had seen. Then they asked for the diagnosis. I thought they meant of the *optic atrophy* and the *choroidoretinitis*. So I said: 'Toxoplasmosis!' They laughed and said: 'No, the patient went suddenly blind'. I then offered a diagnosis of temporal arteritis. The examiner obviously did not know about the choroidoretinitis. I saw the patient afterwards and he told me that they had had another look. I hope they saw it!

The examiners were very pleasant. I know my examination technique was fine but sometimes I was a bit hesitant when answering their questions. (Pass)

'I thought the examiners were probably a little the worse for lunch but don't be fooled by their jovial attitude (if they are like that) into becoming frivolous yourself.'

14 The first patient had bilateral *polycystic kidney disease* and I was asked to examine the abdomen. I went straight to the hands and the examiners asked what I was looking for. They wanted to know if I had found any of these features and before I could say that they were in fact normal. I was jovially accused of not having really looked but I firmly stated that I had! When I asked the patient if he had any pain in the tummy, they said: 'He soon will have!' I was then told: 'We have to get our entertainment this afternoon somehow'. There was eventually a discussion on how polycystic kidneys present.

I was then asked to: 'Examine this woman's chest from the cardiovascular point of view'. She had *mitral stenosis* and *aortic regurgitation*. Again the examination was interspersed with quips from the examiners. They expected me to have felt the trachea to check the position of the mediastinum. I had not and was told: 'Naughty, naughty'. A look of horror must have crossed my face as they said: 'Don't worry, you're doing very well'.

The third patient had *diabetic retinopathy*. It was fairly uncomplicated except that the examiners fell around laughing when, having asked the patient if I could look in the right eye, I then asked if I could look in the left eye. The instruction had been: 'Examine this patient's eyes' (while they were handing me an ophthalmoscope), so I had asked if they only wanted fundoscopy and they had said: 'Yes'.

The next patient had *titubation* and *nystagmus* in all planes. The instruction was: 'Examine this patient's eyes'. I had the Snellen chart from this book and they were delighted, clapping their hands and saying: 'Bonus points for that!' The rest of the examination of this patient was unremarkable and there was a brief discussion on possible causes.

The fifth patient had a *spastic paraparesis* and I was asked to examine the legs. It was uneventful until just before the plantars. I was asked which way they were likely to go and I said: 'Up'. He said: 'OK, make them go up like a real neurologist'. They went up and at that point I could not resist a broad grin! There was a brief discussion on possible causes.

The last patient had *clubbing, pigmentation* and *kyphosis* and we talked about a possible aetiology.

I thought the examiners were probably a little the worse for lunch but do not be fooled by their jovial attitude (if they are like that) into becoming frivolous yourself. When I started the exam they said: 'What are you good at? Don't tell me, everything.' I said: 'Well, I

have been practising', and they roared with laughter. (Pass)

'The delayed fundal question ploy I thought—I was ready for that!'

15 'What do you think the skin lesion is on this leg?' (discoloured, purple/pink with marked scaling). 'Psoriasis', I said, 'but there are no other plaques'. 'No—think again', 'Drug reaction?' 'No', said the examiner who appeared exasperated. 'How about infection?' 'Well it could be *cellulitis*', I said. 'Yes, at last. Well perhaps you'll do better on the others.' (I had never imagined they would put a case of cellulitis in, especially an atypical one.)

'Examine this man's leg and talk as you go through it. You may ask him questions.' I grappled with demonstrating a *paraplegia* while speaking (which was difficult). 'What do you think of his speech?' (Heck! I realized it was not the content but the speech character they wanted me to note.) I asked a question and noted his *dysarthria*. 'Would you like to demonstrate the plantars!' I said that I would normally do them and showed they were upgoing. (By this time I was despondent but determined.)

'Examine this girl's cardiovascular system quickly.' It went smoothly. I presented it clearly and discussed the *ventricular septal defect* (VSD) or mitral regurgitant murmur. 'Do you think the VSD is significant?' 'Well, no, because there . . .' I said. 'Don't say why, just say yes or no' (exasperated examiner). 'No'. 'Fine', he said.

'Look at this man. Perhaps it is easier if he stands up. Tell me what you think.' 'He has a *Marfanoid appearance*, sir.' 'Yes, what would you look for?' 'Aortic and mitral regurgitation', I replied. 'Which valve is most likely to be affected?' '*Aortic regurgitation.*' The examiner pulled back the shirt triumphantly to demonstrate the aortic valve replacement scar (Bingo!).

'Examine this fundus.' There was background *diabetic retinopathy*. I confidently presented my prepared speech. 'Yes', he said and we walked away. *Then* he said: 'And were there any laser scars?' 'No', I said. 'And were there cotton-wool spots?' 'No'. 'Correct.' (The delayed fundal question ploy I thought—I was ready for that!)

'Examine the abdomen of this girl.' There was a palpable *liver and spleen* so I gave these signs succinctly. We moved away and the examiner, noticeably relaxed, was filling time. 'What do you think is the cause?' 'Hodgkin's disease is most likely', I said. 'Yes, anything else—how about biliary cirrhosis?' 'There are no signs of chronic liver disease and the palpable spleen goes against this', I said. 'Yes, but it is *biliary cirrhosis*', and he shrugged his shoulders! (Pass)

'I have already made a diagnosis. Do you want me to continue?'

16 I was asked to examine the arms of a man who was complaining of weakness. He had the facial appearance of *myotonic dystrophy*. I shook hands with the patient and said: 'I have already made a diagnosis. Do you want me to continue?' I then had to demonstrate how to examine power in the arms. I was asked if I wanted to ask the patient any questions. I asked him about family history and the effects of cold.

I was then asked to examine a patient's fundi. He had grade II *hypertensive retinopathy* with marked arteriovenous nipping.

The instruction for the next patient was, 'Examine the respiratory system'. He had dyspnoea, cyanosis, clubbing and the fine, inspiratory, basal crackles suggestive of *fibrosing alveolitis*. I was asked to give the causes and differential diagnoses of fibrosis of the lungs. I was then shown the patient's chest X-ray and asked to comment. It showed bilateral lower zone fibrotic changes.

Next, I was asked to examine a patient's abdomen. There were bilateral *polycystic kidneys* and an arteriovenous fistula in the arm. I was asked to demonstrate one of the kidneys. The examiner seemed satisfied, and asked me the single most useful investigation. I answered: 'Ultrasound', and he nodded.

I was taken to the next short case and asked to examine the heart and to tell the examiner what the diagnosis was. The pulse was of normal character and there was a long *systolic murmur* all over the precordium, maximal at the left sternal edge. I said I was unsure of the diagnosis and gave a differential of mitral regurgitation and aortic sclerosis. He asked me what the heart sounds were like. I could not remember them clearly and said 'Normal'. He then said he thought the second sound was quiet. I wondered whether I had missed aortic stenosis. We then got into a discussion between aortic sclerosis and stenosis. I admitted that I thought aortic sclerosis was a bad term and wished I had never mentioned it! He asked me what I would do in the clinic if presented with such a murmur, so I said an ECG, chest X-ray and an echocardiogram. He nodded.

My advice is to stay as calm as possible and hope that the first case goes well. Always look at the patient's surroundings and general appearance before starting your specific examination. It is impressive if you can make the diagnosis, for example, of myotonic dystrophy from the end of the bed. (Pass)

'What they really wanted me to notice were the old-fashioned controls of a wheelchair.'

17 I was asked to examine a patient's abdomen. I thought I could get over the mass in the left hypochondrium and so I said the diagnosis was of polycystic kidneys. I then looked for dialysis marks on the arms. In retrospect, it was so clearly *hepatosplenomegaly*. In fact, I can still feel my fingers jumping over the sharp edge of the liver. I really do not know why I said polycystic kidneys. If I had been the examiner I would certainly have failed myself!

We then moved on to the next patient. The examiner said: 'What do you notice about this woman?' There was half a minute's pause. 'She's in a wheelchair', I said. 'What does that tell you about the chronicity of her disease?' 'If it's an NHS wheelchair then she will have been waiting some time!' (They liked this.) What they had really wanted me to notice were the old-fashioned controls. They went on: 'Examine her fundi'. She had the whitest discs that I have ever seen. 'What would you like to test next?' They obviously thought I was not extending my examination quickly enough. What they really meant was: 'Examine her gait', which I eventually did and she was grossly ataxic. 'What is your diagnosis?' '*Multiple sclerosis*'. It had taken a long time to drag me through this case! (Pass)

'She must have had cystic fibrosis presenting with a cerebral abscess.'

18 For my next case I was asked to examine a lady's abdomen. She was about 40 years old. I performed a standard abdominal routine and found that she had a large mass on the right side which I could get above. It moved with respiration and was hollow to percussion. I thought it was most likely to be a polycystic kidney but, because I could not feel one on the other side, I suggested that I would investigate it further. The examiner said: 'Well it is a *polycystic kidney*, and I wouldn't worry too much about not being able to feel one on the other side'.

The next short case was a 30-year-old lady. I was told that she had come to casualty last week having had several fits. She had papilloedema and the examiners told me that she had had a CT scan. They then asked me to examine her chest. She had clubbing with a Hickman line *in situ* and she also had a left thoracotomy scar. There was a left pleural effusion with thickening and a right pleural rub. The examiner said: 'Can you piece it all together?' I went: 'Um, um, um', and then the bell went. The examiner said: 'Come on'. I went: 'Uhh . . . uhh . . .' He said: 'OK, forget it!' I think she must have had *cystic fibrosis* presenting with a cerebral abscess.

One must look interested in the cases themselves and take time to be nice to the patients. I said: 'Excuse me' to one of the examiners while pointing to an open curtain behind him before examining a young lady's chest. He said: 'Sorry' and closed the curtains! (Pass)

You never know you've failed until the list is published

The following examples illustrate the extent to which the candidate's assessment of what is happening can be very different from that of the examiners. Although the examiners may appear rude and hawkish, and you may feel that you are doing badly, you may in fact be performing well enough.

'They then both walked off muttering, "Well, I would never employ this woman—would you?". If I had been nervous before, I was even worse now and felt certain that I had failed.'

19 For my first case I was asked to examine the abdomen of a 60-year-old woman. I found a large *mass on the left side of the abdomen*, there was no anterior notch, I could not get above or below it. I thought it was probably a kidney or a spleen but to this day I do not know what it was. I told the examiners I thought it was probably a renal mass and gave good reasons why, but I think I was probably wrong. They said nothing and looked displeased.

For the next case, they took me to a 70-year-old man and asked me to, 'Listen to the back of the chest only'. There were bilateral, basal, fine, expiratory crackles and clubbing. I told the examiners that there was *pulmonary fibrosis* and that it was probably idiopathic. This was followed by: 'For goodness sake, woman, calm down!' 'What is the diagnosis?' I told them the same diagnosis again. 'What does he have?' I told them again! 'What is the cause?' I told them again and got upset and said 'I'm sorry but . . .' The examiner said: 'Look at him again'. I looked and could see nothing so I said that. He eventually hinted at connective tissue diseases so I asked the patient to open his mouth—he had *scleroderma*! In retrospect, I feel that this was not obvious and that the examiner was unduly harsh in his attitude.

The next patient was a 35-year-old woman and I was asked to examine the cardiovascular system. I heard *some sort of murmur*. I noticed a sternotomy scar and a funny pulse. I was still shaking from my experience in the second case and was by now even more nervous. It was either mitral valve disease or combined aortic valve disease—I obviously got it wrong as the examiner listened and looked cross. The examiners muttered be-

tween themselves and I felt completely useless by this stage. The only saving grace was that I had examined the cardiovascular system of the patient efficiently.

The next patient was a 50-year-old man and I was asked to look at his fundi. The room was light and the pupils were not fully dilated. I used my own ophthalmoscope which was a great help. I reported early background *diabetic retinopathy* in the left eye only and they moved on. In the meantime, in a loud voice, the first examiner said: 'Well, I would never employ this woman—would you?'. If I had been nervous before, I was even worse now and felt certain that I had failed.

The next patient was a 60-year-old man with a harsh *pansystolic murmur* at the left sternal edge and a displaced apex. I again examined thoroughly and described what I had heard in response to the instruction, 'Feel the pulse, listen at the apex'. I was asked the diagnosis and said ventricular septal defect because of the apex and the harsh quality of the murmur. He wanted to know the differential diagnosis and how I would differentiate them clinically. The examiner was still unhappy. I think it must have been mitral regurgitation.

The next patient was a 60-year-old woman. I was asked to: 'Look at this face—what do you see?' '*Cushingoid*', I responded. 'Name three causes in a woman of this age.' I gave three. 'Anything else you notice?' '*Basal cell carcinoma*.' 'What else?' I could see nothing else so I pointed out a second basal cell carcinoma which I had already seen. They then both walked off muttering.

The examiners were rude and unpleasant. My only advice to future candidates is to pretend you are in the casualty department and ignore the examiners. (Pass!)

'The examiners looked surprised when I said the tone was increased. I was asked to demonstrate and therefore withdrew my rash and foolish remark and finally concluded with possibilities for combined upper and lower motor neurone lesions.'

20 'Examine this lady's *legs and gait*': a disaster! Gait: partly obscured by a long nightgown—steppage or right foot-drop? Examination on the bed: tone (patient nervous) seemed increased but reflexes and plantars could not be elicited, the power was reduced, and the testing of sensation was laborious and inconclusive. I was uncertain when to say I had finished. There were pitying looks from the examiners. I blurted out some findings. The examiners looked surprised when I said the tone was increased. I was asked to demonstrate and then withdrew my rash and foolish remark and finally concluded with possibilities for combined upper and *lower motor neurone lesions.*

We passed on with much relief but scarcely more success. 'Examine this patient's knees.' On inspection, the knees were clearly swollen, left more than right, and the quadriceps were wasted. On palpation, the knees were warm but I failed to elicit fluid even though effusions were obviously present. The examiners raised their eyebrows as I recounted my findings. 'Please show me how you look for fluid.' On this second attempt, I clearly elicited the patella tap sign. Causes for the *swollen knees* were not discussed. We passed on with increasing confusion on my part.

'Listen to this man's heart!' I heard and reported *aortic incompetence,* having noted the cannula in the patient's arm. I was asked for the aetiology and suggested subacute *bacterial endocarditis* which seemed to be what they wanted—at last (!) but surely I was beyond redemption.

'Look at this lady's neck.' I inspected the plucked chicken skin and gave the diagnosis of *pseudoxanthoma elasticum.* I was not asked any further questions.

'Examine this man's chest.' On inspection he was blue, bloated and very breathless and I proceeded with palpation, percussion and auscultation although the examination was punctuated by bouts of severe coughing which I thought would lead to his death at any moment! The examiners seemed understanding as I asked if he wished me to continue. My diagnosis of exacerbation of *chronic obstructive airway disease* was accepted.

I was grateful to get to the next patient. 'Examine this man's abdomen.' I was going through my normal procedure when the bell sounded, which is always off-putting and I sought to reach a hasty conclusion. I suggested that there was a non-tender 2 cm *liver edge* and then hazarded that there was a mass in the right iliac fossa. The examiners eyebrows were raised again in response to this. I am not sure whether there was a mass. A colleague, who also saw this patient, told me later that he had only felt a liver edge. The short cases ended with ears ringing and I was convinced of failure.

Of my six short cases, two went smoothly, two were barely mediocre (not least because the bronchitic patient threatened to expire at the end of every breath) and two were terrible and I had to repeat the parts of the examination which I got wrong. So, I strongly emphasize that the odd calamity need not mean failure. The candidate is probably very poorly placed to decide how he or she is doing. (Pass)

'*The examiners were continually unnerving me and making me feel that my answers were wrong.*'

21 I was asked to examine the hands of a patient. They looked rheumatoid but the patient also seemed to have tophi. There were no nodules at the elbow and I eventually said it was inactive rheumatoid arthritis. One examiner asked what I would think if told that his uric acid was 0.6 mmol/L. I said that was because he had *gout* as well! On walking to the next case, they asked me about treatment and I managed to discuss this satisfactorily.

I was asked to talk to an elderly man with a nasogastric tube *in situ.* He had dysarthria. They stopped me before I got any further and asked what I thought. I said that with dysarthria and nasogastric feeding, which was probably as a result of dysphagia, that he had a bulbar palsy. They asked me how I would differentiate pseudobulbar from bulbar palsy—I said I would look at his tongue—it was small and fasciculating. I therefore decided on *bulbar palsy.* As they moved away, they asked me the cause—I could only think of multiple cerebrovascular accidents. I forgot this would not do for the bulbar palsy I had just diagnosed!

For the next case, I was asked to look at the fundi. I could see lots of *laser burns* but no signs of diabetic retinopathy and so I said so. They asked me what I thought of the vessels. When I was looking, I did think there was arteriovenous nipping but thought that I would be better not to mention this. However, as they were actually asking me, I said that there was arteriovenous nipping which I had not mentioned before because I thought it was a 'soft sign'. They did not seem to like this. I then said that there may be hypertension as well. They did not respond. I was beginning to get unnerved!

I was then asked to look at a lady's eyes. She had *gross unilateral exophthalmos* and ophthalmoplegia. They soon stopped me and asked me what I thought. The only thing I could think of was thyrotoxicosis. They said she was euthyroid and pointed to a scar just above the nose and eye. I did not have a clue what it was. They asked me what was directly behind the centre of the forehead. I told them the pituitary and that the exophthalmos might be caused by a space-occupying lesion. They asked me what type. I noticed the patient was quite hirsute but by this stage the examiners had walked away and, as I could not think, I did not say anything.

They showed me a man with a *large mole* on his left arm. I did not know what it was. Although it did not look like a melanoma, this was the only thing I could think of so I said that the lesion should be excised and biopsied. They told me that the patient had had the lesion for years and that he had another one on his leg and they asked me what I thought about this. I said that I did not know and that I would still biopsy the lesion! It seemed that I was arguing with the examiner and, as I realized this, it made me feel even worse!

I was then asked to examine the cardiovascular system of a middle-aged woman. She had both a midline and a lateral thoracotomy scar with *prosthetic heart sounds* but with no murmur at the apex — he stopped me before I could listen further. I said that she had a prosthetic valve without any murmurs and with the two scars she had probably had a mitral valvotomy and later a valve replacement. One examiner asked me if this was likely in view of the fact that she was in sinus rhythm. I said that one expects atrial fibrillation but that the sinus rhythm was possible. The examiner laughed! They asked me about the aortic area — I said I had not listened there as I had not had time. The bell went and I was allowed to go. I felt like walking out and giving up.

I thought I did very badly. The examiners were continually unnerving me and making me feel that my answers were wrong. I was made to feel very unsure and I felt that it was very difficult to keep going. By the third and fourth case, I had half given up. As I was told time and time again prior to the exam, I am sure the main thing is to keep going despite what happens — you never know whether you have passed or failed until the letter comes through the door! (Pass)

'I felt like going home there and then but I am glad I didn't.'
22 'Listen to this man's heart — no, go straight to the precordium.' I was not given any history. I was so completely confused by the murmurs which were systolic and diastolic that I could not make head nor tail of them. Some findings were eventually coaxed out of me and a conclusion forced upon me. I felt like going home there and then but I am glad I did not. I was forced into saying that this was *aortic valve disease* with dominant regurgitation. I have not got a clue if I was right or wrong.

I was then asked to look at a man's hands. There was gross *clubbing* with no apparent cause, i.e. he was not cyanosed and there was no Horner's syndrome, etc. I was asked for more possibilities — they eventually told me that this was pachydermoperiostitis — I admitted that I had never seen it before!

'Look at this man's fundi.' I thought I saw a *pigmented lesion in the choroid* which was well demarcated and single. I was asked for more possibilities and to say what it actually was. I plumped for a melanoma.

I was then asked to look at another man's hands. He had *gouty tophi* but there was nothing on the ears or the elbows. They seemed satisfied with this.

The next patient was an 'Examine this man's abdomen'. I felt a *4-cm liver* and they asked me if I could feel a spleen. I said: 'No'.

I was then taken to a lady and asked to look at her — 'What do you see?' She was pigmented and mildly jaundiced with leuconychia and xanthelasma. She also had hepatomegaly and ascites. I was then shown her hands again as I had missed her liver palms — but that was after I had already given the diagnosis of *primary biliary cirrhosis*!

My last short case was another 'Look at this man's hands' and he was another case of *gouty tophi*. The examiners told me that I was correct. I was absolutely convinced that I had made an irretrievable mess of the short cases. I still cannot understand how they passed me! (Pass)

Survivors of the storm

'I found hepatosplenomegaly and told the examiner this. He then turned to the patient and said: "What operation have you just had?" and he answered: "A splenectomy!"'
23 'What's the diagnosis in this patient?' I noticed he had both *neurofibromatosis* and finger *clubbing*. The examiner asked me if I could relate the two conditions. I said: 'No' and the examiner said: 'Neither can I!' I was then asked to examine a fundus. I found *optic atrophy* and *resolving papilloedema*. The examiner suggested that I should look at the patient's neck and I found a ventriculoperitoneal shunt present.

The next patient had an abdomen to be examined. There was a recent midline scar. I found *hepatosplenomegaly* and told the examiner this. He then turned to the patient and said: 'What operation have you just had?' and he answered: 'A splenectomy!'

I was then asked to examine a patient's cardiovascular system. I found atrial fibrillation, *mixed mitral valve disease* (it was a restenosis as there was an old valvotomy scar), *pulmonary hypertension* and *tricuspid regurgitation*. There were pronounced *cv* waves in the neck and a pulsatile liver. I am sure I scored extra marks by feeling the abdomen. I was then asked to discuss the waveforms of the jugular venous pulse and I even had to draw a diagram! (Pass)

'The examiners appeared irritated by all my answers and when we had finished the female examiner shook her head scornfully!'
24 The first two patients were in a dark room. Both had dilated pupils and I was asked to look at their fundi. I did not get the diagnosis with the first patient. I said that the

vessels looked thin and the retina was dark and wondered whether it was *optic atrophy*.

The second patient definitely had a *diabetic retinopathy* and the examiner asked whether there were any hypertensive changes as well.

The third short case was a female patient with a small, smooth *goitre* and eye signs. I was asked to examine the patient and say why I was performing each action. I was then asked if the patient was *euthyroid* or not.

Next I was taken to a 30-year-old patient and asked to feel her abdomen. There was a *mass in the right loin*. I was asked what a horseshoe kidney would feel like, and I was then asked to give my findings before I had finished palpating the kidneys. So I just carried on feeling until I had finished.

I was then asked to examine another patient's heart and again I was asked for the findings when I had only listened at the apex and the left sternal edge. The patient was a lady in her eighties. She had peripheral cyanosis, atrial fibrillation and *right ventricular hypertrophy* but I could hear no murmurs. I said that the diagnosis was probably tight pulmonary stenosis but I should really have said tight mitral stenosis or an atrial septal defect. I was really taken to task on the following points: Was the patient cyanosed? What other signs of cyanosis do you know? How common is pulmonary stenosis in this age group? What is the most common cause of pulmonary stenosis? The examiners appeared irritated by all my answers and when we had finished the female examiner shook her head scornfully!

The last patient was a lady aged about 30. I was asked to examine her pulses and to comment on them. She appeared to have *peripheral vascular disease* and *aortic stenosis*. (Pass)

'I found that if my first answer was incorrect, the examiners continued questioning until I got the right answer; if my first answer was correct, then they took the questioning a little further.'

25 'Look at this patient. What do you notice?' There was pallor, mild jaundice and bruising. I thought the diagnosis could possibly be *pernicious anaemia* and the examiners asked why. 'Because it looks like it', I replied. (Stupid answer!) I tried again and said: 'The patient is of the right sex and age'. The examiner went on to ask me to examine the fundi. There were haemorrhages present which were obviously secondary to the pernicious anaemia but I said it was probably diabetic retinopathy!

My second short case was a *ventricular septal defect* in a 25-year-old but I said I thought he had hypertrophic obstructive cardiomyopathy and we discussed the symptoms and findings, and finally the examiner said: 'What else could it be?' I said a ventricular septal defect and then he seemed happy!

The third patient had *rheumatoid arthritis* with *subluxation of the cervical spine* causing a *spastic paraparesis*. I was asked to examine the legs neurologically. I found this difficult as all the patient's joints were incredibly painful. Therefore, tone and power were hard to test. I had noted the rheumatoid arthritis and the upper motor neurone signs in both legs but failed to put two and two together to come up with subluxation of the spine.

The fourth patient had a complete left *IIIrd nerve palsy*. I demonstrated the findings and suggested all the causes for this but unfortunately failed to see a scar which indicated that she had had an aneurysm clipped!

The fifth patient had finger clubbing and a marked tremor. I noted these findings and suggested *thyroid acropathy*. I was then asked to find whether she was in fact hyperthyroid. I concluded she was euthyroid and found out later that this was correct.

My last patient had *psoriasis* of the hands with an *arthropathy*. I described the nail changes and the skin changes but in my panic forgot to demonstrate the terminal interphalangeal arthritis.

I found that if my first answer was slightly incorrect the examiner continued questioning until I found the right answer; if my first answer was correct then they took the questioning a little further. (Pass)

'I was harassed continually by the examiner saying: "Why are you doing x, y, z?" despite the fact that I was trying to tell him!'

26 'Examine this man's cardiovascular system and talk us through it. You've no need to do the BP.' I was harassed continually by the examiner saying: 'Why are you doing x, y, z?', despite the fact that I was trying to tell him! For example: 'Why did you roll him on to the left side?' My final diagnosis was of *tricuspid incompetence* in a patient with right heart failure. I told the examiner that I would like to look for a pulsatile liver and he said: 'Show me'.

'This gentleman is from Mauritius. Examine his chest.' My findings were of clubbing with bronchial breath sounds at the left upper zone. I said that the most likely diagnosis was a mitotic lesion in the left upper zone. Examiner: 'Tell me where the trachea is'. Whoops, I had forgotten to feel, so I said I had forgotten to look for it. Examiner: 'Would you like to do so now?' I said: 'OK, yes, it's displaced to the left'. Examiner: 'This gentleman has had these signs for 20 years'. I suggested that the most likely diagnosis was of *post tuberculous bronchiectasis with collapse of the left upper lobe.* Examiner: 'Correct. Why, if the upper lobe collapses, do you get bronchial breath sounds but if the lower lobe collapses you only get reduced breath sounds?' I said: 'It depends in either case on whether there is patency of a major airway'. Examiner: 'No, it is because the upper airways are less dependent'. All I could say was: 'Oh!'

I was then taken to a side room with the lights put out. Examiner: 'Examine this lady's eyes with the ophthalmoscope'. I did so and found *background diabetic retinopathy.* Examiner: 'Tell me about the pupils'. (We were in a pitch black room!) I had to tell him that I had not examined the pupils properly as he had asked me to look at the fundi. Examiner: 'Put on the lights and have a look'. I did so. 'The right eye is dilated and the left eye is constricted,' I said. Examiner: 'Look at the eyelids'. I was staring in desperation. Examiner: 'Do you think she has a left-sided ptosis?' I said: 'No'. Examiner: 'Well, she has. She has a left *Horner's syndrome* and midriatics in the right eye.' What a case to end on! (Pass)

'Two stone-faced, non-committal, silent, disapproving examiners! Despite expecting this, it still threw me a bit.'
27 Two stone-faced, non-committal, silent, disapproving examiners! Despite expecting this, it still threw me a bit. The first case was *hepatosplenomegaly* in a patient with *polycythaemia rubra vera.* I got the signs, then was asked for a differential—was then told he had polycythaemia rubra vera and then asked the symptoms. This unnerved me.

I was then asked to look at a patient's right fundus. At first, all I could see were a couple of haemorrhages. They said: 'Would you like another look?' I was convinced I had failed. I then asked if I could use my own ophthalmoscope (with a beam just down from a laser!) and found a *branch retinal artery occlusion* which I described, although I had never seen one before. This satisfied them and they asked me to test his visual fields which was easy and I demonstrated the *unilateral left lower quadrantanopia.*

Still convinced I had failed, I was taken to another patient and told to examine the legs as quickly as possible. I checked the foot pulses, then did a neurological examination. I demonstrated a mixed motor and sensory distal neuropathy, but the plantars kept going up! I said this was probably *subacute combined degeneration of the cord* in an elderly lady, and said why it was not motor neurone disease or Friedreich's ataxia but that syphilis was also a possibility. They asked how else I could demonstrate a plantar response. I did Oppenheim's test but they still looked vexed as the toes went up. They asked how else I

could demonstrate plantars but I could not think of another answer.

Even more convinced I had failed, we went to a lady with a malar flush. I was asked to examine the pulse and I found slow atrial fibrillation. I described the face and then they asked me to auscultate. I picked up *mixed aortic* and *mixed mitral valve disease.* They asked me the cause, and I said rheumatic heart disease. They gave no impression that I was right but asked if she was in heart failure. I replied that they had not allowed me to listen to the lung bases or to look for ankle oedema, but that her pulse was not fast and there was no third heart sound. I looked at the jugular venous pressure and pointed out the systolic waves of *tricuspid incompetence.* Then the bell went.

Presumably I passed because I had my routines completely 'off pat', so I did not hesitate while examining; I got the signs because I had been to so many practice sessions and had seen everything except retinal artery branch occlusion before. Also, I had always practised presenting cases in a loud, clear voice on the grounds that if I was wrong, I might as well sound good and that if I was right I would come across as being confident in my diagnostic ability! (Pass)

'Nothing else was said and they didn't introduce themselves.'
28 At the start, the examiners said very little and they did not introduce themselves.

The first patient was a young woman with a long laparotomy scar, which was pointed out to me, and a distended abdomen. I was asked to examine the abdomen and to suggest an explanation. She had a *palpable liver.* I suggested it was a staging laparotomy but in fact it was a splenectomy scar. They wanted to know the reason so I suggested haemolytic anaemia.

I was then asked to examine the cerebellar system of a man who was unable to sit up. He had nystagmus, past pointing, dysdiadochokinesis and internuclear ophthalmoplegia. They wanted a cause so I gave *multiple sclerosis.* They wanted to know what one would look for in the lower limbs so I suggested pendular knee jerks but only after they had discarded my original suggestion of looking at the gait.

The next patient was a young woman with a *palpable thyroid* and a nodule at the isthmus (it was also diffusely enlarged, according to the examiner). She was clinically euthyroid with exophthalmos. However, when I examined her I thought she had a staring appearance without exophthalmos. The examiner wanted to know the histology of Graves' disease!

I was then asked to examine a man who was short of

breath, and to look particularly at the cardiovascular system. He had a collapsing pulse, was in sinus rhythm, had a carotid pulse, a displaced heaving apex beat with an early diastolic murmur and an ejection systolic murmur at the aortic area radiating to the carotids. So I suggested *mixed aortic valve disease* with predominant incompetence. They did not say anything and moved straight to the next case.

I was asked to examine the man's abdomen. He had *hepatosplenomegaly* and they asked me how big the spleen was. I said it was 8 finger-breadths but they made me go back and measure it. I made it 15 cm but they made it 8 cm! (Pass)

'For some perverse reason, my mouth said pseudobulbar palsy.'

29 The first case was a young lady with *multiple sclerosis*. I had to examine her legs, gait and fundi. The examiners interrupted me continuously and wanted firm, quick decisions and some common sense. The case was easy and went well.

They then gave me a little case history. 'This gentleman was admitted as an emergency with newly diagnosed diabetes mellitus. Would you feel his abdomen.' I was given all of 30 s to feel his abdomen and they wanted to know what I would put my money on as the cause of the firm *mass in the epigastrium*. I do not think they really cared if it was correct but just that I had logically reached a reasonable differential.

We then went on to the next patient. The examiner said: 'This is a quick one. Just look at this fundus.' In retrospect, he had *senile macular degeneration* but I did not get it at the time. The chap was very restless indeed, thus making the examination tricky. I described what I had seen but said that I could not make a diagnosis.

I was then shown a gentleman with an *axillary vein thrombosis*. This was easy as he had a heparin pump. The examiners laughed about this when I came straight out with the diagnosis. They then wanted a few investigations that I would do and this was really quite straightforward.

The next case was a disaster! They gave me a short history of the man's symptoms. He had classical *bulbar palsy* because of the nasal regurgitation and dysphagia, etc. However, for some perverse reason, my mouth said pseudobulbar palsy although I immediately corrected myself. I then got mixed up over which way the uvula deviates with a unilateral palsy. The examiner then corrected me and I just kept smiling!

The last case was my redemption. We only had a few minutes left so I was asked to 'quickly auscultate' a patient. She had *mixed aortic and mitral valve disease* which I diagnosed almost immediately. They slowed me down and asked me to explain which murmurs I had heard. Looking back on it, I am sure that I had got them right. I actually overheard the examiners discuss me as I walked away (I have very acute hearing!). They were agreeing that my general performance was OK and excusing the pseudobulbar disaster as nerves! (Pass)

Some 'fail' experiences

Examiners rarely let the candidate know whether their diagnosis is right or wrong, or whether their clinical examination technique is professional. In the same way that candidates may perceive they have performed poorly and yet pass, as illustrated above, candidates may also think that they have performed well and yet fail. Such candidates may feel that the exam is unfair without being aware of the imperfections in the performance they gave, or that some of their diagnoses were wrong. In the following accounts, some of the candidates recognized that they should have failed but some did not.

'If she had Huntington's at that age, would she be doing the crossword puzzle in the newspaper?'

30 The first patient that I was taken to see was an elderly woman. The examiner said: 'This woman came to the thyroid clinic. What would you write in the notes after examining her eyes?' I tried to test visual acuity but was told to examine the eye movements. I thought she had a left VIth cranial nerve palsy but the examiner seemed unhappy with this. I then said that she had a thyroid ophthalmoplegia. He asked whether it bothered me that the *proptosis* was in the other eye? I was not sure!

The next patient was a middle-aged woman with *eruptive xanthomas* over the elbows and knees.

We then moved on to the next case. This was an elderly woman who was constantly fidgeting with either choreiform or athetoid-type movements. I was asked to have a few words with her. She sounded a bit dysarthric. I was asked for the diagnosis and I wanted to say Huntington's chorea but did not wish to say so in front of the patient. So I tried to say a hereditary chorea. The examiner said: 'Like what?' So I said: 'Huntington's'. He said if she had Huntington's at that age, would she be doing the crossword puzzle in the newspaper? I said: 'No'. I had not actually noticed that she was doing this beforehand. He asked me for another diagnosis. I hesitated but eventually got *drug-induced dyskinesia*.

I was then shown a man with very *deformed arthritic hands*. I pushed up his sleeves and showed the *psoriatic plaques* on the forearms and elbows. The disease looked burnt out so when she asked me what I would treat this man with, I said non-steroidals. She looked irritated and said: 'What else?' I suggested coal tar or dithranol for the skin. She was still not satisfied and walked off to the next case.

'Examine the cardiovascular system.' I examined the patient in silence and she then asked for my findings. Initially, I just said *mitral incompetence*. So she said: 'As manifest by . . .?' I then gave her my findings. The other examiner asked me if the pulse was in atrial fibrillation and I said it was not.

The next patient was a respiratory system case. I thought the percussion was a bit dull at the left base and said that there was a small, left, pleural effusion. They made me examine the *trachea* again but I still did not think it was *displaced*. She then told me to percuss out the chest again. By this time the bell had gone. They did not seem at all pleased about this last case. The senior registrar who led me away said: 'Don't worry about the chest — it's a tricky one'. (Fail)

'If I were examining the examiner, he would have failed!'
31 The examiner asked me to look at a woman's neck. She was sitting in a chair and she had obvious *proptosis and a goitre*. I went straight to the neck and told the examiner that she had a visible goitre. He seemed irritated by this, but I thought he was just trying to put me off my stride, so I continued with what I thought was a faultless presentation.

The same rotten examiner, who was young and abrasive, then asked me to examine a woman's cerebellar system. I asked for her address and he shouted: 'What are you doing?' 'Examining her speech, sir', I replied. 'But we have quotes for that', he retorted. Again I thought he was just seeing if I would crack up. So I replied: 'Yes, sir, but I can hardly walk up to the lady and say, "Hello Mrs J., I am Dr S. and can you say hippopotamus?"!' I moved on to finger–nose testing which demonstrated *gross ataxia*. I looked for nystagmus which I could not find but was asked about vertical nystagmus. I also demonstrated dysdiadochokinesis. He asked me to examine her legs so I began with: 'May I see the lady walk?' He gave me a curt reply: 'She can't walk'. I then tested power, tone, heel–shin test, and he stopped me again abruptly. 'This lady has had some injections years ago, what other system do you want to examine?' I confessed that I had no idea as I thought that I was looking at the cerebellar problem. He then said: 'Posterior columns'. I still do not know what the connection was. First I examined joint position sense — I thought I would get some extra marks here as I had demonstrated the technique to the patient and she com-

plied well. Then I tested vibration sense — I examined sternal sensation first and then the sensation peripherally. 'What else?', he said. I retorted: 'Two-point discrimination, sir'. 'Yes, yes, what else?' He was obviously irritated and I said I did not know what he meant. So he said: 'Deep pain', and then he grabbed the woman's heels. If I were examining the examiner, he would have failed! However, I still felt he was trying to rile me so I continued, still believing I was doing well.

The next two cases were a *mixed mitral valve disease* and *psoriatic arthropathy* and I had no problems with either of these.

The final case was a patient with *hepatosplenomegaly* and nodes, which was possibly chronic lymphatic leukaemia and again I had no problems here.

Overall, I felt that I had coped with the examination and I went home feeling fairly confident that I had passed. However, I failed. I wrote to the College and they told me that I had failed on my neurology case. I talked to a local examiner and when I told him what had happened he said that the examiner must be new and that it all sounded very unfair. I still feel that he was unfair and now having passed the exam on the fifth attempt without doing anywhere near as well as on this attempt I still say that the whole exam is very unfair! (Fail)

'I was asked about the severity of the lesion (aortic incompetence), how long it had been present and whether an operation was indicated. I was totally unprepared for this.'
32 I was initially taken to a young, well-looking patient and was asked to listen to the heart. He had a systolic murmur at the apex, normal heart sounds and no click. I volunteered a *mitral valve prolapse*. The examiner asked about the heart sounds which I said were normal. I think I was right on this case.

I was then asked to look at a patient's fundus having been told that he was completely blind. I found a *cataract* and *retinitis pigmentosa*. I stood up and the examiner asked if I had a diagnosis. I told him my findings and he asked about *optic atrophy* — I had not even looked! I said the discs were normal but they cannot have been.

The next case was: 'Please examine this man's chest from the front'. There was a slightly red patch on the right side of his chest. I watched him take a deep breath and was stopped and asked for my findings. All I had found was the red area which I suggested might be caused by radiotherapy for a bronchial neoplasm. I then found that the trachea was deviated to the left. Also the left hemithorax expanded poorly and the percussion note was impaired. I was then stopped and asked for the diagnosis. For some reason I said neoplasia. I am sure he had *old tuberculosis* at the left apex, and the mark on the right was incidental.

I was then taken to the next patient and was told that his GP had referred him to the clinic because he had a heart murmur and wondered about mitral incompetence. I found signs of lone *aortic incompetence* and thought that the diagnosis alone would satisfy the examiners. The signs were so straightforward that 99% of candidates would get them right. I was asked about the severity of the lesion, how long it had been present and whether an operation was indicated. I was totally unprepared for this and answered badly.

I was told that my next patient had been referred with anaemia and that I should examine her abdomen to find out why. The examiners 'tutted' as I looked at her hands, mouth, neck glands, etc., and impatiently hurried me on. She had *hepatosplenomegaly* and, although I was exceedingly gentle and explained what I was doing, she winced repeatedly. I appealed to the examiners — should I carry on? — but they remained impassive! I gave a list of different lymphoproliferative disorders to the examiners as I had also found numerous *lymph nodes in her axillae*.

I was taken to my last patient and was instructed to ask her some questions. I asked her for her name and she replied with a *cerebellar dysarthria*. I was asked for one other sign that I would like to look for and I proceeded to demonstrate that she had finger–nose ataxia. I volunteered cerebellar disease and suggested demyelination as the cause. One examiner grunted and the other wandered off! (Fail)

'The last patient had polycystic kidneys which I called hepatosplenomegaly. This was probably the final nail in the coffin.'

33 For my first patient I was asked to look in the eyes and I found *optic atrophy*. It was the first time I had ever seen it and I nearly said so! However, I had failed to notice the white stick and the aphakic spectacles.

I was then asked to look at a lady's face. I found a *Horner's syndrome* and again it was the first I had ever seen. I just managed to give a few causes.

For my third patient I was asked to examine a chest. I had no idea what the diagnosis was so I re-examined the front. There was dullness to percussion with reduced expansion and *coarse crepitations at the right upper zone*. I suggested fibrosis, tuberculosis or asbestosis. However, the patient also had an *ataxia*. I was hampered by the examiners asking for my findings at 10-second intervals!

I was then taken to a patient and asked to: 'Listen here' (they pointed to the left sternal edge, fifth intercostal space). There was *mixed aortic valve disease* and I had

been asked to auscultate only. There were no problems here and I was not asked for any causes or investigations or treatment.

The last patient had *polycystic kidneys* which I called hepatosplenomegaly. This was probably the final nail in the coffin. (Fail)

'I felt it was tapping and said so. This was a big error as it wasn't.'

34 'This man has been referred by his GP because of a heart murmur. Examine his cardiovascular system and say what you think.' I was allowed to make a full examination and diagnosed *aortic stenosis*. They did not seem happy and asked: 'Did you hear any other murmurs?' I had not and said so.

I was given the same history for the second patient. I was only allowed to feel the pulse briefly before being told that it was normal and to proceed to feel the *apex beat*. This was abnormal and slightly *displaced*. I felt it was tapping* and said so. This was a big error as it was not. On auscultation I had to amend my diagnosis. There followed a discussion about the different types of apex beat. I was able to answer all their questions quite well but I knew I had done badly on the first two cases.

I was then asked to look at a man's hands. He had classical *dermatomyositis* and I described it as such. However, I had to be prompted to test for muscle power which was much reduced.

For the next patient I was asked to examine the abdomen. It was a young man with *massive splenomegaly* and no other abnormalities. I was asked for a possible diagnosis so I said that it was possibly a myeloproliferative or lymphoproliferative disorder. They told me that it was not and asked for other diagnoses. I started to say: 'In a tropical country . . .' but was stopped. The examiner suggested that hepatic disease might cause such splenomegaly. I answered that it would be unusual to cause such massive splenomegaly and they agreed. I subsequently found out that the diagnosis was *sarcoid*.

I was then asked to examine a patient's fundi. The first retina showed scarring that did not really look like laser burns. I gave a differential diagnosis of diabetes with laser

---

* The expression 'tapping apex beat', commonly used even by some cardiologists and sadly in some books, is a contradiction of terms. The apex beat is a distinct, localizable impulse caused by the recoil of the left ventricle during systole, whereas the tapping impulse is the sharp, indistinct and non-localizable palpable first heart sound caused by the forcible closure of the mitral valve and the rocking of the left atrium. In fact, in severe, lone mitral stenosis with a pronounced tapping impulse (in the left parasternal area), the left ventricle is underactive and the apex beat impalpable.

treatment or choroidoretinitis. They asked me to look in the other eye but not to take so long about it this time. The second retina showed similar scarring but also small haemorrhages giving the diagnosis of a *diabetic retinopathy*. I was asked what I thought of my differential diagnosis of choroidoretinitis and answered that I thought it had been a mistake!

The last patient was a complicated one with heart failure, a raised jugular venous pressure and a pleural effusion. I know now that the diagnosis was *constrictive pericarditis* (from my college tutor). I badly muddled this short case and knew that I had failed the short cases outright. (Fail)

'They asked for a diagnosis. I tentatively said subacute bacterial endocarditis (I later found out it was hereditary haemorrhagic telangiectasia).'
35 Probable *diabetic fundus*. The patient had very thick glasses on and the examiners asked me to take them off. The ophthalmoscope was one I had not come across before and I could not focus it. I was too nervous to remember I had brought one with me in my handbag! (Incidentally, I would advise all female candidates not to take a handbag—they are just a nuisance.) I saw a few exudates and haemorrhages but was very unsure. This was a very bad start.

Then I was asked to examine a young man's chest. In retrospect, I found that it was *ankylosing spondylitis*. However, I managed to convince myself that he had unilateral signs consistent with an effusion and so I presented them. The examiners just said: 'Ummmm . . .', and moved me on!

I was asked to examine a man's cardiovascular system. He had atrial fibrillation, *prosthetic heart valve sounds* and also I thought he had a systolic murmur. However, I was very unsure what it all was. They said: 'So you don't think there is a diastolic murmur?' I said: 'No', and we moved on (in retrospect I found out that he had *aortic valve disease*!).

I was asked to examine a man's abdomen. They did not let me look at hands (see p. 23, *An Aid to the MRCP PACES*, Volume 1), etc. and I found that he had *hepatomegaly*. However, I could not palpate a spleen although I did not turn him over or palpate bimanually. In retrospect, he was deathly pale and presumably had a myelo- or lymphoproliferative disorder. They then showed me what I thought was senile purpura—they dragged out of me that he might be on steroids and asked the mechanism for the discoloration. I talked about capillary fragility but he said: 'No, no, it's all to do with macrophages', in a tone of voice that made me feel really stupid for not knowing.

I was asked to examine a frail-looking lady with *ascites* and *deep jaundice*. I was asked just to assess what I thought was the most important sign from a practical point of view. So I looked for a *liver flap*. They asked about other causes for a flap.

I was shown a lady with cyanosis, clubbing and multiple petechiae and splinter haemorrhages (I thought!) and they asked for a diagnosis. I tentatively said subacute bacterial endocarditis and they gave me another chance but I could not come up with anything else so we moved on. I later found out it was *hereditary haemorrhagic telangiectasia*.

I was shown a young woman with a burn on her hand and an amputated finger. I suggested a sensory problem but they then gave me a clue by telling me that she was unable to move her hand away from trauma in time. I then asked her to grip my hand and she had obvious *myotonia*.

The next patient was a young boy with a *Horner's syndrome*. I was asked what question I would like to ask him and I enquired if he had had any neck surgery. (Fail)

'I said: "Demyelinating disease". The examiner asked me what I meant by that so I said: "Multiple sclerosis". The other examiner who was just approaching us at that moment said: "Never say that, say demyelinating disease!".'
36 My first patient looked as if she was of Mediterranean origin but I thought she had *polycystic kidneys*. The examiners asked me why it was not a large spleen and had I thought of thalassaemia as she looked Greek. I was uncertain after this but said to the examiners that I thought I could get above the masses. Most of the candidates who I spoke to afterwards thought this was polycystic disease but the registrar on duty would not comment.

The second patient was a young, fit man who had a corrected *Fallot's tetralogy*. There was a mid-systolic murmur loudest all along the left sternal edge. Initially, I said it was aortic stenosis despite the fact that there was an easily visible sternotomy scar. I was asked if it was usual to have a stenotic murmur after a cardiac operation and the penny eventually dropped!

The third patient had *diabetic retinopathy*. It was a simple background retinopathy and the pupils had been dilated.

The fourth patient had *rheumatoid hands*. I was just asked to describe the findings and not to examine. I began saying that she had a symmetrical deforming polyarthropathy and was then dragged off to the next patient who had pulmonary fibrosis.

I was asked to list the possible causes and what was the most likely cause in this patient. I said idiopathic *fibrosing alveolitis.* The patient was a fit, middle-aged woman with no other problems. 'What one question would you ask?' I suggested asking what her occupation was and they said that would be more appropriate if the patient was male. 'Anything else?', they said. I asked her if she kept any animals and they led me away.

The next patient had a *spastic paraparesis*. I was asked to examine the legs and the examiners were very pleased when I asked to see the patient walk first but I then got myself into a discussion about the various types of gait. 'Would you like to do anything else?', they asked. 'I would like to examine the fundi and the spine', I replied. 'Good', they said. They asked me what the most likely cause was, so I said: 'Demyelinating disease'. The examiner asked me what I meant by that so I said: 'Multiple sclerosis'. The other examiner who was just approaching us at that moment said: 'Never say that, say demyelinating disease!'

Once again the short cases were late. The examiners seemed very fed-up and annoyed right from the start. I was questioned *en route* between patients while I was trying to keep up with them. At one point the examiner in the front turned abruptly to look at the examiner coming up behind me and said: 'What did she say?' The examiner behind me (who was really fed-up) said: 'How should I know?'. I said: 'Shall I start again?' and they both roared: 'No time!' (Fail)

'*During auscultation one examiner pulled me from the patient by the back of my suit!*'
37 'This patient is breathless, find out why as quickly as possible.' I did not spot the *flattening of the apex on the right* and was asked to look again. I thought that the trachea was central, even on re-examination, but then said that I would not argue with the chest X-ray! The examiner seemed displeased.

The next case was: 'Examine the patient cardiovascularly'. There was fast atrial fibrillation at a rate of approximately 120 beats/min together with *mitral facies and a thoracotomy scar*. There was also a median sternotomy scar. The jugular venous pulse was difficult to see and I was told to move on. During auscultation one examiner pulled me away from the patient by the back of my suit! I described the findings and said that I did not know what the underlying diagnosis was. I was told to give a diagnosis: 'Come on — three, two, one, going, going, gone!'.

The next patient had a large spleen with no lymphadenopathy or hepatomegaly. The diagnosis, I thought, was *myelofibrosis*. The examiner wanted a list of the other possible diagnoses which I gave them.

When we got to the fourth patient the examiner said: 'Examine this patient's eyes'. We were in a darkened room so I asked whether just to look at the fundi. They said: 'Look at everything'. I asked for the lights to be turned up in order to check acuity, fields, pupils and movements. There was no abnormality found. However, the patient had classic *optic atrophy* in the left eye on fundoscopy. I was asked for a differential diagnosis and the possible significance of the field defect. (Apparently he had a *bitemporal hemianopia* and a *pituitary tumour*.)

For the last patient I was again asked to examine the cardiovascular system. There was a collapsing pulse. I was stopped and asked what the diagnosis was. I said this could be *aortic regurgitation* and listed the findings that I would expect. I finished examining the patient and confirmed the findings of aortic incompetence. We then discussed the Austin Flint murmur.

The examiners were quite rude. Even if my examination technique was not good enough to pass the exam, I do not expect to be grabbed by the back of the suit. The examiners should not use their unfair advantage to behave in a way which would be completely unacceptable in public! (Fail)

Four months later I re-sat the exam. My first short case was: 'Examine this man's abdomen'. I said I would like to move the bed in order to examine him from the correct side. Their response was: 'Extra marks for moving the bed in Part II!' When the bed came apart in their hands and I had re-assembled it and then moved it, the examiner said: 'Extra marks for knowing how the bed works!' Eventually, the findings were of *hepatosplenomegaly* and a small amount of *ascites*. There were no stigmata of chronic liver disease or lymphadenopathy. I said that the possible diagnoses were . . .

When we arrived at the second patient the examiner said: 'Examine this patient's hair'. She had a full head of hair and eyebrows but little on her forearms and none in her axillae. I was then allowed to ask if she had ever had hair here, and she said: 'Yes'. She looked mildly Cushingoid and the skin was fine and thin. I thought the diagnosis was of *panhypopituitarism* in a patient who had been given steroid replacement. I said: 'The possible causes are . . . and would you like me to check the visual fields?'

The third patient had proliferative retinopathy and maculopathy.

For the next patient the examiners said: 'This man is breathless. Would you examine him?' He looked as though he had *ankylosing spondylitis* so I asked him to look up but he could not. I said this was likely to be the diagnosis and described the possible associated features of kyphosis and upper lobe fibrosis with a restrictive deficit. The examiner then asked me to examine his eyes. I found *proptosis* with no lid-lag or exophthalmos. He was clinically euthyroid with no goitre and I said the most likely diagnosis was of dysthyroid eye disease. The examiner asked if there was any connection and I said: 'No'.

I was then asked to listen to a patient's heart. I felt the apex and the carotid pulse which I then used to time the murmur at the same time as assessing its character. I found *mitral stenosis* and sinus rhythm. I said that the patient had mitral stenosis because of the loud first heart sound and the mid-diastolic murmur with a presystolic accentuation. There was no evidence of pulmonary hypertension.

I was then taken to a patient with a *skin rash*. I described it and said it did not have the characteristics of psoriasis, eczema or lichen planus, etc. I said I really did not know what it was. The examiners said they did not either and were going to biopsy it!

The last patient had an asymmetrical oligoarthropathy in the small joints of the hands. The examiners seemed to like the quick routine I had been shown which assessed function of all joints, grip and power, pincer and opposition, and fine finger movements. She was a West Indian girl with patchy depigmentation on the face. I said the differential diagnosis of oligoarthropathy included *systemic lupus erythematosus* which turned out to be the actual diagnosis.

On this occasion the examiners were very pleasant and no one grabbed me by the back of my suit! (Pass)

Downward spirals

'I completely collapsed when one of my short case examiners introduced herself as Dr X.'

38 I had heard the previous day from a colleague who had also been examined at Newham General that he had encountered a woman examiner who had given him a really difficult time. My anxiety about this was increased when someone else reported: 'I hope it isn't Dr X., she fails everyone!' followed by a few other stories. I completely collapsed when one of my short case examiners introduced herself as Dr X.

Short case 1: cardiology—a young West Indian woman. 'Examine the cardiovascular system.' I thought she had mixed *mitral and aortic valve disease*. There was absolutely no feedback from the examiners as to whether this was right or wrong.

Short case 2: neurology—a young Asian man. 'Examine these legs.' There was a *spastic paraparesis* and a *peripheral neuropathy*. I was heavily criticized for attempting to demonstrate cerebellar signs in someone who was obviously very weak but I attempted to defend this. I then became very flustered when asked to list the causes of this combination of signs. I handled all this very

badly and even when pushed on the issue of the man's ethnicity and what I should be considering (presumably tuberculosis causing a cord compression) I remained pretty inarticulate. From here on there was a complete loss of confidence and everything was badly handled.

Short case 3: abdomen—an elderly, wasted, ill-looking lady. 'Examine the abdomen.' I found a *hepatic mass* and *1 cm splenomegaly*. There was no ascites. I described the findings as above. The examiner started pushing me on the causes of the mass (which was attached to, but discrete from, the liver). I felt uncomfortable as he had not moved away from the patient's bed and to my horror I ended up saying what I had kept avoiding saying—the word 'tumour' in front of the patient. I knew this was a disaster.

Short case 4: chest—a middle-aged, obese man. 'Examine the respiratory system.' I found *clubbing* as well as very traumatized nails (multiple peripheral splinters). There was poor chest wall movement bilaterally with inspiratory and expiratory crepitations. I suggested *fibrotic lung disease* with an intercurrent infective exacerbation. There was no feedback at all from the examiners. (Fail)

'The examiner was aware I was bluffing and asked for more and more detail.'

39 I was first taken to a gentleman and asked to examine his abdomen. I grabbed for his hand after introducing myself but was told firmly, but politely, to stick to the abdomen. I found a *small spleen* and at this point the examiner stopped me and asked for my findings. He then requested me to ask the patient three questions to elucidate a cause. I asked about alcohol abuse and travel abroad (in particular, malaria) and then I was stumped so I asked a daft question about rheumatoid arthritis (thinking of Felty's syndrome). This was silly because I had already had a look at the gentleman's hands! It annoyed the examiner because it was at the bottom of his differential diagnosis!

I was then led to a fully dressed lady and asked to listen to her aortic area and to decide whether she had aortic incompetence. They did not like it when I tried to take her sweat shirt off to examine her properly. They expected me to examine her around her clothing. I was not sure whether I could hear an aortic incompetent murmur because I had never been convinced by one in the past! So I did a daft thing again and said I thought there was one. He then asked me what other features I would look for on general examination. We went through all of these and of course she did not have any of them. At this point he asked me to look at her generally and it was then that I noticed her malar flush and peripheral oedema. He suggested these were more in keeping with mitral valve disease and asked me to listen for this. I heard a *mitral incompetent murmur*. I was very uptight over my errors from the last case and annoyed because I felt I had been deliberately misled.*

I was then taken to the one case I particularly dread, *diplopia*, and was asked to examine the visual movements. I totally went to pieces and did this very badly. I was unable to establish what the lesion was even after the examiner tried to help. He seemed particularly interested in the *nystagmus* and the direction in which it was maximal. I wondered if I had missed ataxic nystagmus and the diplopia of multiple sclerosis.

I was then taken to a lady and asked to examine her fundi. She had definite *diabetic retinopathy* and after stepping back ready to say this, the examiner said to me that there were no prizes for the diagnosis. It was obviously diabetic retinopathy but could I describe in detail what I saw and where each feature was! I should probably have admitted defeat but instead I strung together what I had seen and made up the position of these relative to the disc. The examiner was aware I was bluffing and asked for more and more detail.

He then took me to a lady and announced that she had had atrial fibrillation and asked me to suggest a cause. I noticed a *thyroidectomy scar* and so offered thyrotoxicosis. I was asked to examine for this and found her clinically euthyroid but with *exophthalmos*. Presumably, she had had thyrotoxicosis treated in the past. He then asked for another cause so I suggested mitral valve disease and then noticed a mid sternal scar. He asked me to listen to her mitral valve which I did literally. At this point I got a sarcastic comment: 'Can you pretend this is the MRCP and examine the heart properly?' By now exasperated, I retorted that he had asked me to *listen* to the mitral valve and he did concede this. I proceeded to listen to the precordium and heard a *prosthetic valve* but was unable to remember how to distinguish between mitral and aortic prostheses. Again, I bluffed and probably got it wrong. With very little comment I was dismissed.

I was thrown in this attempt by the fact that although the cases were relatively straightforward, either the questions or the approach to each case was not. There seemed to be the deliberate attempt to confuse me and to lead me astray. I found it useful the second time round to think about the different ways a short case could be presented other than the straightforward, 'Examine this cardiovascular system'. I also learnt by experience that it is helpful to have some 'answers' ready relating to lists of common causes of, for example, splenomegaly. (Fail)

'I forgot to assess her speech and only knew one way to demonstrate dysdiadochokinesis.'

40 I was taken to the first patient and the examiner said: 'Examine this lady's cardiovascular system'. After I presented my findings of lone *mitral incompetence,* he said: 'Did you hear mitral stenosis?' My reply was: 'No'. He said: 'Did you hear aortic valve disease?' Again my reply was: 'No'.

We went to the next patient. The examiner said: 'Examine this lady's *cerebellar signs* from the waist up'. This was the start of the downward spiral syndrome. I forgot to assess her speech and only knew one way to demonstrate dysdiadochokinesis. The examiner was *not* impressed.

For the third case he said: 'Look at this lady's hands'. She had *rheumatoid arthritis* and I even remembered to look for, and noticed, the Cushingoid facies. However, the follow-up question was a 'killer'. 'Outline your surgical options here'. I was stuffed!

The fourth case was: 'Look at this *fundus*'. I could not see a thing! She was middle-aged and therefore I went for diabetic retinopathy. I still do not know whether I was right or not.

The examiner led me on. 'Look at this lady's hands.' She had *hereditary haemorrhagic telangiectasia*. We talked about inheritance, presentation and management. At last I had a decent case!

The final patient was: 'Examine this man's abdomen'. He had massive *splenomegaly and lymphadenopathy*. All my examiner wanted to know was what I knew about *Waldenström's macroglobulinaemia*! (Fail)

'The examiners were very upset and so was I.'

41 I was asked to examine a lady's chest and I hurt her during the examination. The examiners were very upset and so was I. The whole exam went downhill from there onwards. This particular patient, however, had a *right lower lobe fibrosis* from tuberculosis.

The examiners then said to me: 'What does that man have?' They were pointing to a gentleman who was disappearing through a door at the time. I correctly replied *ankylosing spondylitis*.

I was then taken to another gentleman and asked if he needed treatment. He had a definite *parkinsonian tremor* with rigidity and a little bradykinesia but was walking very well. I said, 'Not at the moment' and explained why.

---

* The examiner would argue that your houseman would not be unfair in asking you to check if a patient had aortic incompetence, even if he had not heard the early diastolic murmur himself. This is, after all, the most missed valvular lesion.

I was then asked to comment on another patient's rash. It was of fading *erythema nodosum* on the legs of a girl of about 20 years. They asked about the most common cause in this age group. I said Crohn's disease and ulcerative colitis and the examiners replied: 'Good'.

I was then taken to the next patient and asked to examine his eyes. I really muddled this up! I asked to test his visual acuity but he had not brought his reading glasses with him. I then missed a *central scotoma* and *optic atrophy*!

The next patient was an 'Examine this lady's abdomen'. She had a 2-cm liver and a 4-cm spleen. They uncovered her chest and asked the diagnosis. She had multiple spider naevi so I suggested *chronic liver disease*. At last the examiners seemed happy!

I was taken to the next patient. 'Your house officer thinks this man has had a *cerebrovascular accident* (CVA), do you agree?' I thought he had had a CVA affecting the left side but they were not happy that the right side was normal. I did not look for fasciculation and I wondered if he actually had motor neurone disease.

The last patient was a spot diagnosis and I was asked to just look. It was a girl who was covered from her shoulders downwards. She had a positive Corrigan's sign and I said that she probably had *aortic regurgitation*. They asked if she needed surgery so I said: 'Yes', after feeling a collapsing pulse. (Fail)

Anecdotes

The examination setting brings into play its own circumstances and idiosyncrasies which may influence, or even interfere with, the process of the examination. The examiner may wilfully or unknowingly hide a crucial clue and the patient may volunteer a helpful suggestion, all of which enrich the candidate's experience. In this section we present a collection of short anecdotes which reflect the varied and often unexpected scenarios of the exam. The pass/fail conclusion at the end of each anecdote should not be attributed to the anecdote alone; it reflects simply whether the candidate passed or failed the whole exam.

1 A candidate was asked: 'Examine the back of this man's chest'. He found a left thoracotomy scar in a man in his thirties. Even though the examiners were standing in front of it, trying to stop him seeing it, he managed to spot the sputum pot and diagnosed bronchiectasis. (Pass)

2 While examining the fundi, the candidate pressed the wrong button on the new type of ophthalmoscope that he had been given and the batteries fell out! The examiners handed him an older ophthalmoscope with which he was more familiar and he went on to diagnose proliferative diabetic retinopathy with a lot of fibrosis. (Fail)

3 A candidate was asked to examine the abdomen. She started with the hands but was told: 'No, just the abdomen'. There was a 15-cm spleen palpable with an obvious notch and liver just palpable on deep inspiration. After presenting her findings, she was asked why she had auscultated. She said that listening to bowel sounds was part of her normal examination of the abdomen. They asked if it was relevant to the patient in question and she answered: 'No'. They then asked that if she had auscultated over the spleen what might she have heard. She was then asked about the significance of a splenic rub! The likely diagnosis was discussed although it is not clear whether or not the patient actually had a splenic rub. (Pass)

4 A candidate was asked to feel a patient's abdomen. He found a mass in the left hypochondrium which felt like a polycystic kidney but was dull to percussion, moved medially with respiration and was not ballottable. The examiners asked him what he thought it was. The candidate said that he was unsure and expressed his dilemma, based on the signs he had found. The examiners said: 'If you could ask one question, what would it be?' The candidate said: 'Does anyone in your family have kidney disease?' The patient answered: 'Yes'. The candidate then went on to ask 'Is it polycystic kidneys?' The patient answered: 'Yes'. The candidate turned to the examiners and said: 'I'm sorry, I asked two questions'. The examiners laughed and at that moment the bell went. (Pass)

5 A candidate was asked: 'Examine this young lady's abdomen'. She found a 20–30-year-old woman with obvious abdominal distension who otherwise looked well. There was slight hirsutism, no lymphadenopathy, no mouth signs and a mass arising from the pelvis. There was no spleen on palpation or percussion and no palpable liver or kidneys. The examiners asked: 'What do you think this is?' The candidate summarized the findings and said she thought that the patient might be pregnant. 'Do you think we would include a pregnant woman in the MRCP exam?', asked the examiners. 'You might', the candidate replied. The other examiner said: 'Yes, we might, its an unfair exam! Would you like to re-examine her to see if there is a spleen?' The candidate demonstrated again that there was not. The candidate reports that she was led away feeling unsure of what she had missed. She later rang the organizing registrar who said that the diagnosis was not known but that she had a pelvic mass and an enlarged spleen on ultrasound. (Pass)

6 A candidate was shown a West Indian lady who had a wig and a Bell's palsy. He got the Bell's palsy and was then

asked to look at her head. She had severe, scarring alopecia and he was asked to give some possible causes. He suggested trauma and/or autoimmune disease but was not really sure what the correct diagnosis was. When he got home his mother told him that she believes she would have got that one right — it follows attempts to straighten the hair! (Pass)

7 A candidate was asked to examine the chest of a patient 'from the front only'. She found all the findings compatible with a left, upper zone fibrosis/collapse and suggested that this could be caused by previous tuberculosis. She was then allowed to inspect the patient's back which revealed a thoracoplasty scar. The candidate was told that she was correct. (Pass)

8 A candidate was asked to examine a chest from the back only. He noticed a left lower thoracotomy scar but failed to mention it or to put any of the other clinical signs he found together. He told us the examiners took the opportunity to hang, draw and quarter him! (Fail)

9 A candidate was asked to examine a woman's legs and found erythema ab igne. The examiners then asked for the differential diagnosis of reticular rashes on the legs and for the different skin biopsy appearances! (Pass)

10 A candidate was asked to examine a patient's cardiovascular system. He found several murmurs and suggested patent ductus arteriosus but he is still not sure whether that was correct. He commented that the examiners were irritated because he felt the pulse first. They seemed to want him to go straight to the precordium, even though they had asked for a 'cardiovascular system' examination. (Pass)

11 While giving her findings for a patient with aortic regurgitation, a candidate mentioned Corrigan's pulse. The examiner asked: 'Who was Corrigan?', although she thought he was not too serious when asking this! They then went on to ask her for the causes of aortic regurgitation and they felt that she should have mentioned degenerative valve disease higher up on her list. (Pass)

12 A candidate was asked to examine a patient's eyes and then the neck. He found unilateral proptosis and a goitre and diagnosed thyrotoxicosis. However, he did not notice the proptosis until he looked from above. (Pass)

13 A candidate was asked to examine a lady's left fundus as she had deteriorating vision in the left eye. He started to examine the right eye and the examiner said: 'Actually, I have told you that the problem is in her left eye!' The diagnosis was a branch retinal artery occlusion. (Fail)

14 A candidate was asked to examine an abdomen. He found a palpable left kidney which he suspected to be either polycystic or hydronephrotic. There was also a

mass in the right iliac fossa which he thought was probably a transplanted kidney. (Pass)

15 A candidate was asked to look at a man's hands. He found purple, swollen fingers with no arthritis, nail involvement or evidence of scleroderma but he noted some telangiectasiae on his face and lips. He was told that he could ask the patient some questions to determine the cause. He said he thought the patient had Raynaud's disease but wondered retrospectively if this may have been a case of CREST syndrome. He reported: 'The examiners wanted the causes of Raynaud's phenomenon and for me to look for evidence of diseases such as scleroderma, systemic lupus erythematosus, etc. They wanted me to ask the patient if he worked with vibrating tools and what happened to his hands if he put them into cold water.' (Pass)

16 'Look at this man's abdomen and describe what you see.' The candidate found a distended abdomen in a middle-aged man who had tattoos, an everted umbilicus, reduced body hair and purpura. The examiners asked 'What else would you look for?' He said: 'Jaundice, spider naevi, Dupuytren's contractures and leuconychia'. He was then asked to look for these signs which were all present. Then he was requested to examine his abdomen. This revealed marked ascites and a tender, 2 fingerbreadths liver but no splenomegaly. As they were walking away they asked him the likely cause of his signs and he answered, 'Alcohol-related liver disease'. The examiners asked him why he thought this and he replied that the patient was wearing a T-shirt advertising Foster's beer! They smiled! (Pass)

17 A candidate was asked to examine a patient's abdomen. He found hepatosplenomegaly. The examiners then showed him the arteriovenous shunt and asked him to re-examine the abdomen. His diagnosis then became polycystic kidneys! He was sure he had failed outright but tried to keep his head, remembering that it was possible to get by with one disaster! (Pass)

18 A candidate was asked to examine the abdomen of a woman with jaundice and hepatosplenomegaly. The examiners got annoyed when he started with examining her hands. (Pass)

19 A candidate reported that his examiners started 5 min late and he was not given any extra time. He had to undress three of the patients and get them positioned correctly. He also found explaining his findings as he went along difficult as one of the examiners appeared very deaf! (Pass)

20 A candidate was asked to examine the respiratory system of a patient with chronic bronchitis and emphysema. He was asked if there was loss of cardiac dullness. He examined for this and found that there was. (Pass)

21 A candidate was asked: 'Look at this rash in a 16-year-old girl'. There was a maculopapular rash on the limbs but not on the trunk. There was no involvement of the eyes, nails, joints or mouth. He was asked what the diagnosis was and if he would like to ask the patient some questions. The condition had been present for 5 years and the joints were painful. He offered the differential diagnosis of juvenile chronic arthritis or systemic lupus erythematosus. In retrospect, he feels it was the former (Still's disease). (Pass)

22 A candidate was asked to examine the abdomen of a woman who weighed 'about 20 stone'. He found two subcostal masses and diagnosed hepatosplenomegaly. In retrospect, he was sure that they were polycystic kidneys and that arguing the case for hepatosplenomegaly made matters worse and wasted a lot of time. (Fail)

23 The examiner said: 'This gentleman is icteric, please examine his abdomen'. He found hepatomegaly and a midline laparotomy scar. He presented these findings. 'Does he have ascites?' He told the examiner that his findings were equivocal and that an ultrasound was needed to define this. 'Does he have splenomegaly?' He replied that he could not feel a spleen but there was a dullness to percussion over the splenic area. He was counselled after he had failed the exam. Apparently the liver that he had felt was a palpable gallbladder. The examiner's comments were: 'He refused to commit himself as to the presence of ascites and hedged on the presence of splenomegaly'. (Fail)

24 A candidate was asked to examine a patient's left eye with the ophthalmoscope provided. He reported that he found optic atrophy, a detached retina, laser photocoagulation scars and aphakia. He suggested that the patient had had a diabetic cataract previously. The examiner asked about primary and secondary optic atrophy and then asked about the refractive error of the patient — covering the head of the ophthalmoscope with his hand as he did so! (Pass)

25 A candidate was asked to look in a patient's eye. He could find no abnormality and said so. He was then informed that he had looked into the left eye, whereas he had actually been asked to look into the right eye! The examiners were both laughing, although the candidate was embarrassed and very apologetic. The right eye showed obvious optic atrophy and he was then asked for a list of possible causes. (Pass)

26 A candidate was asked to examine a patient who had a right pleural effusion — the patient was very deaf and every time he asked him to say '99' he took a deep breath instead! (Pass)

27 A candidate was told: 'Examine this rash but don't rub it'. He found a brownish, macular rash on a young, healthy-looking woman. He had no idea what the diagnosis was. In retrospect, he thinks it must have been mastocytosis. (Fail)

28 A candidate was told that a patient had a chronic cough. On examination, he found right upper lobe consolidation and offered a differential diagnosis of tumour or tuberculosis. He was then shown the patient's chest X-ray which showed a cavity with a crescentic upper border and he diagnosed a mycetoma. (Pass)

29 In his second attempt a candidate was asked to listen to a heart. He heard a mid-diastolic murmur and came up with the diagnosis of mitral stenosis. The examiner asked him to auscultate again; on doing this he thought he could also hear an early diastolic murmur. (Fail)

30 A candidate was asked to examine the pulse of a patient and found a right brachial artery aneurysm. He reports that the examiner expected him to find the right radial pulse reduced in volume compared to the left but that he could not confirm this. The possible causes he offered were traumatic, iatrogenic or mycotic and, in retrospect, feels that it was most likely to have been a mycotic aneurysm caused by subacute bacterial endocarditis many years before. (Pass)

31 A candidate was asked to look at a man's face. He found herpes zoster in the left ear and in the distribution of the mandibular division of the trigeminal nerve. He also reported a left facial nerve paralysis and wasting of the left side of the tongue with deviation of the protruded tongue to the left. He diagnosed Ramsay Hunt's syndrome plus herpes affecting the Vth and XIIth cranial nerves. He was asked if such extensive involvement was possible and he answered: 'It appears so!' (Pass)

32 A candidate was asked to examine the fundus of a patient. He found that the lens had been removed because of a cataract. It was very difficult to see the fundus so he guessed the diagnosis of diabetic retinopathy which he still believes was probably correct. (Pass)

33 After being asked to examine the heart on his first short case, a candidate reported that he found mitral stenosis with an opening snap. The examiners asked him to point out the second left intercostal space. 'That's too high', said one examiner — 'It's here!' 'No it's not, it's here', said the second. 'Well it's a silly landmark anyway', said the first. 'I agree' said the second, 'Let's move on!' (Pass)

34 A candidate was asked to examine a man's abdomen. The patient had several of the signs of chronic liver disease and ascites. After much deliberation, the candidate said he could not feel the liver although he expected it to be there. He was criticized for his technique of examining the spleen (which the candidate says had been taught to him by an experienced examiner) and the examiners told him that the cyanosis was not a sign of liver disease. The candidate commented, 'This all proves that examiners are only human'.* (Pass)

35 A candidate was brought to an elderly lady with an obvious left hemiparesis and with a catheter *in situ*. He offered the diagnosis and explained why. He then had to examine the legs neurologically. He found this very difficult as she was demented and would not cooperate. However, he managed to demonstrate some findings in keeping with the left hemiparesis. They were about to dismiss him when he commented on the marked tibial bowing (sabre tibia) and volunteered a differential diagnosis. The examiners looked pleased. He felt that by making his comments on the tibia he may have made the difference with regard to passing or failing. (Pass)

Some anecdotes in the first person

36 I was asked: 'Look at this man's hands'. He had clubbing and the examiner asked me the causes. I looked at his feet but could not see any clubbing there. However, I noted abnormalities in the left tibia and diagnosed osteomyelitis. The patient nodded encouragingly but the examiner looked really cross! (Pass)

37 'This man has some strange feelings in his feet and legs, would you examine them.' The patient was totally bald and was wearing some sort of corset around his waist. He had a peripheral neuropathy but I had expected to find a dermatome pattern because of the corset. I really got into a mess! The examiner told me that the corset was for an incisional hernia following a splenectomy. I suggested he had pernicious anaemia as a cause for the splenomegaly and neuropathy, then possibly that he had diabetes in association with the alopecia. I eventually worked out that he had had vincristine for leukaemia! The examiners were very good-natured throughout all of this. (Fail)

38a 'Please examine this abdomen.' I did so and found definite splenomegaly. 'What is the diagnosis?', the examiner asked. I replied that he most likely had chronic myeloid leukaemia (CML) but the examiner blew a fuse and said that he had just wanted me to say that he had a 'large spleen'! (Fail)

---

* The candidate did not give the details of the technique that was criticized. We have known some examiners to get exasperated if a candidate, after having found no large splenomegaly at a preliminary light palpation, starts palpating from the right iliac fossa. They argue that this technique is to look for a spleen that is large enough to cross the midline, but it is also large enough for detection on light palpation! The examiners were also right to point out that cyanosis is *not* a sign of liver disease.

38b 'Ask this lady some questions and find out what the problem is' was the instruction addressed to a candidate. He found a rather garrulous lady with senile dementia. He did not ask her questions very well and the examiner stepped in to help. The diagnosis was discussed and the examiner apparently agreed that it was difficult. After wards the candidate was told by the organizing registrar that they had had difficultly finding good cases—otherwise this dementia case would probably not have been included in the examination. (Pass)

39 I was asked to examine the abdomen of a 60-year-old man. I found polycystic kidneys and an enlarged liver and I demonstrated the scars of the dialysis fistula. The examiners laughed when I went on to test for a spleen as they said that to find a patient with polycystic kidneys, liver and spleen was an examiner's dream!† (Pass)

40 I was asked to examine the legs, neurologically, in a 50-year-old man. I was told that he had a burning sensation in his feet but he did not drink. The patient then said that he did drink until he had got diabetes! We all laughed and they then said: 'Show us how you would have proceeded anyway!' (Pass)

41 The neurological case that I was asked to examine would not initially come out from under the bedclothes! I think that most people would have panicked but, given appropriate coaxing, the patient was eased into a suitable position! (Pass)

42 On arriving for the exam, I encountered an old chap who I thought was a caretaker from the hospital. I said to him: 'I'm fairly nervous. Is there a toilet nearby?' So he laughed and pointed me in the right direction. I later discovered that he was one of my examiners! However, I felt there was a friendly atmosphere. He asked me to examine a woman's legs neurologically. He said that she had become very weak but was now getting better. The unfortunate lady was totally deaf and I was almost shouting to make her hear my examination requests.‡ At each point during the examination I was stopped and asked what I had thought, and what I would do next. The sensory testing was an absolute nightmare. She seemed to have a fairly global weakness with absent reflexes and a patchy sensory loss. I thought the diagnosis was probably Guillain–Barré syndrome. The examiner agreed and then held my arm and said that he appreciated that it was very difficult! (Pass)

43 I was asked to look at a man's chest. 'What do you

---

† and a patient's nightmare!
‡ It is often advisable to face the deaf person and lower your voice to a bass tone, because many deaf persons can hear bass notes better than higher pitched ones, and many can lip read as well.

see?', asked the examiner. There was bilateral gynaecomastia. He said: 'If you were in the clinic what would you want to examine next?' 'The liver', I said. 'Go on then.' I struggled to demonstrate a normal-sized liver. 'What would you examine next?', he said. 'His testes', I answered. 'Go on then.' He had bilateral flaccid testes the size of peas. 'What's the diagnosis?', said the examiner. There then followed a nasty discussion about testosterone replacement and its relation to hair, skin texture and gonadal size! (Pass)

44 I was asked to examine a patient's abdomen. I started at the hands but was told to go straight to the abdomen.* There was a renal transplant in the left groin and a left radial fistula with tenderness in the left loin, and I thought there was a palpable kidney. I did not palpate too firmly because it was painful and they did not mind this. The patient was also Cushingoid. I felt the diagnosis was a left renal transplant with a ?polycystic kidney and that he was Cushingoid as a result of the steroids. At this stage the patient put his thumbs up! We then went on to the next patient and I was asked to examine her cranial nerves. It was an elderly lady with a complete right ptosis and her eye was looking down and out. Before I had completed the examination of the IIIrd, IVth and VIth cranial nerves she started to vomit. Therefore we left her! However, we continued to discuss the causes of a IIIrd nerve palsy. I said that diabetes was the most common cause and they said multiple sclerosis was. We then went through the entire list! They asked for investigations and I offered a blood glucose and a CT scan. (Pass)

45 'This man has been short of breath recently, could you examine his chest to find out why?' The expansion seemed reduced on the right side but the breath sounds were reduced at the left base. I could not recover from this conflicting information and completed my examination not having a clue what I was going to say. I could not go back over the findings as they were rushing me. I stood up and confidently gave the signs for a left pleural effusion. They said: 'Some people, when they say "left" really mean "right", are you sure this is left?' I realized I had got the wrong side but I could not retract what I had said so I repeated that I had carefully examined the patient and felt the signs were on the left. Then the bell went. The moral of this is that whenever they tell you to speed up—slow down. (Pass)

---

* It is useful when this happens because it indicates that there are no signs in the hands because you would not be stopped if there were. It also reduces the likelihood that the condition is one which might have signs in the hands such as chronic liver disease.

46 Examiner: 'Feel this woman's pulse and tell me what you find'.
Answer: 'There is atrial fibrillation'.
Examiner: 'and . . .? This is the MRCP, not finals'.
Answer: 'The pulse is of good volume and possibly collapsing in character'.
Examiner: 'and . . .?'
Answer: [Long silence—you could hear a penny drop!] 'I did not count the rate'.
Examiner: 'No you didn't, but what is it approximately?'
Answer: '80 beats/min'.
Examiner: 'Now continue to examine the precordium and tell us what you find'.
Answer: 'There are no thrills, nor a palpable heart sound. The apex beat is displaced to the anterior axillary line and there is a loud pansystolic murmur of mitral regurgitation. There are no clinical signs to suggest mitral stenosis but this could be silent so I would arrange for an echocardiogram.' (Pass)

47 The examiner handed me an ophthalmoscope. 'This patient is having trouble with her vision. Would you examine her eyes?' I commented on the cataract and then described hard exudates, both blot and flame haemorrhages, arteriovenous nipping and microaneurysms. I said that the features were consistent with both diabetes mellitus and hypertension. This did not please one of the examiners who said that hypertensive retinopathy should have more superficial flame haemorrhages. I stood my ground and said that she did in fact have quite numerous flame haemorrhages, but otherwise the appearances suggested diabetes. He finally asked me what her refractive index was. When my answer was rather quick at 14 dioptres, he tried to trip me up by saying that I had not included my own refractive error. However, I was able to point out that I had contact lenses and so I was perfectly corrected! (Pass)

48 I was asked to examine a man having been told that he had weak hands. On inspection, he had wasted small muscles bilaterally in a distal rather than a proximal distribution. There was no Horner's syndrome or fasciculation of the tongue and there was no sensory loss. The feet were also involved. There was a discussion then about findings that looked like a pure motor neuropathy. It could have been Charcot–Marie–Tooth but I opted for porphyria as this was Professor Goldberg's unit in Glasgow! The examiners smiled for the one and only time—either in absolute amusement at the ridiculous answer, or because I was correct! (Pass)

49 My last case would have been an easy cardiovascular system case except for the patient's stomach which must have been the loudest rumbling stomach in history—audible at 100 paces! I think she had atrial fibrillation, mixed mitral valve disease and aortic regurgitation. It would have been OK if I could have heard the blessed murmurs without the orchestrations from her gut! (Pass)

50 I had to examine a lady with Graves' eye disease who also had a VIth cranial nerve palsy. I found trying to examine her pupils and eye movements rather difficult because she was silhouetted against the backdrop of a bay window—perhaps I should have turned her round. (Pass)

51 I lost the membrane off my stethoscope during my respiratory case. It was a patient with a pleural effusion. I was very puzzled at finding a completely quiet chest—something which I had never seen beforehand. I suspected a pleural effusion from the percussion and vocal resonance. However, I discovered the faulty stethoscope at the very end of the examination. The examiners wanted to hear first what I thought, but did eventually agree to a second listening! (Pass)

52 'What's the diagnosis?' I was given no history. However, the diagnosis was obvious as there was evidence of psoriatic plaques together with arthropathy and nail changes. I was asked what was atypical about the patient and so I mentioned that the plaques did not have any scales. The examiner asked why and I suggested that it had been treated. The examiner then said something to me in Latin and asked what it meant.* I did not have a clue. The examiners both laughed but said nothing, except that the exam was now over! (Pass)

53 I was asked to examine a patient's fundi. They were very abnormal but goodness knows what the diagnosis was! I said hypertensive retinopathy because no laser burns were present, and I could not imagine someone having such terrible diabetic retinopathy without having had photocoagulation! (Pass)

54 After my first three cases the 'dove' took over. I was taken to a man and told that he recently had a problem with his eyesight but that things were now improving. 'Would you like to examine his fundi?' I did not have a clue what was going on. He seemed to have a mixture of disc swelling and atrophy but I said that I was very unsure about the degree of swelling. The examiner said that if he told me that the disc was definitely swollen what would be my differential diagnosis. At this point the head of my ophthalmoscope fell off! I said that partially treated benign intracranial hypertension or a tumour treated with

radiotherapy would both give this appearance. As we walked to the next patient the head of my ophthalmoscope fell off again. I said how awful it must be for them to take candidates like me around! (Pass)

55 The short cases went very well. The examiner were extremely pleasant and they even carried my ophthalmoscope box for me! I felt confident and very much in command. However, for my fifth short case I was asked to examine a chest. I could find no physical signs at all and I said so. The examiner said: 'That's very honest'. I was devastated. Whilst walking away the other examiner whispered to me 'Never mind, we couldn't hear anything either when we listened this morning!' In fact it was an upper lobe collapse that had resolved. (I passed the short cases but failed the exam.)

Miscellaneous

56 A candidate was asked to examine the heart. He could find no abnormality and said so because he thought he had to be honest. He has no idea what the diagnosis was. He failed.

57 A candidate was asked to examine a man's abdomen. He could find no abnormality and diagnosed a normal abdomen. In retrospect he is not sure if he missed something. Though he failed the clinical he felt he had passed the short case section.

Useful tips

Novice candidates preparing for MRCP pick up tips from their tutors, senior colleagues and other candidates who have 'already been there'. Then through their own experiences they develop their own. Some have been passed to us through our surveys and we present a selection of them here.

1 Practise, again and again, on 'short case patients' and when you think you have done enough—do more!

2 Practise being harassed. Get some 'mock' examiners to put you under stress. Nervousness gets no credit; the examiner is more likely to think that in a real emergency you would not rise to the challenge.

3 In every spare moment practise talking short case *records* (not just reading them) and talking lists (not just writing them). Get the order of lists right—give the common and uncontroversial ones first. Avoid controversial causes completely.

4 Practise presenting cases as much as examining them. If you can present clearly and quickly it is as impressive as examining well.

5 You have got to really practise doing short cases with SpRs, consultants, friends—even the dog or a doll! You have got to be able to examine without thinking and to

---

* The patient probably had guttate (from Latin for 'spots that resemble drops') psoriasis in which salmon pink plaques with minimal scales appear on the face and trunk.

then come up with sensible diagnoses from your clinical findings.

6 Dress smartly and conservatively.

7 Take to the examination a stethoscope, a pen torch, red-headed hat pin (dip a white-headed one in red paint if necessary), a tape measure, some cotton wool and some orange sticks.*

8 Be polite to the patient and the examiners; say 'Please' and 'Thank you'. The occasional use of 'Sir' will not do any harm.

9 You will have read the instructions outside the room and on entering you will be introduced to the patient. Do not ask the examiners to repeat the instruction but read the instruction carefully—it may contain a clue which you will miss without care. Greet the patient politely and get on with the task in hand.

10 Do not hurt the patient, especially during the abdominal examination. Look at the patient's face during deep palpation.

11 Make sure that during the examination of the patient you let the examiner see that you are doing the correct things—as one does in a driving test.

12 Do not be put off by any of the examiner's mannerisms.

13 Think *while* you are examining. Extend the end of the examination by a few seconds, if necessary, to give you time to put the findings together, and to prepare what you are going to say before you turn to the examiner.

14 Do not panic if you find very few signs in a patient. It is better to miss something subtle than to make up something that is not there.

15 Practise having to comment on your findings as you proceed through any clinical examination of a patient.

16 Do not let your tie or hair dangle in the patient's face. When you have finished be sure to leave the patient adequately covered up.

17 Present cases to the examiner as if you are speaking to an equal about an easy case.

18 Be confident—but not overconfident. A supercilious attitude is fatal.

19 Look at the examiner rather than at the patient or the floor when answering. Speak clearly and fluently. Do not mumble.

20 Take time to think before opening your mouth.

21 Keep cool, even when interrupted, and have a systematic examination technique to fall back on if you cannot make a spot diagnosis at the start.

22 Be aware that the stress of the examination can cause you to 'blurt out' things you do not really mean. Keep calm and think before you speak.

23 Remember common things are common. Beware of thinking that because it is the MRCP it is likely to be rare, although there will be the rarer cases (the usual suspects) as well.

24 Do not talk while the examiners are talking and be wary of arguing with them. If you say something which is definitely wrong then be prepared to say: 'I withdraw that', rather than try to defend it. Remind yourself that the examiner is the judge and the jury!

25 Do not try to pull the wool over the examiner's eyes. He or she is eminent and intelligent or he or she would not be an examiner, and will resent it if you treat him or her as a fool.

26 Do not guess or waffle. Cut your losses and admit if you do not know.

27 Avoid strange mannerisms of speech and action including using your hands excessively when speaking. Avoid 'ers' in your speech as much as possible.

28 Do not be casual. Say 'myocardial infarction' rather than 'heart attack' or 'MI'. Stand properly without leaning on the bed or putting your hands in your pockets.

29 Avoid using trade names of drugs—always use the proper pharmacological name.

30 Do not mention in your presentation that a physical sign is dubious or 'slight', e.g. starting your presentation on a case of mitral stenosis with: 'The pulse is slightly collapsing'.†

31 At the end say: 'Thank you', in a sincere manner.

32 Be careful in your choice of hotel for the night before the exam. A candidate recalls: 'For my first attempt, I booked a random hotel and ended up with a room in a cheap hotel overlooking a road which was busy all night, with burglar alarms going off. The walls were thin and the televisions and other loud noises of the neighbours could be heard going on throughout most of the night. For subsequent exam visits, I was very careful with my choice of hotel and always rang up to plead for a room in

---

* Equipment is provided but it is so much easier to use one's own. You may wish to take your own tendon hammer, sterile pins and ophthalmoscope. At least with the latter you know how to use it and you will have put in new batteries and have the lens set for your own lens correction.

† You should know that mitral stenosis does not have a collapsing pulse and if there is aortic incompetence then you would have heard the appropriate additional murmur. If it is not present then *do not mention* a 'possible collapsing pulse'. Leave out what does not fit. The examiners would tear you to shreds!

a corner, well away from any roads or other sources of noise, explaining to the hotelier that I had an exam to do. I believe this important strategy is essential.'

Quotations

These quotations are valuable suggestions and remarks derived from candidates' own experiences in the exam, and they have crystallized them in one or two sentences. We have grouped them under suitable headings which highlight their main points. It is no surprise that the chief lessons one learns from them is to practise, adopt good bedside manners and wear a confident and caring countenance. We have put our remarks in the footnotes wherever we felt a comment was warranted.

Adopt good bedside manners

1 The examination is not really very different to the final MB but obviously set at a higher level and with no help or encouragement from the examiners. Your approach to the patient is *very* important.

2 Do not panic; be kind to the patient and do not let the examiners hassle you.

3 Always introduce yourself by name to the patient and explain what you are going to do (in lay terms). Position the patient correctly and check whether the area to be examined is painful. Do not be afraid to ask the examiner if you can examine another but relevant part of the body if you consider this necessary (he can always say 'no').

4 For women, I would suggest that you wear something comfortable which will accommodate your stethoscope and to leave your handbag in a cloakroom. There is enough stress without worrying if your blouse buttons are undone or whether you have left your handbag by the previous patient!

5 Remember to suggest moving away from the patient when having to use words like 'tumour' or 'multiple sclerosis'.

6 Play the game. Introduce yourself to the patients and explain what you are going to do. Always expose the patient fully and then stand back and look at them before starting. There is plenty that can be missed if you do not take the time to 'observe'. It is also said that you always fail the exam if you hurt the patient. In my exam, I grabbed a patient by the hand—it was obviously sore and they shouted out. However, I apologized profusely and got away with it.

7 The short cases went well. However, the lack of feedback was very difficult to cope with. The examiners, though, seemed happy with my simple but confident answers. I think I appeared caring and was polite to the patients. I smiled a lot at the examiners and tried to be relaxed yet professional. It all seemed to work!

Practise clinical examination and presentation

8 Do not try the MRCP too soon. See as much general medicine as possible in a busy job—'cushy' jobs are not helpful in the end.

9 Be very professional in your presentation. I agree it's an easy exam—it's easy to fail!

10 Senior colleagues and consultants had prepared me for the psychological torture I was about to endure!

11 Go to as many clinical courses for MRCP as possible. Work out the best method for the examination of each system and practise it until it is second nature to you. Be as direct and positive in your answers as possible (even if they are wrong!).

12 I failed badly on the short cases. Do not take the examination unless you can properly prepare for it. I was very anxious and was not thinking while I was examining. I kept imagining that the cases were supposed to be difficult, rare or complex, but on the day they were very straightforward.

13 Talk through as many short cases as possible before the exam with someone who has been through it recently or with someone who is used to teaching. Preferably do this on a one-to-one basis or in a small group.

14 Practising the technique of examination is essential so that it becomes second nature under stress. Persuade colleagues to grill you mercilessly on short cases and with the differential diagnoses. Certain 'favourite' topics seem to recur so make sure you know these. Also, in the exam, do not make any statements unless you can back them up.

15 The most important point is to look professional— as if you have done it quickly and thoroughly a hundred times before. You do not need to know that much theoretical knowledge. Every clinical station has the necessary equipment but you will probably prefer to take your own as you will be much more familiar with it.

16 Before the examination I spent 6 weeks getting registrars to take me on short cases and then questioning me under examination conditions. Be meticulous about examination technique and do not be fooled by the apparent relaxed nature of the examiners—examine everything properly. Do not listen to tutors saying that one mistake makes a failed exam—it is not true.

17 Get together with someone else doing the exam and practise until you are bored with reciting the appropriate litany. I only just practised enough and wished I had

started 2 months earlier. It is the only way, especially if you can get someone senior (and preferably nasty!) to put you through it!

18 The more practice at presenting short cases the better.

19 I had a lot of practice presenting short cases to a 'hawk' of a senior registrar. This experience was invaluable.

20 Adopt a systematic approach to the examination of all the major systems and have the features of the common clinical conditions at your fingertips, e.g. upper and lower motor neurone lesions, the auscultatory findings of various valvular lesions, etc. A well-integrated, comprehensive system is needed for presenting the findings to examiners. Do not rush the presentation and omit important points.

21 It is important to have a method for examining each system. I do not think the examiners necessarily want you to make a definitive diagnosis in every case but you should be able to describe adequately the physical signs and offer some logical diagnostic possibilities.

Get it right

22 Do not rush a case—the examiners were very keen to stop me once they considered that I had enough information to make a diagnosis.

23 If you are unsure of the diagnosis then describe the findings and give them a differential diagnosis.

24 Do not be afraid to allow a few seconds of silence to pass before answering a question. Use this time to collect and organize your thoughts so that your answer comes in a logical order.

25 Know the diagnosis before you finish examining the patient and then state it confidently. Be prepared for further questions about the physical signs and on the management of the disease.

26 When examining fundi do not stop until you have finished and have thought of what to say.

27 Do not make comments that cannot be substantiated. Everything will be challenged if you are on the borderline.

28 The examiners already had in their mind what answers they would accept and they kept on until they got the actual wording they wanted.

29 Try not to be obtuse in the short cases or to pick on unimportant details, as the examiners may then draw you into a frustrating and often irrelevant discussion as to what you mean and sidetrack you away from the main issue.

30 If you know the diagnosis from just observing the patient (e.g. scleroderma), there seems to be a ritual series of questions and answers (swallowing, etc.) that you should anticipate and be prepared for.

31 I missed optic atrophy on one of my short cases. The moral is, if the fundus looks normal, to always ask yourself, 'Is there optic atrophy?'

32 In general, I found that getting the diagnosis right was not as important as I had been led to believe. Examining the patient with a systematic plan in mind and having a good differential diagnosis at each stage was much more important.

33 The examiners were very pleasant all the time and, as I got more cases right, I became more confident—and then I even started to enjoy myself. The examiners did not harass me but seemed concerned to let me get as much right as possible.

34 The short cases went really well. After the first case they did not ask any more aggressive questions. I think I had already satisfied them. Start well and look confident even if you do not know anything!

Listen, obey and do not stray

35 Just stick to what they ask and do not mess around. For example, do not start checking the temperature just because you hear a murmur. It seems to irritate them.

36 Do only what is asked of you. Give positive and concise answers to questions, unless a differential diagnosis is requested.

37 Always do a full examination of the system asked for—show off your technique. Do not be put off by 'dead-pan' examiners. The result comes as a particular shock when you have been sitting exams for many years *without* failing them.

38 I think I passed because I took the examiner's instructions one step further, e.g. I felt the pulse of someone with a dysphasia. Perhaps that is the secret!

39 Look at the patient as a whole and not just the system you are examining. So much useful information can be obtained by good observation.

40 They may ask you just to listen to the heart so that you cannot get clues from the pulse and palpation. In this case, one just has to do the best one can.

41 I think that they liked the way I examined the first patient, which was a neurological case in which I extended the examination beyond the legs, and then decided that I was probably competent.

42 Perform the physical examination and answer questions as requested. Try asking patients as much as possible; I had to look at a fundus so I asked him if he was diabetic and my examiners made *no* attempt to stop me. I was left with the impression that the exam, although difficult, is fundamentally *fair*.

One wrong does not make one fail

43 Treat each short case individually and put your apparent disasters behind you.

44 Do not be put off if you get a few things wrong. I made a lot of mistakes (that I know of!) and still passed.

45 Do not be distracted by mistakes made (or imagined) in preceding cases or by an examiner's mannerisms or approach.

46 I was put off right from the beginning after they stopped me during the examination of the first case—a vague, non-specific instruction was given and I had not found enough to be sure of. I was on the downward slope from then on. I might have passed had I pulled myself together and put the experience of that case behind me.

47 At the time and until I received my result, I was convinced I had failed. I think the experience of my previous attempt helped considerably, because I consciously reminded myself to put each bit behind me after I had done it, and not to dwell on my mistakes.

48 Never, never, never give up. I made many mistakes and thought I had had it but I still passed. You do not have to get it all (or even mostly) right if you can appear logical, *caring** and reasonably sensible. The examiners were *totally* non-committal and obviously trying to see how confident I was. I nearly failed myself!

If you say less they want more

49 After my first case there was a long silence as if they were waiting for me to say more—I went to pieces after this.

50 Be prepared for supplementary questions and for examiners who disagree or argue with your comments, but do not fall into the trap of arguing back. Just try and justify yourself and retract a statement if you know you have said something stupid.

51 Be complete in your examination—examine everything even if it does not seem relevant. For example, all hearts need to be listened to for early diastolic and mid-diastolic murmurs even if you think you already have the diagnosis. Every possible aspect of eyes needs to be looked at if asked to 'examine the eyes', unless something in the instruction suggests otherwise.

52 I was shown a patient with a IIIrd cranial nerve palsy (and possibly a IVth) following transfrontal surgery. I was asked why the eye was down and out.† I was a bit shaky on this—one takes it for granted that the pupil is dilated without asking why! I got really hot under the collar with this one.

Humility is more persuasive than self-righteousness

53 Be kind and confident but humble in the short cases.

54 By far the major problem was keeping my head and holding my ground *politely* when we disagreed.

55 Learn good examination techniques for all systems. Do not argue with the examiners and be polite to the patients.

56 If you know you have made a glaring error retract the remark and start again—if you are right (or at least think you are) stick to your answer.

57 The MRCP short cases are not a test of your medical knowledge. Mine is not profound. It is simply a test of whether you are competent at your job. If you think that you are and can convince the examiners of that then you will pass.

Keep cool: agitation generates aggression

58 'Panic not.' This is greatly helped if you have practised a lot of short cases under stress and seen most things before.

59 A good start is a great help. It is like skating on thin ice—if you keep going and do not fall through, then you make it.

60 The most off-putting aspect of each case is the lack of feedback from the examiners as to whether you are right or wrong. This is much more disconcerting than outright criticism.

61 Stay calm and talk sensibly even when the diagnosis appears unclear (easy to say—difficult to do!).

62 At the end of the exam I was sure I had failed as I did not have a clue what was wrong with one of the patients and did not do very well on another. However, I was wrong in my pass/fail self-assessment. A factor in my pass mark must have been that I did not lose my nerve and I remained calm, even after the mistakes. After all, it is as much a test of your nerve as your knowledge.

63 I did not feel confident enough to think I had passed, but I thought I had a reasonable chance. It is so important to start well, keep calm, score points when you can and treat each case independently. I did not do that in my first attempt and failed as a result; I maintained my concentration (with a supreme effort of will!) in the second attempt and it paid off.

64 Relax—and enjoy what are predominantly easy but beautifully classical signs.

---

* Our italics. It is the *raison d'être* of being a doctor.
† Because of the unopposed actions of the lateral rectus (abduction) and superior oblique (depression and abduction) muscles.

Simple explanations raise simple questions

65 Very simple, straightforward answers seem to prompt straightforward questions.

66 They appear to be satisfied with a good physical examination and interpretation of simple basic signs but I am sure they penalize heavily if obvious signs are missed. They seemed quite happy for me to ask the patient questions.* It is a great relief when the answers are what you want and also gives one time to think while the patient is answering.

67 The examiners seem to be impressed by short definitive answers and not with long lists of differential diagnoses. I think it is best to answer questions as directly as possible and get on to the next patient.

68 Always be honest—it pays in the end.

Think straight, look smart and speak convincingly

69 If the diagnosis is obvious then focus down and elicit all the relevant signs, regardless of the generality of the instruction. If the diagnosis is not immediately obvious, examine the relevant parts systematically and hope for the best. Do not be put off by mistakes or be paranoid about your performance. I was, and suffered for it.

70 Be definite about the positive findings; do not hedge your answer with 'possibly', 'almost', 'perhaps'. If there is no obvious first-choice answer then give a sensible and relevant differential diagnosis.

71 I think I failed because of hesitancy; I gave no impression of confidence and blurted out statements without thinking.

72 You must be quick and comprehensive in your examination; it looks bad if you need to go back to do something which you had forgotten.

73 Do not change your mind half way through—as long as you are sure you are right.

You have seen it all before

74 My cases were more straightforward than I had been led to expect. In fact, nothing was particularly rare.

75 It is easy to be daunted by the feeling that there will be conditions you have never heard of and that the cases will be difficult and rare. After my experience in four attempts it seems that in most cases the same old conditions keep recurring and they are mostly straightforward if only you can keep calm.

76 The cases are simple (the ones I saw were!). It is the candidate who makes them difficult and he or she may fail him or herself.

77 This was a much more enjoyable and interesting exam than Part I. With a single-minded approach to passing an exam rather than learning everything about medicine it is much more straightforward than people think. Remember that the majority of the examiners' knowledge outside their own field is unlikely to be much greater than your own (after revising!) and particularly about details. As long as you can justify your answers it will be difficult to fault you. After all, what more is the exam for than to reassure consultants that they can stay at home while you are looking after their patients!

78 When you come out of the exam you realize that after months and months of hard work and swotting the amount of knowledge you actually used could be written on a postage stamp!

Use your eyes first and most

79 One of the short cases—pretibial myxoedema—was given away by the eyes. I think, from talking to other people, there is often an obvious 'clue' in the short cases.

80 Spend at least 10–15 seconds just looking at the patient before even attempting an examination. When presenting, speak slowly and clearly and look the examiners in the eye.

81 Always look at the patient as a whole as well as the part in question. In one case (skin lesions in a black person) my first impulse was to suspect a tropical disease (?cutaneous leishmaniasis!) but the presence of exophthalmos gave me the diagnosis (pretibial myxoedema). Do not be put off by examiners who are (as mine were) totally non-committal.

82 Do exactly what is asked but give yourself a second or two to look at the whole patient from the end of the bed.

83 Remember to look at the bedside for clues—in my case I missed the tablet containers which would have suggested hypertensive retinopathy. When examining fundi, keep looking until you have covered all areas and try not to panic if you think you are taking too long.

Doing and forgetting

84 I examined the patient in an orderly sequence looking for the right things but for some reason, when I came to present the case, I could not recall my findings with regard to the stigmata of chronic liver disease. I could not even remember whether she was jaundiced!

---

* Asking the relevant but not the forbidden questions ('What is the diagnosis?') may be appreciated by some examiners, as part of developing a good rapport with the patient.

85 The examiners were fair and did not try to unsettle me. I fell down on presenting my findings and should have practised this more. In the heat of the moment, I went through the examination routine and then discovered I could not remember what I had found! I had also had a car crash driving up to the exam so that did not help to steady the nerves! Advice — do not drive there!

Examiners are different

86 The examiners were very pleasant and wanted to see how confident I was when faced with a problem. They could have failed me on many things but appeared to be wanting to see how my mind worked. They like you to be slick, thorough and to present your findings precisely without dithering. Stay relaxed and be honest.

87 I felt that the examiners unnecessarily rushed me. Some patients were not undressed and not on their bed. This seemed to frustrate them as well as myself though I didn't let it show and I tried to take it all in my stride. I had very little indication from their expression as to whether I was saying or doing the right thing. I found the lack of feedback to be very disconcerting but I knew it was to be expected and therefore I did not let it upset me.

88 Some of my examiners were very aggressive and sarcastic in their approach. Also the way they interrupted and corrected me made me feel completely incompetent and stupid.

89 It was very unnerving not getting any feedback and on one or two occasions they said: 'I see', which always sounds very ominous!

90 Do not get flustered. If you say something silly retract it quickly and continue to talk. The examiners can be aggressive and try to hurry you. Do not let them! Look smart in what you wear and be nice to the patients.

91 Try to be calm and imagine that you are seeing the cases in a clinic and carrying out a routine examination. The examiners made me very nervous especially with their comments which, in retrospect, I should have tried to ignore. They were only trying to test my knowledge and physiological comprehension of the physical signs I had elicited.

92 There was nothing difficult. The examiners were polite, unobtrusive, to the point and clear about their requirements. They were also amazingly expressionless throughout.

93 I wish the examiners were a little more friendly and did not interrupt every 10–15 s!

94 Do not be bullied by the examiners. There is no substitute for experience. You can pass even if you make a mess of one short case.

95 Do not let them rattle you. Never think you have failed until you get the letter.

96 Do not let the examiners rush you as you are then likely to make mistakes and this just surrenders all control to them. They cannot fail you for a methodical clinical examination.

97 The examiners kept asking me if I was sure of my findings as though they were trying to put me off. I wish I was this good always!

Additional comments and quotes from candidates

1 I had no time for my central nervous system examination and I thought that the ethics station was much easier than any practice sessions that I had had on previous courses. I found that on courses the actors were fairly horrible in so far as they cried and shouted. This never happens in the real exam or even in real life.

2 I thought the exam was bizarre but I passed!

3 The few minutes break that is given in between each station is very useful. For example, if you have a bad case or a bad examiner (or both as in my case) it gives you time to compose yourself.

4 Know your basic information really well. Therefore, it is useful to revise material from the written exam. You need to know lists for causes of things and it is important to know them in a logical order.

Appendices

1 | Website links

Resuscitation Council (UK)
http://www.resus.org.uk

US Centre for Disease Control and Prevention (CDC)
http://www.cdc.gov/

CDC HIV website
http://www.cdc.gov/hiv/pubs/facts.htm

General Medical Council (GMC)
http://www.gmc-uk.org/

GMC standards of practice
http://www.gmc-uk.org/standards

Department of Health
http://www.doh.gov.uk/

Department of Health guidelines on consent
http://www.doh.gov.uk/consent/index.htm

Driver and Vehicle Licensing Agency (DVLA)
http://www.dvla.gov.uk

DVLA at a glance guide to current medical standards of
the fitness to drive
http://www.dvla.gov.uk/at_a_glance/content.htm

International Huntington Association
http://www.huntington-assoc.com/

International Huntington Association guidelines for
the molecular genetics predictive test in Huntington
disease
http://www.huntington-assoc.com/guidel.htm

Unrelated Live Transplant Regulatory Authority
(ULTRA)
http://www.doh.gov.uk/ultra/index.htm
http://www.doh.gov.uk/ultra/ultrareview.htm

British Medical Association (BMA)
http://web.bma.org.uk/

BMA ethics
http://www.bma.org.uk/homepage.nsf/
htmlpagevw/ethics

BMA guidelines on withholding and withdrawing life
prolonging medical treatment
http://www.bmjpg.com/withwith/ww.htm

Royal College of Pathologists
http://www.rcpath.org/

Royal College of Pathologists guidelines for the
retention of tissues and organs at post-mortem
examination
http://www.rcpath.org/resources/pdf/
tissue_retention.pdf

Multiple Sclerosis Society (UK)
http://www.mssociety.org.uk/

Department of Work and Pensions
http://www.dwp.gov.uk/index.asp

Blood Transfusion Service (UK)
http://www.blood.co.uk/

Department of Health guidelines on Hepatitis B
infected healthcare workers
http://www.doh.gov.uk/nhsexec/hepatitisb.htm

Action on Smoking and Health (ASH)
http://www.ash.org.uk/

Department of Health MRSA guidelines: what nursing
and residential homes need to know
http://www.doh.gov.uk/mrsaguid.htm

Medical Defence Union (library of contents)
http://www.the-mdu.com/oms/library/contents.html

2 | Detailed contents of Section F

Index

Readers are advised that Section F (experiences and anecdotes) has not been included in the index.